Healthcare Delivery in Surgery

Scientific Principles and Practice

Healthcare Delivery in Surgery

Scientific Principles and Practice

Justin B. Dimick, MD, MPH
Frederick A. Coller Distinguished Professor
Chair, Department of Surgery
University of Michigan Health System
Ann Arbor, Michigan

Lesly A. Dossett, MD, MPH
Associate Professor
Chief, Division of Surgical Oncology
Vice Chair for Faculty Development
University of Michigan
Ann Arbor, Michigan

Amir A. Ghaferi, MD, MSc, MBA
Professor of Surgery
President & CEO, Physician Enterprise
Senior Associate Dean for Clinical Affairs
Froedtert & Medical College of Wisconsin
Milwaukee, Wisconsin

Andrew M. Ibrahim, MD, MSc
Maud T. Lane Research Professor of Surgery,
 Architecture & Urban Planning
Co-Director, Center for Healthcare Outcomes
 & Policy
University of Michigan, Ann Arbor.
Chief Medical Officer and Senior Principal, HOK
Chicago, New York, St. Louis, Washington, DC

Dana A. Telem, MD, MPH
Associate Professor
Associate Chair for Quality and Patient Safety
Department of Surgery
University of Michigan Health System
Ann Arbor, Michigan

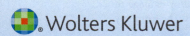

Philadelphia • Baltimore • New York • London
Buenos Aires • Hong Kong • Sydney • Tokyo

Acquisitions Editor: Keith Donnellan
Development Editors: Ashley Fischer and Barton Dudlick
Editorial Coordinator: Remington Fernando
Marketing Manager: Dan Dressler
Senior Production Project Manager: Alicia Jackson
Manager, Graphic Arts & Design: Stephen Druding
Senior Manufacturing Coordinator: Beth Welsh
Prepress Vendor: Lumina Datamatics

First edition

Copyright © 2024 Wolters Kluwer.

All rights reserved. This book is protected by copyright. No part of this book may be reproduced or transmitted in any form or by any means, including as photocopies or scanned-in or other electronic copies, or utilized by any information storage and retrieval system without written permission from the copyright owner, except for brief quotations embodied in critical articles and reviews. Materials appearing in this book prepared by individuals as part of their official duties as U.S. government employees are not covered by the above-mentioned copyright. To request permission, please contact Wolters Kluwer at Two Commerce Square, 2001 Market Street, Philadelphia, PA 19103, via email at permissions@lww.com, or via our website at shop.lww.com (products and services).

9 8 7 6 5 4 3 2 1

Printed in Singapore

Library of Congress Cataloging-in-Publication Data available upon request

ISBN-13: 978-1-9751-9637-0

This work is provided "as is," and the publisher disclaims any and all warranties, express or implied, including any warranties as to accuracy, comprehensiveness, or currency of the content of this work.

This work is no substitute for individual patient assessment based upon healthcare professionals' examination of each patient and consideration of, among other things, age, weight, gender, current or prior medical conditions, medication history, laboratory data and other factors unique to the patient. The publisher does not provide medical advice or guidance and this work is merely a reference tool. Healthcare professionals, and not the publisher, are solely responsible for the use of this work including all medical judgments and for any resulting diagnosis and treatments.

Given continuous, rapid advances in medical science and health information, independent professional verification of medical diagnoses, indications, appropriate pharmaceutical selections and dosages, and treatment options should be made and healthcare professionals should consult a variety of sources. When prescribing medication, healthcare professionals are advised to consult the product information sheet (the manufacturer's package insert) accompanying each drug to verify, among other things, conditions of use, warnings and side effects and identify any changes in dosage schedule or contraindications, particularly if the medication to be administered is new, infrequently used or has a narrow therapeutic range. To the maximum extent permitted under applicable law, no responsibility is assumed by the publisher for any injury and/or damage to persons or property, as a matter of products liability, negligence law or otherwise, or from any reference to or use by any person of this work.

shop.lww.com

CONTRIBUTORS

Janet Abbruzzese, BS
Associate Chief Operating Officer
Department of Operations and Ancillary Services
University of Michigan Health
Ann Arbor, Michigan

Mohamed Abdelgadir Adam, MD
Assistant Professor of Surgery
Department of Surgery
University of California, San Francisco
San Francisco, California

Sapan N. Ambani, MD
Associate Professor; Associate Medical Director of
    Ambulatory Surgery
Department of Urology
Michigan Medicine
Ann Arbor, Michigan

Erika Arndt, MPA
Administrator
Department of Surgery
University of Michigan
Ann Arbor, Michigan

Michael Barringer, MD, FACS
Medical Director Surgical Affairs
Atrium Health Cleveland
Shelby, North Carolina

Ian Berger, MD, MSHP
Resident
Department of Surgery, Division of Urology
Duke University Medical Center
Durham, North Carolina

Nicholas L. Berlin, MD, MPH, MS
House Officer
Department of Surgery, Section of Plastic Surgery
Michigan Medicine
Ann Arbor, Michigan

Karl Y. Bilimoria, MD, MS
John B. Murphy Professor of Surgery
Department of Surgery
Northwestern University
Chicago, Illinois

Sidra N. Bonner, MD, MPH, MSc
General Surgery Resident
Department of Surgery
University of Michigan
Ann Arbor, Michigan

Ryan A. J. Campagna, MD, MEd
Fellow, Cardiothoracic Surgery
Department of Surgery
University of Michigan
Ann Arbor, Michigan

Brenda Carlisle, MSHA, BSN, RN, CENP
VP Clinical Operations
Department of Hospital Administration
University of AL Hospital (UAB)
Birmingham, Alabama

Pooja Chandrashekar, AB
MD/MBA Student
Harvard Medical School and Harvard School of Business
Boston, Massachusetts

Alvin Chang, MD, MHA
Resident Physician
Department of General Surgery
Geisinger Medical Center
Danville, Pennsylvania

Andrew C. Chang, MD
Professor
Department of Surgery
University of Michigan
Ann Arbor, Michigan

Karan R. Chhabra, MD, MSc
Resident
Department of Surgery
Brigham and Women's Hospital
Boston, Massachusetts

Leeanna Clevenger, MD
Surgical Critical Care Fellow
Department of Surgery
Medical University of South Carolina
Charleston, South Carolina

Patricia C. Conroy, MD
Resident Physician
Department of Surgery
University of California, San Francisco
San Francisco, California

Matthew Corriere, MD, MS
Frankel Professor of Surgery & Associate Professor
    of Surgery, Section of Vascular Surgery
Michigan Medicine
Ann Arbor, Michigan

Steven R. Crain, MD
General Surgeon
Department of General Surgery
Kaiser Permanente
Woodland Hills, California

Christopher L. Cramer, MD
Resident Physician
Department of Surgery
University of Virginia
Charlottesville, Virginia

Mihir S. Dekhne, MS, MD
Resident Physician
Hospital for Special Surgery
New York
Gerard Doherty, MD
Moseley Professor of Surgery
Harvard Medical School
Boston, Massachusetts

Lesly A. Dossett, MD, MPH
Associate Professor
Chief, Division of Surgical Oncology
Vice Chair for Faculty Development
University of Michigan
Ann Arbor, Michigan

Shukri H. A. Dualeh, MD
General Surgery Resident
Department of Surgery
University of Michigan, Michigan Medicine
Ann Arbor, Michigan

Sunil Eappen, MD, MBA
Chief Medical Officer and Senior Vice President for
     Medical Affairs
Department of Administration/Anesthesiology
Brigham and Women's Hospital/Harvard
     Medical School
Boston, Massachusetts

Michael Englesbe, MD
Professor of Surgery
Department of Surgery—Transplant
University of Michigan
Ann Arbor, Michigan

Heather L. Evans, MD, MS
Vice Chair of Clinical Research and Applied
     Informatics
Department of Surgery
Medical University of South Carolina
Charleston, South Carolina

Liane S. Feldman, MD, CM
Edward W. Archibald Professor and Chair
Department of Surgery
McGill University
Montreal, Quebec, Canada

Alexandra Gangi, MD
Assistant Professor
Department of Surgery
Cedars Sinai Medical Center
Los Angeles, California

Amir A. Ghaferi, MD, MSc, MBA
Professor of Surgery
President & CEO, Physician Enterprise
Senior Associate Dean for Clinical Affairs
Froedtert & Medical College of Wisconsin
Milwaukee, Wisconsin

Caitlin Halbert, DO, MS
Chief Surgical Services, Wilmington Campus
ChristianaCare
Wilmington, Delaware

Geoffrey E. Hespe, MD
House Officer
Department of Surgery
University of Michigan
Ann Arbor, Michigan

Ronald B. Hirschl, MD
Professor of Surgery
Department of Pediatric Surgery
Michigan Medicine/CS Mott Children's Hospital
Ann Arbor, Michigan

Melissa E. Hogg, MD, MS
Director of HPB Surgery
Department of Surgery
NorthShore University Health System
Evanston, Illinois

Ryan Howard, MD
Surgery Resident
Department of General Surgery
Michigan Medicine
Ann Arbor, Michigan

Kakra Hughes, MD, PhD
Professor & Chief of Vascular Surgery
Department of Surgery
Howard University and Hospital
Washington, DC

Tasha M. Hughes, MD, MPH
Assistant Professor of Surgery
Department of Surgery
University of Michigan
Ann Arbor, Michigan

Andrew M. Ibrahim, MD, MSc
Maud T. Lane Research Professor of Surgery,
     Architecture & Urban Planning
Co-Director, Center for Healthcare Outcomes & Policy
University of Michigan, Ann Arbor.
Chief Medical Officer and Senior Principal, HOK
Chicago, New York, St. Louis, Washington, DC

Contributors

Sachin H. Jain, MD, MBA, FACP
President & CEO, SCAN Group and Health Plan
Adjunct Professor of Medicine, Stanford University
 School of Medicine
Los Angeles, California

Deborah R. Kaye, MD, MS
Assistant Professor
Department of Surgery, Duke-Margolis
 Policy Center, Duke Clinical Research
 Institute
Duke University
Durham, North Carolina

Lawrence Lee, MD, PhD
Assistant Professor of Surgery
Department of Surgery
McGill University Health Centre
Montreal, Quebec, Canada

Cynthia Lewis Kavanagh, MBA
Executive Director
Department of Strategy, Planning & Intelligence
Mass General Brigham
Boston, Massachusetts

Jimmie Loats Jr., MBA
Senior Director—Financial Operations &
 Analytics
Department of Finance & Clinical Operations
The University of Alabama at Birmingham
 Hospital
Birmingham, Alabama

Alisha Lussiez, MD, MSc
General Surgery Resident
Department of Surgery
University of Michigan
Ann Arbor, Michigan

Mariam Maksutova, BS
Medical Student
Department of Vascular Surgery
University of Michigan Medical School
Ann Arbor, Michigan

Kelly Michelle Malloy, MD, FACS
Associate Professor of Otolaryngology—Head and Neck
 Surgery
Fellowship Director of Head and Neck Surgical
 Oncology & Microvascular Reconstruction
Associate Chief Officer for Surgical, Preoperative, and
 Rehabilitation Services
Department of Otolaryngology—Head and
 Neck Surgery
University of Michigan
Ann Arbor, Michigan

Jayson S. Marwaha, MD, MSc
General Surgery Resident; Postdoctoral Fellow
Department of Surgery; Biomedical Informatics
Harvard Medical School
Boston, Massachusetts

Brent D. Matthews, MD
Professor and Chair, Surgeon-in-Chief
Department of Surgery
Atrium Health Carolinas Medical Center, Wake Forest
 University School of Medicine
Charlotte, North Carolina

Ayako Mayo, MD
Assistant Professor
Department of Medicine
Oregon Health & Science University
Portland, Oregon

Melanie S. Morris, MD
Professor
Department of Gastrointestinal
 Surgery
University of Alabama at Birmingham
Birmingham, Alabama

Hari Nathan, MD, PhD
Associate Professor
Department of Surgery
University of Michigan
Ann Arbor, Michigan

Erika A. Newman, MD
The Michael W. Mulholland Distinguished
 Professor
Department of Surgery
University of Michigan
Ann Arbor, Michigan

Vanessa S. Niba, MD
General Surgery Resident
Department of Surgery
University of Michigan
Ann Arbor, Michigan

Vahagn C. Nikolian, MD
Assistant Professor of Surgery
Department of Surgery
Oregon Health & Science University
Portland, Oregon

Nabeel R. Obeid, MD
Clinical Assistant Professor
 of Surgery
Department of Surgery
Michigan Medicine
Ann Arbor, Michigan

Contributors

Sean Michael O'Neill, MD, PhD
Clinical Assistant Professor
Department of Surgery
University of Michigan
Ann Arbor, Michigan

Nicholas Osborne, MD
Chief of Surgery
Charles S. Kettles VA Medical Center
Ann Arbor, Michigan

Kavya Pathak, BA
Harvard Medical School
Boston, Massachusetts

Anthony T. Petrick, MD
Chief Quality Officer, Inpatient
    Services
Department of Surgery
Geisinger Medical Center
Danville, Pennsylvania

Melissa Pilewskie, MD, FACS
Associate Professor
Department of Surgery
University of Michigan
Ann Arbor, Michigan

Scott E. Regenbogen, MD, MPH
Associate Professor
Department of Surgery
University of Michigan
Ann Arbor, Michigan

Caroline E. Reinke, MD, FACS
Associate Professor
Department of Surgery
Atrium Health
Charlotte, North Carolina

Malcolm K. Robinson, MD
Vice Chair for Clinical Operations
Department of Surgery
Brigham and Women's Hospital
Boston, Massachusetts

Christina L. Roland, MD, MS
Associate Professor of Surgery
The University of Texas MD Anderson
    Cancer Center
Houston, Texas

Andrew J. Rosko, MD
Assistant Professor
Department of Otolaryngology—Head and Neck
    Surgery
University of Michigan
Ann Arbor, Michigan

Ashley E. Russo, MD
Complex General Surgical Oncology
    Fellow
Department of Surgery
Cedars-Sinai
Los Angeles, California

Devdutta Sangvai, MD, MBA
VP, Population Health
Duke University School of Medicine
Durham, North Carolina

Nicole M. Santucci, MD, MA
Medical Student
Oregon Health & Science University
Portland, Oregon

Abhishek Satishchandran, MD, PhD
Fellow
Department of Gastroenterology, Internal
    Medicine
University of Michigan
Ann Arbor, Michigan

Robert S. Saunders, PhD
Senior Research Director, Health Care
    Transformation
Margolis Center for Health Policy
Duke University
Washington, DC

Christopher P. Scally, MD, MS
Assistant Professor
Department of Surgical Oncology
University of Texas MD Anderson Cancer Center
Houston, Texas

Allison R. Schulman, MD, MPH
Associate Professor of Medicine & Surgery; Director
    of Bariatric Endoscopy
University of Michigan
Ann Arbor, Michigan

Erika D. Sears, MD, MS
Associate Professor of Surgery
Department of Surgery, Section of Plastic
    Surgery
Michigan Medicine and VA Ann Arbor Center for
    Clinical Management Research
Ann Arbor, Michigan

Kyle H. Sheetz, MD, MSc
Clinical Instructor and Fellow, Abdominal
    Transplant Surgery
Department of Surgery
University of California, San Francisco
San Francisco, California

Andrew Shin, JD, MPH, MBA
Senior Vice President, Strategy
Mass General Brigham
Somerville, Massachusetts

Casey M. Silver, MD
Surgical Outcomes and Quality Improvement Center
Northwestern University
Chicago, Illinois

Jeffrey W. Simmons, MD, MSHQS, FASA
Professor
Department of Anesthesiology and Perioperative Medicine
UAB Medicine
Birmingham, Alabama

Lauren Smithson, MD, MPhil, FACS, FRCSC
General Surgeon
Charles S. Curtis Memorial Hospital
Labrador Grenfell Health
St. Anthony, Newfoundland, Canada

Christopher J. Sonnenday, MD, MHS
Transplant Center Director
Department of Transplant Surgery
Michigan Medicine
Ann Arbor, Michigan

Julie Ann Sosa, MD, MA, FACS, MAMSE, FSSO
Leon Goldman, MD Distinguished Professor and Chair of Surgery
Department of Surgery
University of California, San Francisco
San Francisco, California

John H. Stewart IV, MD, MBA
Director, LSU-LCMC Cancer Center
Louisiana State University
New Orleans, Louisiana

Dana A. Telem, MD, MPH
Associate Professor
Associate Chair for Quality and Patient Safety
Department of Surgery
University of Michigan Health System
Ann Arbor, Michigan

Thomas C. Tsai, MD, MPH
Assistant Professor of Surgery
Department of Surgery
Brigham and Women's Hospital
Boston, Massachusetts

Chandu Vemuri, MD
Assistant Professor
Department of Surgery
Michigan Medicine
Ann Arbor, Michigan

Brooke Reeves Vining, MNA
Senior Director, Anesthesia Services UAB Hospital
Department of Anesthesia Services
UAB Hospital
Birmingham, Alabama

Pratyusha Yalamanchi, MD, MBA
Resident Physician
Department of Otolaryngology—Head and Neck Surgery
University of Michigan
Ann Arbor, Michigan

Anthony D. Yang, MD, MS
Professor
Department of Surgery
Indiana University School of Medicine
Indianapolis, Indiana

Victor M. Zaydfudim, MD, MPH
Associate Professor of Surgery
Department of Surgery
University of Virginia
Charlottesville, Virginia

Herbert J. Zeh, III, MD
Professor and Chair of the Department of Surgery at UT Southwestern
UT Southwestern
Dallas, Texas

Biqi Zhang, MD
Resident Surgeon
Department of Surgery
Brigham and Women's Hospital
Boston, Massachusetts

Randall Zuckerman, MD, FACS
HPB Surgery
Renown Health
Reno, Nevada

PREFACE

HEALTHCARE DELIVERY IN SURGERY: SCIENTIFIC PRINCIPLES AND PRACTICE

We believe this book represents a resource unlike other existing books on the topic of healthcare management or health systems science. We sought to bring together cutting-edge ideas in health system science and to place them in the context of real-world challenges with practical solutions. This book uses a *case-based* approach to make the material easy to engage with. Each case covers a common challenge in improving the delivery of surgical care.

Each of the editors has deep experience in health services research combined with practical experience, working as leaders in different areas of healthcare delivery, including roles such as department chair, division chief, president of a medical group, and chief medical officer for an architecture firm. We have used our networks to select authors with other areas of leadership experience in healthcare systems.

We wrote this book for surgical leaders and health system administrators at all levels who seek to understand how to improve the delivery of surgical care. We believe this unique book will help leaders understand the strategy and operations of delivering surgical care with the goal of building clinical programs, improving access for patients, optimizing the use of resource-intensive facilities, and ensuring the highest quality of care.

Justin B. Dimick, MD, MPH
Lesly A. Dossett, MD, MPH
Amir A. Ghaferi, MD, MSc, MBA
Andrew M. Ibrahim, MD, MSc
Dana A. Telem, MD, MPH

CONTENTS

Contributors v
Preface xi

SECTION 1: IMPROVING ACCESS TO CARE

1 Rural Patients Who Need Complex Surgical Care 3
   Randall Zuckerman and Lauren Smithson

2 Imbalanced Clinic Utilization Across the Workweek—Balancing Low Space Utilization, Patient Access, and Provider Workflow 8
   Tasha M. Hughes

3 Emergency Department Visits With Semi-Urgent Problems 14
   Matthew Corriere and Erika Arndt

4 High Inpatient Capacity and Unable to Accept Specialty Transfers 19
   Lesly A. Dossett

5 Aligning Surgical Care Delivery With Population Health Needs 24
   Ryan Howard, Alisha Lussiez, and Michael Englesbe

SECTION 2: EFFICIENCY OF INPATIENT OPERATIONS

6 Building a Hospital-at-Home Program to Reduce Length of In-Hospital Stay in Surgery . . . 33
   Nicole M. Santucci, Ayako Mayo, and Vahagn C. Nikolian

7 Postoperative Patients Come to the Emergency Room Because They Do Not Have Urgent Access to Surgical Clinics 42
   Heather L. Evans and Leeanna Clevenger

8 Efficiency in the Operating Room: Get the Data, Make the Change 48
   Melanie S. Morris, Brenda Carlisle, Brooke Reeves Vining, Jimmie Loats, and Jeffrey W. Simmons

9 Ensuring Access to Operating Room for Complex Time-Sensitive Cases 55
   Christopher L. Cramer and Victor M. Zaydfudim

SECTION 3: SITE OF CARE OPTIMIZATION

10 "Right Case, Right Place": High Number of Outpatient Cases at an Inpatient Facility 63
   Pratyusha Yalamanchi, Sapan N. Ambani, Amir A. Ghaferi, and Kelly Michelle Malloy

11 Avoiding Life-Threatening Complications at an Ambulatory Surgery Center 69
   Pratyusha Yalamanchi and Andrew J. Rosko

12 Low Acuity Inpatient Cases at High Acuity Hospital 75
   Nabeel R. Obeid and Dana A. Telem

13 Home Monitoring for Surgical Home Hospital 79
   Biqi Zhang, Jayson S. Marwaha, Kavya Pathak, Malcolm K. Robinson, and Thomas C. Tsai

14 Service Line With Low Operating Room Utilization at Ambulatory Surgery Center 86
   Andrew M. Ibrahim, Geoffrey E. Hespe, and Amir A. Ghaferi

SECTION 4: BUILDING REGIONAL NETWORKS

15 Hospital Losing Market Share: Is Joining a Hospital Network the Answer? 95
   Andrew Shin and Cynthia Lewis Kavanagh

16 Low-Volume Surgery Within One Site of a Hospital Network 101
   Kyle H. Sheetz and Hari Nathan

xiii

xiv   Contents

17 Disseminating Quality Standards Across a Hospital Network 107
Caroline E. Reinke and Michael Barringer

18 Ensuring Quality while Exporting Brand to New Network Affiliates 116
Ronald B. Hirschl

19 Outreach and Referral Building at New Network Affiliates 121
Brent D. Matthews

20 Coordinating Care and Referrals Across Affiliates 131
Ryan A. J. Campagna and Andrew C. Chang

21 Investing in Health Outside the Hospital: Public and Community Infrastructure 137
Pooja Chandrashekar and Sachin H. Jain

22 Working With Employers to Build Destination Programs for Complex Surgery 141
Caitlin Halbert

SECTION 5: ENSURING QUALITY AND SAFETY

23 Ensuring Quality and Safety When Building a New Clinical Program 149
Anthony T. Petrick and Alvin Chang

24 Monitoring Quality and Safety Early in the Adoption of New Technology............... 157
Herbert J. Zeh and Melissa E. Hogg

25 Negotiating Turf Battles Between Specialties 165
Nicholas Osborne

26 Addressing Low Performance Outliers in Outcomes Monitoring Programs 170
Casey M. Silver, Karl Y. Bilimoria, and Anthony D. Yang

27 Managing a Surgeon With Demonstrated Poor Outcomes 176
Gerard Doherty

28 High-Volume Hospital With Low-Volume Surgeons................................ 183
Patricia C. Conroy, Mohamed Abdelgadir Adam, and Julie Ann Sosa

29 High Variability in Surgical Teams 189
Sapan N. Ambani

30 Provider Burnout Impacting Clinical Care Delivery 195
Liane S. Feldman and Lawrence Lee

SECTION 6: BUILDING MULTIDISCIPLINARY SERVICE LINES

31 Establishing Service Lines in a Competitive Market 205
Melissa Pilewskie

32 Efficient, Comprehensive Patient Care for Multidisciplinary Visits 212
Christopher P. Scally and Christina L. Roland

33 Ensuring Multidisciplinary Access Aligns Across Disciplines........................ 217
Ashley E. Russo and Alexandra Gangi

SECTION 7: HEALTHCARE EQUITY

34 "Top" Hospital Is Bypassed or Avoided by Minorities in the Community Who Feel More
Comfortable at Other Hospitals: Distrust of Medical System and Minority Health Care 225
Kakra Hughes and John H. Stewart IV

35 Inadequate Diversity in Hospital Committees Charged With Review
of Clinical Operations and Quality 231
Shukri H.A. Dualeh, Vanessa S. Niba, and Erika A. Newman

36 Dismantling Capacity Management Policies That Prioritize Highly Reimbursed
Specialty Surgery Over Caring for Uninsured Patients................................ 236
Sidra N. Bonner and Christopher J. Sonnenday

SECTION 8: POLICY-RESPONSIVE LEADERSHIP

37 Enrolling in Voluntary Bundled Payment Programs in Surgery 243
Nicholas L. Berlin and Scott E. Regenbogen

38 Considerations in Accountable Care Organizations (ACOs) 250
Ian Berger, Robert S. Saunders, Devdutta Sangvai, and Deborah R. Kaye

39 Out-of-Network Billing: The Surgical Leader's Perspective 256
Karan R. Chhabra, Mihir S. Dekhne, and Sunil Eappen

SECTION 9: IMPROVING VALUE OF CARE

40 Overuse of Preoperative Testing in Low-Risk Patients 263
Nicholas L. Berlin and Erika D. Sears

41 Incorporating New Technology That Is Not Reimbursed 269
Abhishek Satishchandran and Allison R. Schulman

42 Consolidating OR Supply Chain to a Single Vendor 275
Mariam Maksutova, Janet Abbruzzese, and Chandu Vemuri

43 When Healthcare Systems Become Their Own Insurer 281
Sean Michael O'Neill and Steven R. Crain

Index   289

SECTION 8: POLICY-RESPONSIVE LEADERSHIP

27. Enrolling in Voluntary Bundled Payment Programs in Surgery 243
    Thomas C. Tsai and Scott E. Regenbogen

28. Considerations in Accountable Care Organizations (ACOs) 250
    Ian Soriano Roberts, Sounders, Devendra Sahay, and Rebecca Minter

39. Out-of-Network Billing: The Surgical Leader's Perspective 256
    Karen E. Chabes, Mark S. Dekkus, and Sara Scarlet

SECTION 9: IMPROVING VALUE OF CARE

40. Overuse of Preoperative Testing in Low-Risk Patients 263
    Nicholas B. Elianb, and Eric B. Rosero

41. Incorporating New Technology That is Not Reimbursed 269
    Katherine Kelley Gallagher and Melissa A. Coleman

42. Consolidating OR Supply Chain to a Single Vendor 275
    Ann Ann Maksuova, Janet Abbruzzese, and Shanda Varon

43. When Healthcare Systems Become Their Own Insurer 281
    Sean Monahan O'Neill and Steven R. Craig

Index 285

SECTION 1

Improving Access to Care

1 Rural Patients Who Need Complex Surgical Care
Randall Zuckerman and Lauren Smithson

2 Imbalanced Clinic Utilization Across the Workweek—Balancing Low Space Utilization, Patient Access, and Provider Workflow
Tasha M. Hughes

3 Emergency Department Visits With Semi-Urgent Problems
Matthew Corriere and Erika Arndt

4 High Inpatient Capacity and Unable to Accept Specialty Transfers
Lesly A. Dossett

5 Aligning Surgical Care Delivery With Population Health Needs
Ryan Howard, Alisha Lussiez, and Michael Englesbe

Rural Patients Who Need Complex Surgical Care

RANDALL ZUCKERMAN AND LAUREN SMITHSON

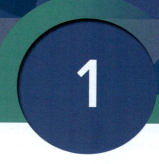

Clinical Delivery Challenge

A 64-year-old man presents to a rural emergency room because his wife felt like he looked yellow. He complained of itching at night and an unintentional 10 lb weight loss in the last month. A laboratory panel drawn in the emergency room showed a bilirubin of 14. Transaminases were one and half times normal, and alkaline phosphatase was in the 200s. White blood cell count and other labs were within normal limits. Right upper quadrant ultrasound did not reveal gallstones, though the common bile duct was markedly enlarged. Noncontrast CT scan was performed and showed a vague mass in the head of the pancreas with a common bile duct and intrahepatic biliary dilatation. You were consulted as the surgeon on call for further management.

The delivery of surgical care in rural environments is complex and challenging. The reasons for this are multifactorial and relate to the heterogeneity of rural hospitals across America. This heterogeneity is based on definitions of rural as well as unique hospital capabilities. There are many medical and surgical problems that can be safely cared for in rural environments; however, it has become increasingly apparent over the last 20 years that for a certain subset of highly complex operations, institutional and personal volume factors and expertise directly affect outcomes.

● WORKUP

The presumptive diagnosis in this patient is pancreatic cancer. Standard workup would include a pancreatic protocol CT scan with contrastas as well as the serum expression of the tumor marker CA 19-9. These are typically easy to obtain in a rural setting, provided that a CT scanner and laboratory studies are available. A magnetic resonance imaging/magnetic resonance cholangiopancreatography (MRI/MRCP) would be required to further delineate the anatomy of both the biliary tree and the mass. Additionally, this patient would benefit from endoscopic ultrasound (EUS) as well as endoscopic retrograde cholangiopancreatography (ERCP) to decompress his biliary tree. Both procedures can also provide tissue diagnosis, which is critical for determining the next steps in management. The patient also needs referral to hepatobiliary surgery or surgical oncology, discussion at a multidisciplinary meeting, and likely involvement of medical oncology, radiation oncology, and pain management (pain service or anesthesiology). This is where the requirements of the patient outstrip the capabilities of most rural surgical practices.

Although MRI scanners are becoming more commonplace in many rural hospitals, it is not standard and represents a large investment for institutions and administration. ERCP is not a procedure typically found in most rural hospitals, as it is typically performed by gastroenterologists. ERCP is performed by some general surgeons with advanced endoscopic training or fellowships; however, they do not practice in rural areas. Gastroenterologists, who do have this additional training to perform an ERCP, are even more scarce in a remote setting. Even if the proceduralist is available, the procedure requires a particular endoscope with a side-viewing camera, various instruments (brushes, balloons, cautery needles, and stents) that are not used in regular endoscopy, and a skilled nursing department trained to perform the endoscopic procedure. EUS is also surgeon dependent and requires unique equipment. If the cost and necessary staff were not a deterrent, then the frequency of preforming these procedures in a rural setting may be the rate-limiting factor. Most training programs that specialize in advanced endoscopy require a minimum of

50 procedures to obtain certification. Clinical studies suggest that to maintain standards and patient safety, a minimum of 50 ERCP should be performed per year, and at least 100–200 ERCP procedure should be performed annually for achieving competency in managing complex problems.[1]

With regard to additional treatment, the advantage of a rural setting is limited travel, lower cost to the patient, and the comfort of one's own surroundings. Telehealth or videoconferencing from home or a rural clinic is a benefit of the current technological age. This is a form of infrastructure that hospital administration can invest in, wisely. Unfortunately, in the complex surgical patient presented here, the additional needs, such as medical and radiation oncology, multidisciplinary teams, pain management, cancer support groups, and interventional radiology, are found in the tertiary centers. What rural hospitals can do, after the initial imaging and blood work point toward this diagnosis, is to prepare their patients for what is to come by having a knowledge of the changing management of hepatobiliary cancers and likely direction therapy will take.

● DIFFERENTIAL DIAGNOSIS

In this case, the differential diagnosis would include the following:

- Pancreatic cancer
- Distal common bile duct cancer
- Duodenal cancer

  Less likely would be:

- Common bile duct stones
- Pancreatitis pseudocyst at the head of the pancreas
- Main-duct intraductal papillary mucinous neoplasm
- Lymphoma of the pancreas

● DIAGNOSIS AND TREATMENT

The authors believe that the patient in this clinical scenario would benefit most from an expeditious referral to a hepatobiliary surgeon. The receiving hepatobiliary team would direct further workup, such as the MRI/MRCP, ERCP, or EUS described in the "Workup" section. As the patient is feeling fine except for some fatigue and itching, it would be safe to discharge the patient home from the rural emergency room, with some options for medical management of pruritus. A follow-up in the local rural surgical clinic should be established so that the patient's progress can be monitored and he does not lost to follow-up. Ensuring care progresses is another area where the rural surgeon/physician can affect change: In order for the patient to be expedited, phone contact from physician to physician should be done, followed by a formal referral or letter.

● SCIENTIFIC PRINCIPLES AND EVIDENCE

Rural hospitals are a diverse group of institutions with varying capabilities. Rurality alone does not dictate the level or complexity of care that can be provided. There are many large rural hospitals that provide a full spectrum of care including complex surgical oncology. There is also incredible diversity among critical access hospitals. There are many critical access hospitals that provide minimal or no surgical services, contrasted by critical access hospitals with robust surgical programs including robotic surgery. Geography also plays a big role in this equation. A critical access hospital that is 10 miles away from an academic Medical Center in New England functions very differently than a critical access hospital in Montana or Alaska where transport to larger facilities is lengthy and difficult in poor weather.

There are many diseases that can be safely cared for in a rural critical access hospital. There are even data suggesting that for certain select procedures, outcomes might be better than those at academic medical centers.[2-4] It is important to recognize the limitations of your facility and recognize a core group of procedures that should be done at tertiary or quaternary facilities. These would include pancreatic, esophageal, lung, as well as gastric cancers. Most rural hospitals are not currently caring for vascular diseases. Many colon cancers can be safely cared for in rural hospitals, but there is a growing consensus that rectal cancer should be referred to a high-volume center. This could be revisited if the rural hospital meets the volume criteria (ie, high endemic population) and has a skilled rectal surgeon.

From a patient-centric perspective, the best complex surgical oncolgic includes excellent relationship with a referral center. If the patient is seen in the emergency room with a nonurgent hepatobiliary problem, a generic referral to a tertiary care center often comes with delays in care. These delays can be exacerbated if the patient is not referred to the appropriate physician. Patients with pancreas and liver cancer are often sent to either gastroenterology or oncology department, when, in fact, a surgical oncologist is often best suited to quickly address the problem. If a rural surgeon has close relationships with referring physicians, then care is often streamlined and expedited. With appropriate referral, it is often possible to have the entire workup done over a day or 2. For example, with our patient above, appropriate imaging, EUS, and ERCP with stenting could be done in a single visit over the course of 24–48 hours. The patient then would have a disposition and plan regarding the care of their pancreatic cancer.

A surgeon's ability to perform complex surgical procedures in a rural environment needs to be tempered by multiple external institutional factors.[5] The technical ability to perform an operation is only a small portion of the patient's surgical journey. Institutional capabilities, including operating room personnel, equipment, as well as postop care and recovery, need to be strongly considered. The ability of nurses to care for complex surgical patients when they are not used to seeing such a cohort of individuals can be challenging. Many critical access hospitals have limited or no intensive care units, and the access to interventional radiology and GI is often limited or nonexistent. Other medical subspecialists are often not available as well, including cardiology, epidemiology, and nephrology.

A patient's attributes should also strongly weigh into the decision to transfer even if their surgical problem is not necessarily complex. A patient with a complicated medical history and multiple comorbidities, who has a treatable problem such as right-sided colon cancer or small bowel obstruction but has a high risk of postoperative cardiopulmonary complications, should be considered for transfer to a tertiary care facility. Many critical access hospitals are not capable of providing prolonged intubation and ventilatory management postoperatively. It is often much better to make that decision preoperatively so that the entire spectrum of care can be provided in a singular environment.

Our patient was discharged from the emergency room with surgical oncology follow-up within 48 hours. The patient was seen and underwent a pancreatic protocol CT scan, as well as EUS and biliary stent placement. The patient was found to have a locally advanced pancreatic cancer and was treated with neoadjuvant chemotherapy. At the conclusion of chemotherapy, a pancreaticohepatojejunostomy was performed (the Whipple procedure). Follow-up care was provided locally for a small wound infection though definitive care still took place at the tertiary care center.

● IMPLEMENTING A SOLUTION

As we have suggested, there are some cases where rural hospitals are not equipped to manage complex surgical problems in an ever-changing, advancing world. With the expertise available to us in tertiary centers, it would be deficient of us ruralists not to expediently refer our patients to these services. It is with multidisciplinary care that they will receive the best outcomes.

It has been noted in the literature that rural patients prefer to receive their care nearer to home, even if there is a higher risk of morbidity and mortality.[6] For some situations, that is a factor to consider in the management of a patient's disease. In this case, however, a hepatobiliary cancer, such as pancreatic cancer, has too many needs that we cannot meet. What a rural facility, and rural practitioners, can do is to prepare the patient, offer support, streamline or expedite care, and provide follow-up.

The extent to which a rural facility can add to this type of management depends on personnel, equipment, and volumes. If your rural facility has trained advanced endoscopy nurses, a trained ERCP surgeon who does enough cases a year to maintain standards, and the equipment for the procedure, then this can be done at home. If your facility has the financial ability to invest in an MRI machine and the appropriate technicians, then this could be part of the workup for the patient and may mean less travel time to the tertiary center. The rural hospital can provide as much of the workup for complex surgical care as they are able to do so, if records can be shared, and the receiving team is satisfied with an external practitioner performing tests. Often the hepatopancreatobiliary (HPB) surgeon managing the case in the tertiary center feels more comfortable performing some of these invasive tests themselves, and it would only hamper the patient's care if it were done externally.

Communication with the HPB team and the tertiary center is paramount. Knowing the protocols that are followed for workup and management of advanced surgical problems in the tertiary center will help the rural site prepare the patient. Having a network between rural and tertiary surgical teams, where there is a good working relationship, is one of the ways administrations can ensure good communication.

Potential pitfalls in the solutions listed above would include doubling up on procedures. As was mentioned, if an advanced procedure is done in the rural community, often the tertiary center would want it repeated with their own staff and proceduralists. If the MRI/MRCP in the rural area does not meet the standards that they require, it may have to be repeated. This adds to the stress and frustration of not only the surgical teams in both locations but also of the patient. Involving the hepatobiliary team early is the key to the management of this patient, but it may not be easy on the patient. A potential problem of having to send patients to the tertiary centers may be that they choose not to go, thus forgoing treatment. Rural stoicism is one of the reasons noted in the literature for delay in diagnosis, but it can also affect treatment. A reduced socioeconomic status, also seen in rural populations, can contribute to a patient's unwillingness to travel for treatment. Rural administrations and communities can work together to assist with travel, either through community fundraisers or providing hospital-based transport for patients.

In summary, in a complex HPB patient, such as the one in our scenario, early referral, expedient workup, and support from the physicians, hospital, and community are the best ways to provide the best outcomes. All rural hospitals can prepare their patients for what to expect and offer support and assistance if the means of higher diagnostic tests and workup are not available locally. Networking and communication remain the key to ensure good outcomes for all involved parties.

Key Steps in Change Management and Potential Pitfalls

Key Steps in Change Management

1. Recognize when complex surgical procedures are outside the scope of practice of your entire staff—nursing, physician, ancillary, and multidisciplinary.
2. Establish a network between the rural and tertiary centers and physicians.
3. Know the capabilities of your facility and your staff before implementing changes in practice or technologies.
4. Keep up to date with telehealth and videoconferencing software.
5. If advanced techniques in HPB surgery are available in your facility, make sure it does not interfere with the practices of the tertiary team.
6. Look for providing ways to facilitate patient transport and what care can be given close to home.

Potential Pitfalls

1. Patients may not wish to proceed with care outside their local facility (rural stoicism or low socioeconomic status).
2. Advanced management in the rural facility may double up procedures if there is no good communication with the tertiary team.
3. Plan to manage expectations—of staff and patients.

REFERENCES

1. Guda M, Freeman ML. Are you safe for your patients: how many ERCPs should you be doing? *Endoscopy*. 2008; 40(8):675–676.
2. Ibrahim AM, Hughes TG, Thumma JR, Dimick JB. Association of hospital critical access status with surgical outcomes and expenditures among Medicare beneficiaries. *JAMA*. 2016;315(19):2095–2103.
3. Joynt KE, Harris Y, Orav EJ, Jha AK. Quality of care and patient outcomes in critical access rural hospitals. *JAMA*. 2011;306(1):45–52.
4. Finlayson SR. Assessing and improving the quality of surgical care in rural America. *Surg Clin North Am*. 2009; 89(6):1373–1381.
5. Chappel AR, Zuckerman RS, Finlayson SRG. Small rural hospitals and high-risk operations: how would regionalization affect surgical volume and hospital revenue? *JACS*. 2006;203(5):599–604.
6. Finlayson SR, Birkmeyer JD, Tosteson AN, Nease RF Jr. Patient preferences for location of care: implications for regionalization. *Med Care*. 1999;37(2):204–209.

Imbalanced Clinic Utilization Across the Workweek—Balancing Low Space Utilization, Patient Access, and Provider Workflow

TASHA M. HUGHES

2

Clinical Delivery Challenge

In a busy, tertiary care system comprised of a complex network of 25 ambulatory care units (ACU), we were tasked with addressing the imbalance in the number of visits across outpatient clinics, with the ultimate goal of equilibrating the number of visits across each day of the week. The leadership identified that unequal visits on different days of the week pose a challenge to patient access to specialty and primary care services and provide logistic challenges in a space-constrained care delivery system. Using unit and individual-level data to understand patterns of utilization, we aimed to identify opportunities to achieve a more balanced opportunity to access ambulatory care services across our health system.

Defining the Problem

Over the course of the year preceding our work, our institution saw more than 2 million (N = 2,186,000) outpatient visits, across 25 ACU. Most, but not all, providers see patients in more than 1 ACU, and independent providers included in the analysis are both attending physicians and advanced practice providers. Patients were seen across all 7 days of the week, although the weekend volume was miniscule, and for the purposes of discussion and analysis, we will be describing only the variation between Monday and Friday. The distribution of outpatient visits across the workweek for the preceding fiscal year is displayed in Figure 2.1. Of note, this variation is across all 19 clinical departments in this health system, and the distribution across the weekdays is not the same for each clinical department, which we will reference later in the discussion. Across the institution, more patients were seen on Mondays and Tuesdays than on Thursdays and Fridays, posing challenges for staffing and space (ie, resource allocation), both of which negatively impact access to our health system.

Understanding Institutional Goals

Smoothing of clinic utilization across the workweek was first identified as an institutional goal in 2020, in the months following the onset of the COVID-19 pandemic. Our institution had previously established a program of establishing clinical delivery metrics tied to financial incentives for individual clinic departments. In 2020, our leadership rolled out "group" metrics, where the achievement of specific clinical delivery goals would be evaluated institution-wide, and every department was awarded a financial incentive if the goal was achieved by the institution as a whole. This meant that, while an individual clinical department could look internally and be compliant with any given metric, if the average across the institution did not meet the goal, the financial incentive was not earned by any of the departments. In the first year of this group metric, there was an emphasis on access, which is well established within our health system as an area for improvement.

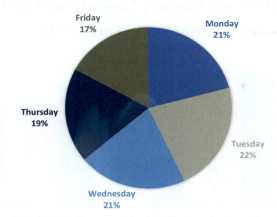

FIGURE 2.1 Ambulatory care visits for fiscal year preceding institutional metric creation.

● WORKUP AND EVALUATION

Defining Our Goal—Equilibrating Clinic Visits Across the Weekdays

Our institution established a goal around clinical utilization to achieve less than a 3% difference between the busiest and least busy outpatient clinic days. In the fiscal year preceding the establishment of this goal, the institution-wide weekday variation was 5%, with Tuesday being the busiest day and Friday the least busy (Figure 2.1). Clinic visits were defined as a visit to a physician or advanced practice provider (including nurse practitioners and physician assistants) across the 25 ACU in our organization. The number of visits was based on in-person, completed visits. All telehealth visits were excluded as were holidays and weekend visits, which were extremely rare as our institution did not have significant established weekend clinic hours at that time.

Key Stakeholders

Identification of key stakeholders in the process was an important first step toward narrowing the gap between the busiest and least busy days. As we were working within a single clinical department, we first needed to understand the relative contribution of each clinical department to the overall visit numbers, and specifically how our department was influencing the overall baseline variation. For example, visits within our surgical group comprise just 5% of the total number of ambulatory care visits across the health system. Changes within the single department, then, would not result in major shifts without consideration of the influence of more ambulatory-focused services. Within our department, key stakeholders include providers, patients, sectional/divisional leadership, and the clinical support staff within each ACU. In particular, providers and leaders were particularly important in thinking through what changes could be made to existing grids that would be least detrimental to a provider's overall productivity and where were the greatest opportunities to narrow this gap within incremental new hires and expected increases or decreases in ambulatory care grids.

Identification of Data Sources

As part of the effort to establish and work toward this and other metrics, our health system generated dashboards to capture progress toward the metric in real time. Figure 2.2 demonstrates an early version of the dashboard corresponding to "visit leveling" in both our health system and our surgical group. Our ability to see both the health system distribution across the workweek and our own microcosm within our group was an essential component to our framing of the problem. All data were provided through

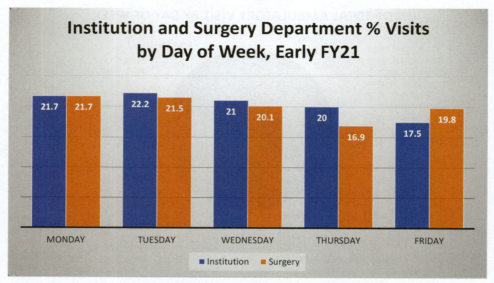

FIGURE 2.2 Institution-wide and surgical practice ambulatory care visits, first dashboard report after metric reporting.

dashboards provided by the health system. The advantage of this form of data acquisition was consistency across departments and a very clear understanding of the "gold standard" in terms of the data used to measure progress.

● DIFFERENTIAL DIAGNOSIS

As we began to think about what may be driving differential uptake of ambulatory care across the workweek within such a large health system, we had more questions than answers. It was these questions that drove our eventual suggestions and actions for improvement. Specifically, was this something likely driven by patients, providers, or staff? Or was it a complex interplay of more than one stakeholder? Were these differences largely historical or were they being perpetuated and exacerbated continuously across the health system with each new hire and each change to the faculty schedule? Finally, were there other system factors and processes in place when new providers were hired that may be influencing this distribution?

● DIAGNOSIS AND TREATMENT

When we began to describe an action plan, it was important to recognize that although the metric posed by our health system was set out as a "group goal," our most immediate sphere of influence was a large group of surgeons (ie, our clinical department) within the health system. Specific to our case and to our clinical influence, it became clear that for surgeons, who were simultaneously being tightly scheduled into operating room and clinic time, the demands of the operating room schedule often took precedence over the clinic and, perhaps more importantly, the restrictive nature of scheduling operating room time made changes in ambulatory care schedules more difficult for many of the providers within our practice. At the same time as this metric was put forth within our health system, we were emerging from the first wave of the COVID-19 pandemic and a new operating room rubric was simultaneously rolled out, largely without consideration of the ambulatory care goals, which made flexibility around the operating room even more challenging.

The other challenge, which was briefly mentioned earlier in the chapter, was the discrepancy between the workweek distribution across the health system and within our group of providers (Figure 2.2). While we had in common one of the least busy days (Thursday), our least busy day was not Friday as it was in the larger healthcare system. As we began to dig deeper into the nuances of this distribution, it became clear that within our surgical group, Thursdays were a designated "late start" day due to educational activities across the group, which provided an additional barrier to expanding services on Thursdays. We did have in common with the overall health system our busiest day (Tuesday) so we were able to think about concrete ways in which we could contribute to off-loading ambulatory care on Tuesdays.

Through our initial analysis, we discussed the ways in which we could leverage the most influence on the desired outcome by contributing to more even distribution of ambulatory care across the practice. We identified two major areas for possible influence. First, we asked that clinical disease group leaders look at the distribution of nonsurgical providers (nurse practitioners and physician assistants employed within our group) for opportunities to move these providers off the busiest clinical day. Second, we made a plea, with the support of departmental leadership, to strongly avoid assigning new hires to the busiest clinic days. At the time of the original discussion, we were in the middle of an institution-wide hiring freeze due to the pandemic, but in anticipation of this being lifted eventually, we were able to garner support at all levels to be thoughtful in the assignment of new hire clinic hours when hiring did resume.

● SCIENTIFIC PRINCIPLES AND EVIDENCE

Unequal distribution of provider scheduling in outpatient clinics has been associated with poor utilization of resources, provider burnout, and increased patient wait times for appointments, all of which may exacerbate the very barriers to access that lead to these variable clinic schedules in the first place. In many ways, within our health system, the unequal distribution of outpatient clinic volume seemed to be both a symptom of low access and a barrier to better access for our patients. One proposed model to address this unequal distribution of clinical care is termed constrained optimization modeling. Constrained optimization modeling is, at its core, a decision-making tool that has been widely used in non-healthcare settings, including manufacturing and production, and recently has been recognized as applicable in the ever-changing face of outpatient healthcare delivery.[1] The model itself requires three elements to be implemented. Namely, these are decision variables, an objective function, and the identification of relevant constraints.[2]

When applied in our case, the decision variables, which can be manipulated, could be considered as the individual provider, the time/days the provider is in a clinic and the number of time units a clinic is open/available. The objective in our case is to minimize the variation in clinic visits across days of the workweek. The potential constraints, in our clinical example, may include the proportion of a provider's time that is spent in a clinic (ie, their full-time equivalent dedicated to outpatient clinic duties), the order/arrangement of clinic hours within a single day (ie, that hours are contiguous), and the weekly schedule of a given provider (ie, do providers see patients on one day per week, skip weeks, alternate sites, or have multiple days of clinic per week). Although beyond the scope of this description, the decision variables and constraints can then be modeled to achieve minimal variance in the objective and provide guidance for optimal scheduling strategies for a health system.[2]

This type of model has been applied practically in a large urological practice, with similar types of constraints to our surgical group. In this group, they defined the optimized function was to maximize patient access and the identified constraints included integration of evaluation and management visits, office and operating room procedures, teaching, trainee mentorship, committee work, and outreach activities, all of which impacted providers' time and availability. This group reports significantly reduced variation in the number of providers scheduled per shift and a significant increase in the number of encounters. Using this example, it is plausible that implementation of such a model would both address our health system metric of equalizing the number of providers on any given shift and would have also independently increased access to ambulatory care in our health system.[3]

IMPLEMENTATION, CHANGE MANAGEMENT, AND POSSIBLE PITFALLS

Implementing a Solution

After establishing a firm understanding of the problem, key stakeholders, and available data, we elected to put forth two main proposals for a solution. First, we worked closely with administrative leadership within our surgical group to focus efforts on new surgeon hires and on existing and new hires in our advanced practice provider pool. For the former, new hires were few in the first year after the metric was proposed due to economic recovery in the wake of the pandemic. However, in the year following, hiring was robust and we were able to recommend that new surgeon hires have clinic days assigned that were complementary to the overall demands on the health system across the workweek. Additionally, we were also able to make several small, incremental changes in advanced practice provider schedules, largely among new hires but also by finding opportunities within existing schedules when such changes were not otherwise detrimental to these providers' other professional demands or workflow.

Change Management

In this real-life example of a clinical delivery challenge, many of the key steps for change management were naturally present and some had to be actively pursued to achieve our goals. To begin, our problem was defined for us by the larger health system. In this case, it was clear numerically what the goal was (<3% variation between the busiest and least busy clinical days) and the data source for measuring progress toward this outcome was provided, in a regularly updated and easy-to-access data dashboard, by the health system leadership. The key factors influencing how providers and patients were assigned variably across workdays were less clear and left some gaps in our analysis. Additionally, the transparency of this process between departments was not easily facilitated by available data. As a group, we spent time with identified key stakeholders, including administrative leaders who had direct influence over the assignment of clinic schedules as well as representatives from both faculty and advanced practice providers who offered insight into the nuances of clinic day and time assignment. Similarly, we were able to utilize our multidisciplinary workgroup to solicit feedback on potential solutions we proposed. Finally, within our clinical sphere of surgical practice, we were able to pilot the placement of newly hired faculty and advanced practice providers on Thursday and Friday clinic days. Solicitation of feedback on this process from both providers and administrative leadership within our department is ongoing and exactly how well we were able to achieve a working schedule that functions harmoniously with other demands, especially the demands of the operating room schedule, is a work in progress. Key steps in change management are summarized below.

Potential Pitfalls and Threats to Equity

Perhaps most notably missing from the above description, and from the framing of the problem of clinical care delivery described above, is the simultaneous rapid expansion of telehealth within the larger health system. At the onset of the COVID-19 pandemic, the use of telehealth across our health system was small, comprising <5% of all visits. At the time of this writing, telehealth visits make up nearly 30% of visits across the health system. This shift to telehealth has been identified, simultaneously, as a sustained and important metric of our health system and there is no intention for this number to decrease with the transition out of the pandemic crisis. As such, access to our physical clinical spaces has been markedly impacted by this change and this was not considered when setting goals for the calibration of clinic utilization across the workweek.

Perhaps also not well considered or incorporated into decisions around clinic utilization was the role of patients as stakeholders in this process. We did not address patient preference toward certain appointment days and, given our large catchment area that often is associated with long travel times, this may have a relevant influence on our patients and their preferences for particular appointment days and times. By pushing more appointment availability to the end of the week (ie, Friday), we may be excluding patients in nonrandom ways depending on their socioeconomics or the distance required to travel to our ambulatory sites. This effect is largely unmeasured in our current approach to change management.

Key Steps in Change Management and Potential Pitfalls

Key Steps in Change Management

1. Identify a clear problem (high variation between busiest and least busy clinic days) with a measurable outcome (<3% variation in clinic utilization between busiest and least busy clinical days).
2. Understand the process and systems in place that determine clinic schedules and clinical scheduling.
3. Spend time on the front line with key stakeholders involved including providers (faculty and advanced practice providers), section administrators, and intake coordinators.
4. Identify sources of quantitative data (eg, health-system-level dashboards) that are used to measure the outcome of interest.
5. Introduce possible solutions to key stakeholders to test face validity and refine based on feedback.
6. Pilot the potential solution (eg, purposeful placement of new hires into underutilized clinic days) and have regular opportunities to solicit feedback. Continue to track outcome measurement in real time.

Potential Pitfalls

1. Not considering a simultaneous rise in telehealth as we seek to calibrate in-person visits across the workweek.
2. Unclear incorporation and influence of telehealth visits on access, which is the underlying driver of our own change strategies.
3. Lack of engagement of patients as key stakeholders in clinic access and utilization.

● MEASURING OUTCOMES

The measurement of variation in clinic visits across clinic days was provided by a robust infrastructure of institution-level data. We were able to monitor this through an accessible dashboard on a regular basis. In the first fiscal year measuring this metric, we were able to achieve a 3% variation, largely through some significant changes made on the part of colleagues in our primary care settings.

● FOLLOW-UP AND MAINTENANCE

Importantly, our health system continued to offer a financial incentive for this metric in the subsequent fiscal year, with an even lower goal for variation (<2.5% variation between the busiest and least busy days). Unfortunately, in the subsequent fiscal year, this metric proved more challenging and the difference between the busiest and least busy days rebounded slightly to just above 3%. This may be due to many factors, including ongoing detrimental effects of the pandemic, increased proportion of practices that were virtual, which limits the impact of changes in in-person care delivery, and the influence of such clinical changes on provider well-being and workplace satisfaction, all of which have been discussed by our group as possible contributors to this rebound to modestly higher variation than we were able to achieve with our intentional efforts described within this chapter.

REFERENCES

1. Capan M, Khojandi A, Denton BT, et al. From data to improved decisions: operations research in healthcare delivery. *Med Decis Making*. 2017;37(8):849–859. doi: 10.1177/0272989X17705636
2. Berg BP, Erdogan SA, Lobo JM, Pendleton K. A method for balancing provider schedules in outpatient specialty clinics. *MDM Policy Pract*. 2020;5(2):2381468320963063. doi: 10.1177/2381468320963063
3. Lobo JM, Ayca ES, Berg BP, et al. Provider scheduling to maximize patient access. *J Urol Urol Pract*. 2020;7(5): 335–341.

Emergency Department Visits With Semi-Urgent Problems

3

MATTHEW CORRIERE AND ERIKA ARNDT

Clinical Delivery Challenge

A 62-year-old woman with a history of diabetes and severe peripheral artery disease undergoes an urgent lower extremity bypass. Her hospital course is relatively uncomplicated, though she had elevated glucose levels immediately postoperatively, which was controlled with the escalation of her home regimen. She is cleared by physical therapy for home discharge despite living alone. She is discharged on postoperative day 5 with a plan for clinic follow-up in 2 weeks. On postoperative day 7, she notices mild incisional erythema at the calf. Though she otherwise feels well, she is cautious of the change in the appearance of her incision. She refers to her discharge paperwork; however, she does not recall all of the instructions provided to her by the nurse, and she has trouble understanding the written instructions. She asks her neighbor to transport her to the emergency department (ED). After a 4-hour triage process, vascular surgery is consulted. She undergoes an arterial duplex that demonstrates the bypass is patent and there is no underlying fluid collection. She is initiated on an oral antibiotic regimen and discharged from the ED 16 hours after her initial presentation. The patient completes her antibiotic course, the redness resolves, and she is seen at her scheduled follow-up visit with her vascular surgeon where she describes recovering well.

Hospital readmissions are a significant burden to the United States healthcare system. Readmissions pose a financial strain, increase unplanned costs and resource utilization, and most importantly, lead to worse patient outcomes.[1] A marker for quality of care, preventing avoidable readmissions has substantial implications for the health system and patient care and thus warrants intensified efforts to reduce rehospitalization.[2,3] While the reasons for postoperative readmissions are multifactorial, postsurgical complications, including surgical site infection or hematoma, postoperative myocardial infarction, and ileus, are common and contribute to unplanned readmissions.[4,5] Recognizing that health outcomes are shaped by the social determinants of health (SDoH)—"the conditions in the environments where people are born, live, learn, work, play, and work, and age that affects a range of health, functioning, and quality of life outcomes and risks"—readmissions for postsurgical complications may also be a direct manifestation of unmet social need.[6,7] Given the prevalence of postoperative readmissions and its disruption to patient quality of life and health system efficiency, developing strategies to reduce readmissions is critical. Eliminating readmissions for all acute postsurgical issues may not be feasible; however, reducing emergency room visits for problems that do not require inpatient management may be an important first step.

● WORKUP

Postsurgical ED visits and readmissions at large are a burden to the health system; however, they are not all equal in their impact on the system. To gain an understanding of the current state, health systems need a widely shared and accepted nomenclature around the different types of readmissions. The Centers for Medicare and Medicaid Services (CMS), which has instituted policies to reduce surgical readmissions, makes a distinction between planned versus unplanned readmissions. For CMS's purpose, there are limited types of care that are always considered planned, such as obstetrical delivery, transplant surgery, and maintenance chemotherapy and radiotherapy, as well as planned readmissions for a scheduled procedure. Unplanned readmissions are presentations for all other acute issues or complications.[8] Unplanned ED visits and readmissions should be characterized by urgent versus nonurgent status, and further stratified by surgical service, procedure, index procedure urgency (elective versus urgent/emergent), and possibly surgeon as readmission rates will likely vary widely across these domains.

Patient-level factors also contribute to postsurgical readmission, which should be considered when collecting and evaluating readmission data. Patients with greater comorbidities are at increased risk for readmission. Comorbid conditions may independently or synergistically increase the risk for surgical complications and readmission; thus, understanding those subsets of patients at increased risk can be useful for targeted interventions. Because surgical outcome disparities associated with specific patient demographic characteristics persist, stratifying readmission rates by race, ethnicity, gender, and socioeconomic status will be important to ensure equitable healthcare delivery and quality improvement. Structural inequities that contribute to outcome disparities are related to SDoH.[9] While most health systems do not integrate SDoH domains into their electronic medical record, finding ways to capture these data could be pivotal in identifying upstream drivers of poor outcomes and strategically directing resources to those at greatest risk.

Stakeholder collaboration has the potential to reduce unplanned readmission rates through coordinated care as patients transition from their in-hospital stay to the outpatient setting. As the recipient of healthcare services, the patient is a key stakeholder. Patient caregivers and other patient advocates are also integral to the patient recovery process. Important stakeholders that predominantly operate in the inpatient setting include residents, inpatient advance practice providers (APPs), nurses, and other members of the clinical care team. Key stakeholders from the outpatient setting include clinic staff/nurses, outpatient APPs, and primary care providers. Emergency medicine physicians are especially critical at the point of care where readmission is being considered. The surgeon holds primary responsibility for outcomes following surgery and is the ultimate facilitator of care coordination. Hospital leadership and other administrators with knowledge of hospital resource utilization should be included.

● DIFFERENTIAL DIAGNOSIS

There are many drivers for unplanned readmissions at the patient, provider, and health system levels. Patients may not have the necessary family or community support or lack adequate health literacy to understand care instructions. At the provider level, there may be a lack of standard discharge processes or ineffective communication of relevant clinical information. Non-coordination between compartmentalized units (eg, inpatient and outpatient teams) may result in a lack of timely follow-up or fragmented postoperative experiences for patients and primary care physicians.

● DIAGNOSIS AND TREATMENT

There is no one-size-fits-all solution to unplanned readmissions for nonurgent postsurgical complications. Solutions should be driven by the needs of the patient population served by the health system. Identifying avoidable readmissions will likely require tailored interventions that consider the patient population and procedure-specific factors (including incisions, wounds, drains, and anticipated posthospital needs). Regardless of the exact intervention employed, those that are proactive, seeking to identify at-risk patients, and those experiencing postsurgical problems early in their recovery process are preferred.

One potential solution is the use of *Transitional Care Programs*. Though the exact nature of the program might vary on specialty, the goal of transitional care programs is to anticipate early post-discharge needs and meet them through direct patient engagement. In a protocol described by Medina et al.,[10] a vascular registered nurse calls patients on post-discharge day 1, followed by a subsequent call on post-discharge day 7. Patients are asked about any symptoms including pain, fever, nausea, vomiting, and ambulatory status, in addition to the assessment of their incision and concerns for bleeding, swelling, or redness. Any concerns regarding patient status are escalated to the surgeon who would then decide whether to bring the patient in for an office visit or recommend an ED visit or inpatient readmission. Though the potential for improvement in care delivery is significant, such a program requires the appropriate infrastructure, including nursing personnel and dedicated appointment slots. In the case of our clinical delivery challenge example, the woman's status post lower extremity bypass, a call from the clinic nurse may have primed the patient to take note of any redness around her incision sooner. Even if there was no redness the day of the clinic call, the initial contact by the clinic nurse may have empowered the patient to call the clinic the following day with her symptoms instead of proceeding to the ED for her care.

Another solution could include a *social needs assessment* in the preoperative and in-hospital phases of care. The assessment would help to identify the most vulnerable patients at risk for postoperative complications and readmission based on unmet social needs, and ideally, in the preoperative setting link them with community resources to optimize conditions outside of the hospital. While addressing social needs is likely to be the most impactful, it is also likely to be the most challenging because it requires health systems to consider healthcare delivery beyond that which is provided within the hospital walls. It also requires building community partnerships, and these relationships may require years to build the necessary trust. From the perspective of SDoH, the woman in the example has trouble interpreting the written discharge instructions. A health literacy assessment in the preoperative setting may have identified this problem and alternative modes of instruction (eg, video) could be provided.

● IMPLEMENTATION OF A SOLUTION

Designing systems to prevent unplanned ED visits and readmissions, especially for nonurgent post-surgical complications, is challenging. Though there have been numerous randomized, controlled trials and observational studies evaluating pre- and post-discharge interventions, they have had varying success. Additionally, even those interventions found to be effective in one setting do not translate to meaningful outcomes in a different set-up. When considering the design and implementation of an intervention, it should be approached systematically. It is worth choosing a framework (eg, *Consolidated Framework for Implementation Research*) to guide intervention development and to ensure all the relevant contexts that would influence barriers and facilitators to the intervention are considered.[11] Stakeholders should be engaged throughout the entire process, and as such decisions should be based on group consensus, acknowledging that due to inherent power differential, hospital leadership will likely be the final arbiter.

The key steps in change management to unplanned readmission reduction include identifying a clear problem with measurable outcomes. One should understand the process and steps leading to a patient being readmitted. This step might require identifying an exemplar patient *and journey mapping* his/her course from the preoperative setting to the point of readmission. One should identify and engage key stakeholders, spending time in the various settings in which care is delivered (eg, inpatient ward, outpatient clinic, and emergency room). By spending time on the front line and through meaningful discussions with stakeholders, one will better identify sources of quantitative and qualitative data to inform the root causes of unplanned readmissions. The problem should be revisited as necessary based on new data. Potential solutions should be developed with the assistance of key stakeholders. The intervention should then be piloted for a high-yield surgical service. It might be easiest to pilot the intervention in the surgical services to which the surgeon stakeholders belong. As part of the pilot rollout, there should be routine opportunities to provide feedback.

Potential pitfalls in the implementation of an intervention include lack of a clearly defined problem or a solution based on the patient's needs and perceptions. Stakeholders with a working understanding of population- and community-level barriers and diverse backgrounds (professionally, gender, racially/ ethnically, etc.) are also needed and should be engaged throughout the process. Arguably, the success of the intervention hinges upon the diversity of stakeholders as the variety of perspectives shapes the design of the intervention and will offer considerations for monitoring unintended and inequitable consequences of the intervention. Broadly implementing the solution without pilot testing, not eliciting routine feedback of those affected by the pilot, and not adjusting processes and outcomes based on feedback are also pitfalls to implementation.

Key Steps in Change Management and Potential Pitfalls

Key Steps in Change Management

1. Identify a clear problem with a measurable outcome.
2. Understand the process and steps leading up to the patient being readmitted. Consider creating a patient journey map to understand the steps in sequence.
3. Spend time on the front line (eg, Gemba Walks) with key stakeholders involved, including patients, patient caregivers, residents, surgeons, nurses, clinic staff, advanced practice providers, and administrators.
4. Identify sources of quantitative data (eg, unplanned versus planned readmissions) and qualitative data (eg, patient satisfaction and patient's perspectives on discharge processes) to bring measurable outcomes to understand your potential sources of readmission.
5. Identify key stakeholders, reclarify the problem as necessary based on new data, and develop potential interventions with their engagement.
6. Pilot the potential solution in high-yield surgical services and have regular opportunities to solicit feedback. Make sure you can track a measurable outcome (ideally what you identified in #1).

Potential Pitfalls

1. Jumping straight to a solution without clearly defining the problem or based on an individual's perceptions of the problem.
2. Not accruing the correct stakeholders with diverse backgrounds (professionally, gender, racially/ethnically, etc.).
3. Forgetting to monitor unintended consequences of your solution.
4. Broadly implementing your solution (eg, new ED readmission triage guidelines) across the whole department, without pilot testing or eliciting routine feedback.

● MEASURING OUTCOMES

The most apparent metric to assess the effectiveness of the solution is to measure the percentage of unplanned readmissions and ED visits stratified by some of the variables mentioned in the workup: urgency status, patient demographics, and surgical services. In addition to measuring unplanned readmission rates, tracking the reasons for readmission might yield new information to focus intensified efforts. Other metrics that may be complementary to readmission rates include changes in the utilization of virtual health, outpatient appointments, clinic calls to patients, and patient calls to clinic or to the on-call resident during off hours. Beyond traditional clinical outcomes, measuring patient satisfaction or other patient-reported outcomes is important to providing patient-centered care, and may reveal some success with the intervention even in the face of stagnant or worsening readmission rates. Specific to the implementation process, measuring fidelity, the degree to which the intervention is delivered as intended, helps to explain why an intervention succeeds or fails, and whether the changes in outcomes are in fact due to the intervention or other causes. Finally, any intervention has the potential for unintended consequences. Minimizing harm requires routine evaluation of outcomes and maintaining transparency of outcomes, especially with key stakeholders.

● FOLLOW-UP AND MAINTENANCE

To achieve lasting outcomes, it is essential to sustain the implementation of the intervention. Ideally, through the implementation framework selected at the onset of the process, potential barriers to sustainability would have been identified and thus strategies to combat the dissolution of the intervention would have been integrated into the implementation process. It is also possible that a different framework might be better suited to managing issues that arise surrounding sustainability, as all frameworks are not suited for every phase of the implementation process. Recognizing that patients, institutions, and the landscape of medicine changes, alterations to the intervention and the measured outcomes should also be expected and welcomed. Ultimately, an organization's culture will have the greatest impact on sustainability if there is a shared belief in its importance and there is support for it.

REFERENCES

1. Duwayri Y, Goss J, Knechtle W, et al. The readmission event after vascular surgery: causes and costs. *Ann Vasc Surg*. 2016;36:7–12. doi: 10.1016/j.avsg.2016.02.024
2. Jencks SF, Williams MV, Coleman EA. Rehospitalizations among patients in the Medicare fee-for-service program. *N Engl J Med*. 2009;360(14):1418–1428. doi: 10.1056/nejmsa0803563
3. Berenson RA, Paulus RA, Kalman NS. Medicare's readmissions-reduction program: a positive alternative. *N Engl J Med*. 2012;366(15):1364–1366. doi: 10.1056/nejmp1201268
4. Pienta M, Fallon B, Wakam GK, Kim GY, Zogaib J, Corriere MA. Identifying low-value inpatient hospitalizations following emergency department requests for surgical consultations. *J Am Coll Surg*. 2021;233(5):e99–e100. doi: 10.1016/j.jamcollsurg.2021.08.265
5. Merkow RP, Ju MH, Chung JW, et al. Underlying reasons associated with hospital readmission following surgery in the United States. *JAMA—J Am Med Assoc*. 2015;313(5):483–495. doi: 10.1001/jama.2014.18614
6. U.S. Department of Health and Human Services. Social determinants of health. *Healthy People 2030*. Accessed June 30, 2022. https://health.gov/healthypeople/objectives-and-data/social-determinants-health
7. Paro A, Hyer JM, Diaz A, Tsilimigras DI, Pawlik TM. Profiles in social vulnerability: the association of social determinants of health with postoperative surgical outcomes. *Surg (United States)*. 2021;170(6):1777–1784. doi: 10.1016/j.surg.2021.06.001
8. Horwitz L, Partovian C, Lin Z, et al. *Centers for Medicare and Medicaid Services—Planned Readmission Algorithm—Version 2.1.*; 2013. https://hscrc.maryland.gov/documents/HSCRC_Initiatives/readmissions/Version-2-1-Readmission-Planned-CMS-Readmission-Algorithm-Report-03-14-2013.pdf
9. Baciu A, Negussie Y, Geller A, et al, eds. The State of Health Disparities in the United States—Communities in Action. *Communities in Action: Pathways to Health Equity*. NCBI Bookshelf; 2017.
10. Medina D, Zil-E-Ali A, Daoud D, Brooke J, Paul K, Aziz F. Implementation of transitional care planning is associated with reduced readmission rates in patients undergoing lower extremity bypass surgery for peripheral arterial disease. *J Vasc Surg*. 2022;75(3):28–39. doi: 10.1016/j.jvs.2021.12.029
11. Damschroder LJ, Aron DC, Keith RE, Kirsh SR, Alexander JA, Lowery JC. Fostering implementation of health services research findings into practice: a consolidated framework for advancing implementation science. *Implement Sci*. 2009;4(1):50. doi: 10.1186/1748-5908-4-50

High Inpatient Capacity and Unable to Accept Specialty Transfers

LESLY A. DOSSETT

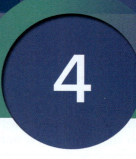

Clinical Delivery Challenge

A large tertiary academic medical center has a distributed transfer management program where numerous physicians can accept patients for interhospital transfers. These physicians are motivated to care for patients, assist referring physicians, and grow their respective clinical programs. This has led to nearly all transfer requests being accepted for inpatient interhospital transfers. Due to high inpatient hospital capacity, many of these accepted patients face long wait times for transfer. At the same time, the hospital faces high levels of admitted patients being boarded in the emergency department and canceled operative cases due to a lack of inpatient beds. Further, the distributed nature of the transfer program creates inefficiencies and delays in identifying and contacting the correct physician teams and collecting the necessary medical records and imaging to inform care decisions. The creation of a new centralized transfer program is hypothesized to improve the management of transfer requests while helping to preserve inpatient capacity for specialty clinical programs.

● WORKUP

The COVID-19 pandemic has highlighted the critical importance of interhospital transfer programs and policies allowing the right patients to be cared for in the right hospitals at the right time. Interhospital transfer can be initiated for several reasons, including to provide patients with access to specialists and technologies not available in their current setting (ie, medical necessity or higher level of care), to provide continuity of care for established patients, and patient or family requests.[1] Interhospital transfers can be declined due to a lack of available inpatient or emergency department capacity, or a determination that transfer is not medically necessary. The goal of transfer management programs is to facilitate appropriate and timely decisions on transfers and to help coordinate the safe movement of patients from one facility to another.

Prior to allocating resources or implementing operational change, the factors contributing to an inability to accept transfers must be fully understood. The key to the implementation of a successful transfer management program is making decisions based on accurate data with a commitment toward continuous quality improvement. In discussion with the transfer center staff, important metrics to consider include daily inpatient and emergency department capacity with particular emphasis on units caring for specialty program patients; the number of daily transfer requests; the number of requests accepted, canceled, or declined; the types of patients (ie, diagnosis and acuity) being considered for transfer; the time required to reach a decision on a transfer; and satisfaction of patients and referring physicians. Partnership with hospital administration is critical to obtain and monitor this data, leverage resources to implement a consolidated transfer program, and communicate with the relevant clinician teams.

Given the broad team involved in caring for patients transferred from one hospital to another, the involvement of all key stakeholders is necessary to have multidisciplinary engagement and coordinated efforts. In this scenario, stakeholders include all members of the transfer center staff tasked with answering initial calls and collecting relevant data, members of the clinical programs most sought out for transfer, hospital capacity management leads, and members of the emergency department as these stakeholders will provide valuable insight into both current barriers to transfer and ideas for improvement.

● DIFFERENTIAL DIAGNOSIS

High inpatient capacity limiting the ability to accept transfer patients may be due to several sources. These include prolonged hospital length of stay for admitted patients, high admission rates from emergency department visits, overallocation of inpatient beds to elective surgical patients, and accepting too many transfers without the necessary capacity to care for them. The specific factors most contributing to capacity issues could be confirmed by measuring data over time on average hospital length of stay and the number and complexity of emergency department visits. For example, changes in the availability of postacute discharge services such as subacute rehabilitation facilities or home health nurses could prolong hospital length of stay and worsen inpatient capacity. Similarly, if a hospital has a policy of accepting all transfer requests (regardless of an ability to offer additional services), capacity may then be limited for other patients who could benefit from the transfer (ie, a patient with liver failure needing urgent transplant).

● DIAGNOSIS AND TREATMENT

To maintain capacity for critically ill patients in need of specialty services or technology, hospitals must look to evolving technologies and novel strategies to improve hospital capacity management where possible. They must further implement transfer programs and policies that facilitate getting the right patients to the right hospitals at the right time.[2]

Options for Improving and Managing Hospital Capacity

Hospitals have several options to improve capacity management, including implementing strategies to reduce the length of stay (eg, enhanced recovery protocols for surgery patients) or avoiding hospital admission (eg, outpatient administration of intravenous antibiotics for uncomplicated cellulitis).

Advanced telemedicine offers hospitals several advantages for capacity management including reduced readmissions of established patients, extended specialist care delivery, and a reduction in unnecessary transfers.

Remote patient monitoring programs can help clinicians manage chronic disease and lower acuity patients at home. For example, the *Care Beyond Walls and Wires* remote monitoring program improved outcomes for patients with chronic diseases in rural communities, reducing hospital length of stay by over 60% and readmissions by over 40%.[3]

Hospitals can also improve capacity management by extending specialist care delivery by providing patient evaluation and specialty consultation to hospitals lacking this access. Examples of these programs include stroke triage, evaluation of transfer requests through review of shared photographs for dermatologic evaluation, and transferred digital radiology images. In some cases, these teleconsultations may eliminate the need for transfer and reduce unnecessary visits and expenses for patients.[4]

Finally, access to on-demand virtual health care may allow patients to avoid emergency department visits for low acuity problems to preserve emergency department and hospital capacity for other patients.

Options for Improving Transfer Center Programs and Policies

Once capacity management has been optimized, improving decisions regarding interhospital transfers requires optimizing the transfer process and investing in the hospital's transfer center. A cornerstone of a well-run transfer center is a communications platform allowing physicians, nurses, and staff to communicate with each other reliably and dynamically.

Second, the center must work to standardize the data collection and decision-making process by providing a single contact center for both transferring and accepting physicians and entrusting transfer decisions to an available and informed clinician who has both the medical knowledge necessary to make informed decisions and up-to-date information regarding current hospital, emergency department, and operating room capacity.

Finally, the center and process should be automated where possible. As many interhospital transfer requests involve critically ill patients, decisions must be made quickly. Utilizing systems avoiding manual data entry can speed up the collection and transfer of information and avoid errors.

● SCIENTIFIC PRINCIPLES AND EVIDENCE

The transfer of patients between hospitals is common with approximately 1.5% of all Medicare patients admitted to the hospital undergoing interhospital transfer with greater frequency occurring among select patient groups.[5] A properly resourced transfer center can help improve transfer quality and efficiency as well as can serve as an important revenue center in both a fee-for-service and value-based payment models. For example, one study has estimated each interhospital transfer contributes over $10,000 in the contribution margin. The Emergency Medical Treatment and Labor Act (EMTALA) requires hospitals to transfer patients needing specialty care unavailable at the transferring institution and directs hospitals that offer these services to accept these patients for transfer.[6] Despite this law, in practice, it is often difficult to define which patients are truly in need of such specialty care. For example, although patients are often transferred to receive specific procedures unavailable at the referring institution, many patients do not actually receive the procedural care for which they were initially transferred.[7] This illustrates that while EMTALA provides general directions for interhospital transfers, it fails to accurately assist in selecting the patients most appropriate for transfer. As a result, the interhospital transfer process remains largely arbitrary and at the discretion of treating clinicians.

Once the decision is made to transfer a patient, the process of selecting a receiving hospital, discussing the case with clinicians and administrators at the receiving hospital, and efficiently and safely accomplishing the transfer also tends to be highly variable,[8] without national, regional, or local standards to direct high-quality transfers.[9] Hospital transfer centers have become increasingly common, particularly in large referral centers accepting a high volume of interhospital transfers.[10] Although the functionality and scope differ between transfer centers, most seek to create a centralized process to streamline various aspects of interhospital transfer. These processes often involve simplifying and standardizing both the transfer request process for referring clinicians and the accepting and admitting processes within the receiving institution. However, the working aspects of each transfer center remain largely distinct across hospitals, including the type of personnel staffing the center and what, if any, specialty training they have had; the roles different personnel have during the transfer process (ie, nurse versus physician acceptance for transfer); what tools are utilized to assist with information exchange (ie, templates, electronic health information exchange, shared electronic health records); what, if any, communication guidelines exist (ie, timeliness of communication prior to transfer, frequency of communication if a transfer is delayed); and the existence of any modalities for feedback and quality improvement with the transfer process.

● IMPLEMENTATION OF A SOLUTION

Implementing solutions requires understanding shared priorities as determined by a review of data and in response to stakeholder engagement. In this scenario, the areas identified as priorities include maintaining transfer capacity for specialty clinical programs which few designated hospitals are equipped to provide (eg, trauma, burn, aortic emergency, and transplant), establishing patients with specialty needs, and avoiding transfers that can be adjudicated through phone consultation or imaging review.

From a hospital administration standpoint, there must be a commitment to a properly resourced transfer center including the proper staff and technology to facilitate safe and efficient transfer. This requires putting in place the correct team of staff with the necessary personalities, skill sets, roles, and training to assess patients and communicate with referring clinicians.

At the clinician level, consolidating transfer decisions into the fewest number of clinicians possible provides a greater line of sight on current capacity limits and patient priorities. Once the team is built, the team must be supported by the technological resources that facilitate the accurate and efficient accessing of relevant data.

Electronic health record-based solutions that auto-populate key data elements and avoid redundant data entry facilitate efficiency and can reduce errors in communication. Additionally, using well-designed, easy-to-use dashboards can give transfer center employees fast access to data with the most up-to-date information about system capacity speeding the time from first contact to appropriate care.

Key Steps in Change Management and Potential Pitfalls

Key Steps in Change Management

1. Identify sources of reliable information for key metrics including hospital census, number of transfer requests, and the outcome of each request.
2. Understand the difference at your institution between opportunities to improve inpatient capacity and improve the efficiency of handling transfer.
3. Identify relevant stakeholders to hospital capacity and transfers including clinical providers and administrators to identify opportunities to increase capacity.
4. Develop strategies for improving hospital capacity, including shorter length of stays, adoption of telehealth or remote monitoring, and increasing specialty access at other sites that otherwise would have to transfer care for that specialty.
5. Outline strategies to improve transfer efficiency including centralizing communication and creating clear dashboards with automated information to allow for rapid decision-making for transfer requests.

Potential Pitfalls

1. Blindly accepting all transfers without a clear strategy to triage them or to ensure appropriate hospital capacity to accept them.
2. Implementing a change to hospital transfer policy without appropriate engagement of relevant stakeholders, including administrators and sites initiating transfer requests.
3. Too decentralized of a transfer process that does not facilitate coordination.

● MEASURING OUTCOMES

Following the implementation of these practices, an ongoing review of implementation outcomes is important. In this scenario, daily capacity management and transfer reports are discussed with leadership and key stakeholders to discuss up-to-date capacity constraints and access to specialty programs. In addition to this data, hospitals should collect data on time to transfer decisions, satisfaction from referring clinicians, and overall costs of the program.

● FOLLOW-UP AND MAINTENANCE

Hospital capacity and transfer management and maintenance is not a static process and will require ongoing attention from the leadership as well as all stakeholders. As one area of improvement is accomplished, the team should continue to identify additional areas to improve the patient and clinician experience. For example, once the unified transfer program is in place, the team can continue to expand services such as offering specialty consultation via telemedicine.

REFERENCES

1. Wagner J, Iwashyna TJ, Kahn JM. Reasons underlying interhospital transfers to an academic medical intensive care unit. *J Crit Care.* 2013;28(2):202–208.
2. Gomez D, Haas B, Larsen K, et al. A novel methodology to characterize interfacility transfer strategies in a trauma transfer network. *J Trauma Acute Care Surg.* 2016;81(4):658–665.
3. Riley WT, Keberlein P, Sorenson G, et al. Program evaluation of remote heart failure monitoring: healthcare utilization analysis in a rural regional medical center. *Telemed J E Health.* 2015;21(3):157–162.
4. Garber RN, Garcia E, Goodwin CW, Deeter LA. Pictures do influence the decision to transfer: outcomes of a telemedicine program serving an eight-state rural population. *J Burn Care Res.* 2020;41(3):690–694.

5. Iwashyna TJ, Kahn JM, Hayward RA, Nallamothu BK. Interhospital transfers among Medicare beneficiaries admitted for acute myocardial infarction at nonrevascularization hospitals. *Circ Cardiovasc Qual Outcomes.* 2010;3(5):468–475.
6. Lulla A, Svancarek B. EMS USA Emergency Medical Treatment and Active Labor Act. In: *StatPearls.* Treasure Island FL: StatPearls Publishing; 2022.
7. Safaee MM, Morshed RA, Spatz J, Sankaran S, Berger MS, Aghi MK. Interfacility neurosurgical transfers: an analysis of nontraumatic inpatient and emergency department transfers with implications for improvements in care. *J Neurosurg.* 2018;131(1):281–289.
8. Bosk EA, Veinot T, Iwashyna TJ. Which patients and where: a qualitative study of patient transfers from community hospitals. *Med Care.* 2011;49(6):592–598.
9. Iwashyna TJ. The incomplete infrastructure for interhospital patient transfer. *Crit Care Med.* 2012;40(8):2470–2478.
10. Hulefeld M. The development of the patient transfer center at ochsner medical center. *Ochsner J.* 2009;9(3):169–170.

Aligning Surgical Care Delivery With Population Health Needs

RYAN HOWARD, ALISHA LUSSIEZ, AND MICHAEL ENGLESBE

> **Clinical Delivery Challenge**
>
> Noor is a 48-year-old woman who presents to the emergency department after repeated episodes of abdominal pain and nausea. In the emergency department, she is diagnosed with symptomatic cholelithiasis and scheduled to see a surgeon in the clinic next week. The surgeon reviews her medical history that includes active smoking, class 2 obesity (body mass index of 38 kg/m^2), and poorly controlled diabetes (hemoglobin A1c 8.1%). Although it does not come up during the visit, she is also unemployed, has difficulty affording food and rent, and is often unable to fill her insulin prescription due to her financial hardship. The surgeon determines that she has no contraindications to surgery, and the following month she undergoes an outpatient laparoscopic cholecystectomy. At her routine follow-up visit, her incisions are healed, she feels well, and her abdominal pain has resolved.
>
> By every current metric, her surgical care was a complete success. However, despite a period of prolonged engagement with the healthcare system (an emergency department visit, 2 clinic visits, and an operation), multiple intervenable risk factors were left entirely unaddressed. These unaddressed medical comorbidities and unmet social needs will likely shorten her life by over a decade. What role could her care have played in addressing these factors?

Efforts to improve surgical care delivery have focused primarily on standardizing perioperative processes, minimizing the costs of care, and improving patient outcomes. While these efforts have shown success, surgical care—and health care in general—has only a modest impact on the overall health of society. Currently, the United States has the lowest life expectancy, the greatest burden of chronic diseases, and the highest rate of preventable death among high-income countries. A person in the United States has a lower chance of living to celebrate their 50th birthday than those living in 17 other peer countries. These poor health outcomes in the United States are driven largely by health behaviors, such as physical inactivity and tobacco use, and social determinants of health, such as food insecurity and limited access to regular health care. These factors account for 70% of all health outcomes and make up 9 of the top 10 risk factors for premature death in the United States.

The abysmal state of population health in the United States requires urgent solutions. Though not traditionally considered part of surgical care, there are opportunities to leverage surgical episodes to address these problems. Tens of millions of surgical procedures are performed each year and patients are often highly engaged and motivated to improve their health around the time of an operation. In many cases, these episodes may represent a patient's only significant interaction with the healthcare system for years. In this chapter, we review evidence and opportunities to capitalize on surgical care to improve population health.

● WORKUP

The conceptual model illustrated in Figure 5.1 juxtaposes the current surgical care delivery pathway with a more longitudinal pathway that could address the issues raised in the above scenario. Currently, patients arrive to the surgical episode with some kind of surgical problem that exists amidst a background of comorbidities, which themselves exist in the context of the patient's health behaviors and social determinants of

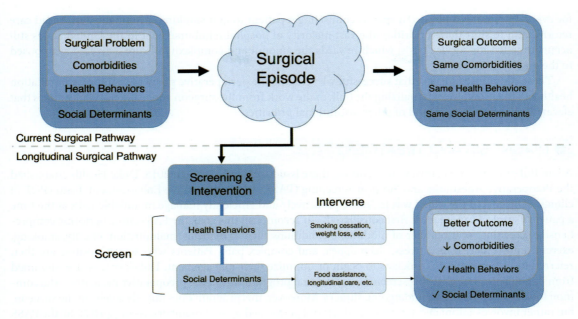

FIGURE 5.1 Conceptual model of the surgical episode.

health. Patients proceed through the surgical pathway and arrive on the other side with their surgical problem resolved, but usually the same comorbidities, health behaviors, and social determinants. Unfortunately, it is precisely these unchanged factors that have the biggest impact on shortening lifespan and impairing quality of life.

Now consider an alternative approach where the surgical episode involves screening for modifiable health behaviors and unmet social needs. Potentially intervenable health behaviors could include tobacco use, alcohol use, physical inactivity, and poor diet. Potentially intervenable social needs could include housing instability, food insecurity, transportation insecurity, financial hardship, and lack of access to regular health care. These interventions would not only improve the immediate surgical outcome but also have the potential to make a lasting impact on patients' longevity. Most healthcare systems have programs in place to address all of these issues, but patients are rarely connected to them at the time of surgery. This is a significant missed opportunity because, as we review as discussed in this chapter, the surgical episode is a time when patients are more likely than ever to make positive health behavior changes.

As an example, the ethos of this approach is nicely captured by a National Health Service England program entitled "Making Every Contact Count."[1] This program views every single interaction a patient has with the healthcare system as a chance to identify and address modifiable risk factors. Patients undergoing anything from a routine eye exam to major surgery are screened for a variety of health behaviors and offered assistance to optimize them. Given the potential impact of this approach, why isn't it more commonplace?

● DIFFERENTIAL DIAGNOSIS

There are multiple reasons this pathway does not typically occur in current practice. First, most surgeons do not view this work as their role. Qualitative interviews reveal that even though virtually all surgeons recognize the overriding importance of health behaviors, such as smoking, most do not engage their patients in these domains.[2] Many cite time constraints, lack of resources, and even the belief that such efforts would simply be futile.

Second, there is a lack of incentive for health systems to prioritize these efforts. Under current reimbursement schedules, a hospital can earn nearly $1 million for every heart transplant it performs but less than $30 for every 15 minutes a physician spends counseling a patient to quit smoking. Although value-based care reforms aim to shift these priorities, the vast majority of hospital reimbursement in the United States still occurs on a fee-for-service basis, which rewards the amount and complexity of care delivered as opposed to the quality of that care.

These root causes suggest that successfully leveraging the perioperative pathway to improve population health will likely involve externalizing the bulk of the work from the surgeon and using novel incentives that elevate these efforts to the level of other institutional priorities.

● DIAGNOSIS AND TREATMENT

A handful of novel care pathways that address these issues currently exist. In 2018, Duke Health established the Preoperative Anesthesia and Surgical Screening (PASS) and Perioperative Enhancement Team (POET) clinics.[3] The goal of this clinic was to "more proactively and efficiently manage modifiable risks at the time a patient's surgical candidacy is first considered." To accomplish this goal, the PASS clinic performs comprehensive screening for a number of modifiable conditions such as diabetes, malnutrition, obesity, smoking, exercise intolerance, frailty, stress, sleep apnea, and complex pain. Patients who screen positive are then referred to the appropriate clinicians to begin or optimize their management. Duke's success has stemmed from its ability to centralize this screening and referral program within the preoperative evaluation, the common touchpoint for patients undergoing surgery. Moreover, this program does not rely solely on the surgeon, but rather involves automated screening and referral performed by staff members. As of April 2020, the PASS program has referred more than 5,000 patients for optimization.

At Michigan Medicine, a number of programs are also underway to address health behaviors and unmet social needs around the time of surgery. The Michigan Surgical and Health Optimization Program is available to any patient scheduled for an operation and engages patients in increased physical activity through step counting, perioperative smoking cession through our institution's smoking cessation service, nutritional diet through healthy recipes, and social work support.[4] We also have a dedicated optimization program for patients referred to our institution for abdominal wall reconstruction. This program provides longitudinal check-ins to help patients lose weight, optimize chronic health conditions, and quit smoking. Both of these programs are eligible for additional reimbursement incentives in order to encourage their prioritization within the health system.

In the context of these examples, we can envision what successful "treatment" would look like by returning to our scenario from above. When Noor presents to either the emergency department or surgeon's clinic, she is automatically screened for modifiable medical risk factors such as obesity, tobacco use, and uncontrolled diabetes, but also nonmedical risk factors such as unemployment, food insecurity, and housing instability. This screening evaluation could result in referral to a number of resources that likely already exist either at the hospital or within her community. For example, she could be enrolled in the hospital's smoking cessation service, referred to a structured exercise and/or bariatric surgery program, and evaluated on the spot by the endocrinology service. Referral to a nonmedical needs assistance program could connect her with resources for financial assistance and alternative insurance options to better facilitate affordable drug prescriptions. Although the coordination involved in these referrals is great, success in just one of these areas will likely have a greater impact on her long-term health and longevity than her surgical care. What is more, these referrals have the potential to establish longitudinal health management that will last long after her surgical care has ended.

● SCIENTIFIC PRINCIPLES AND EVIDENCE

There is an abundance of evidence to suggest that the perioperative period is an effective time to intervene in patients' modifiable risk factors. First, surgery is a "teachable moment." A teachable moment is an event that spontaneously motivates positive behavior change. David Warner described in *JAMA Surgery* how undergoing a laminectomy for acute radiculopathy motivated him to begin an exercise regimen that he still maintained 15 years after the operation.[5] This notion has been corroborated by multiple studies. Smokers have been shown to achieve quit rates of over 50% after undergoing surgery for smoking-related diseases, which far exceeds the average annual quit rate of 7.5%.[6] Longitudinal data from the Health and Retirement Study demonstrate that even patients who undergo nonsmoking-related surgery such as joint replacement are more likely to quit smoking than patients who do not undergo surgery.[7]

Not only can undergoing surgery motivate patients to improve their health behaviors, but there are opportunities that make surgical patients a particularly important population in which to focus these efforts. We found that among patients undergoing surgery in Michigan, the prevalence of tobacco use at the time of surgery was nearly 25%, which is twice the overall prevalence of smoking nationally.[8] We also found that certain vulnerable patient groups such as those with Medicaid or no insurance had a smoking prevalence of 50%. A 50% smoking rate in a group that already faces barriers to receiving regular health care underscores the need for these efforts at every possible opportunity. Other surgical cohorts such as trauma patients have also been shown to have a high incidence of undiagnosed or unmanaged chronic medical or psychiatric conditions.

Finally, interventions do not need to be complex. There is overwhelming evidence that even the most basic interventions around the time of surgery are effective. Randomized trials of smoking cessation efforts, such as simply advising patients to quit smoking, demonstrate that patients who received an intervention are 3 times more likely to quit smoking 1 year after surgery. In Michigan, smokers undergoing vascular surgery had a 43% quit rate after receiving a simple intervention consisting of physician-delivered advice, quit-line referral, and nicotine replacement therapy.[9]

● IMPLEMENTING A SOLUTION

Implementing steps to address population health issues within the surgical care pathway should rely on evidence-based quality improvement strategies. As a representative example, we recently implemented a program that screens patients for smoking and food insecurity as follows.

We began by working to understand the current state. For example, were patients already being referred for these services? This was accomplished by using data from our health system's electronic health record (EHR) system. We found that only 8% of active smokers were referred to smoking cessation around the time of surgery. Although our EHR did not contain information regarding food insecurity among surgical patients, available data suggested that between 4% and 19% of Michiganders were food insecure, and given that screening for food insecurity did not exist when this program was launched, the baseline referral rate was 0%.

Key Steps in Change Management and Potential Pitfalls

Key Steps in Change Management

1. Understand current efforts and resources aimed at addressing social needs during the surgical episode.
2. Spend time with frontline workers in their place of work (eg, "gemba walks") to understand if and how these resources are being used.
3. Ask frontline providers for recommendations on how process or workflow could be improved to allow better uptake of existing resources.
4. Reevaluate after changes are made following key metrics.

Potential Pitfalls

1. Avoid jumping to a solution without spending adequate time with frontline providers.
2. Assume surgical episode of care is "just about the surgery" and not an opportunity for broader care to be improved.

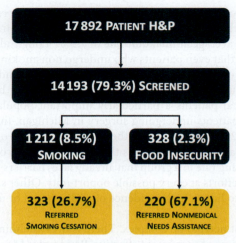

FIGURE 5.2 Preoperative screening and referral pathway for smoking cessation and nonmedical needs assistance.

Next, we met with frontline workers, namely the advanced practice providers (APPs) who staff our preoperative clinic, to understand their current experience and workflow. Importantly, the first two meetings were purely focused on understanding *their* perspective rather than immediately introducing *our* ask. The APPs expressed that they view their job as evaluating and treating the whole patient. They felt strongly that the perioperative period was a crucial time to address unmanaged needs, whether directly related to surgery or not. Consequently, they supported our goal of screening surgical patients for health behaviors and social needs. We engaged in "gemba walks" to observe the steps involved in patient evaluation and understand where screening and referral might fit. Finally, we embraced the principle that those doing the work were the experts, and it was the APPs who designed the screening and referral tool that was incorporated as a checklist into the EHR. The entire process added fewer than 30 seconds to the APP workflow.

To review, we successfully developed and implemented a preoperative screening and referral program using simple quality improvement principles: understand the current state; go and see; understand the people, processes, and technology; and show respect. In the first 12 months of this program's operation, over 14,000 patients were screened, of which 26.7% of smokers accepted referrals to smoking cessation counseling (compared to an 8% baseline referral rate) and 67.1% of patients with food insecurity accepted referrals to nonmedical needs assistance (compared to a 0% baseline referral rate) (Figure 5.2). Among a subset of patients who administered follow-up surveys, 43.6% of smokers reported quitting smoking and 32.1% of patients with food insecurity reported no longer being food insecure. Finally, over 80% of patients agreed that the preoperative appointment was an appropriate time to discuss these issues.

● MEASURING OUTCOMES

A thorough evaluation to understand the impact of any healthcare intervention requires a variety of quality metrics. We recommend the following 5 categories of outcome measures adapted from Gottlieb et al.[10] (Figure 5.3):

1. **Process measures:** understanding whether the program is doing what it intended to do. This includes measures of feasibility and acceptability, which in our pilot was measured by rates of screening and referral, as well as patient-perceived appropriateness of addressing health behaviors and unmet social needs at the time of surgery.
2. **Behavior/social needs outcome:** measuring health behavior change or resolution of unmet social need. Screening and referral are necessary steps, but on their own, they are not sufficient for impact.

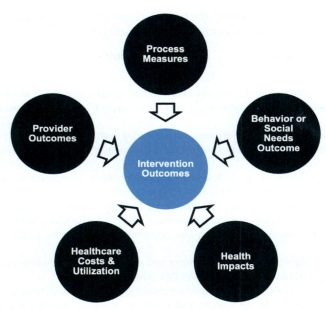

FIGURE 5.3 Outcome measure categories necessary for intervention evaluation.

Understanding intermediate outcomes, such as rates of smoking cessation and resolution of food insecurity after a referral, is essential to determine whether utilized resources are meaningful.
3. **Health impacts:** assessing changes in health outcomes, such as mortality, postoperative complications, and quality of life as a result of behavior modification and resolution of social needs. This requires longitudinal data and rigorous study design.
4. **Healthcare costs and utilization:** measuring changes in hospital admissions, readmission, emergency room visits, and preventative care. This also includes cost analysis to understand the cost-effectiveness of the intervention.
5. **Provider outcomes:** understanding the provider's experience of care. This includes assessing provider satisfaction, confidence in implementation, and potential negative consequences such as burnout.

● FOLLOW-UP AND MAINTENANCE

Delivery of successful interventions to address population health issues is a continuous process requiring iterative testing, evaluation, and subsequent revision. One such guiding framework for this type of iterative process improvement is the Plan-Do-Study-Act (PDSA) cycle. This method provides a systematic approach to developing an initiative (plan), implementing it (do), measuring outcomes (study), and refining the process based on the measured outcomes (act). When applying the PDSA cycle, 3 questions are being asked: (1) What are we trying to accomplish? (2) How will we know if we are successful? (3) What changes can we make that will result in success? As the surgical episode becomes increasingly recognized as an avenue for population health impact, the application of the PDSA cycle will allow complex healthcare systems to understand if perioperative health behavior and social needs interventions are working for patients, providers, and the community.

● DISCLOSURES

Dr. Howard receives unrelated funding from the Blue Cross Blue Shield of Michigan Foundation and the National Institute of Diabetes and Digestive and Kidney Diseases (5T32DK108740-05). Dr. Lussiez receives unrelated funding from the National Cancer Institute (T32CA009672). Dr. Englesbe receives unrelated funding from the Michigan Department of Health and Human Services, the National Institute on Drug Abuse, and salary support from Blue Cross Blue Shield of Michigan.

REFERENCES

1. Lawrence W, Black C, Tinati T, et al. "Making every contact count": evaluation of the impact of an intervention to train health and social care practitioners in skills to support health behaviour change. *J Health Psychol.* 2016;21(2):138–151.
2. Barrett S, Begg S, Sloane A, Kingsley M. Surgeons and preventive health: a mixed methods study of current practice, beliefs and attitudes influencing health promotion activities amongst public hospital surgeons. *BMC Health Serv Res.* 2019;19(1):358.
3. Aronson S, Murray S, Martin G, et al. Roadmap for transforming preoperative assessment to preoperative optimization. *Anesth Analg.* 2020;130(4):811–819.
4. Howard R, Yin YS, McCandless L, Wang S, Englesbe M, Machado-Aranda D. Taking control of your surgery: impact of a prehabilitation program on major abdominal surgery. *J Am Coll Surg.* 2019;228(1):72–80.
5. Warner DO. Surgery as a teachable moment: lost opportunities to improve public health. *Arch Surg.* 2009; 144(12):1106–1107.
6. Mustoe MM, Clark JM, Huynh TT, et al. Engagement and effectiveness of a smoking cessation quitline intervention in a thoracic surgery clinic. *JAMA Surg.* 2020;155(9):816–822.
7. Shi Y, Warner DO. Surgery as a teachable moment for smoking cessation. *Anesthesiology.* 2010;112(1):102–107.
8. Howard R, Singh K, Englesbe M. Prevalence and trends in smoking among surgical patients in Michigan, 2012–2019. *JAMA Netw Open.* 2021;4(3):e210553.
9. Howard R, Albright J, Osborne N, Englesbe M, Goodney P, Henke P. Impact of a regional smoking cessation intervention for vascular surgery patients. *J Vasc Surg.* 2022;75(1):262–269.
10. Gottlieb LM, Wing H, Adler NE. A systematic review of interventions on patients' social and economic needs. *Am J Prev Med.* 2017;53(5):719–729.

SECTION 2

Efficiency of Inpatient Operations

6   Building a Hospital-at-Home Program to Reduce Length of In-Hospital Stay in Surgery
    Nicole M. Santucci, Ayako Mayo, and Vahagn C. Nikolian

7   Postoperative Patients Come to the Emergency Room Because They Do Not Have Urgent Access to Surgical Clinics
    Heather L. Evans and Leeanna Clevenger

8   Efficiency in the Operating Room: Get the Data, Make the Change
    Melanie S. Morris, Brenda Carlisle, Brooke Reeves Vining, Jimmie Loats, and Jeffrey W. Simmons

9   Ensuring Access to Operating Room for Complex Time-Sensitive Cases
    Christopher L. Cramer and Victor M. Zaydfudim

SECTION 2

Efficiency of Inpatient Operations

6 Building a Hospital-at-Home Program to Reduce Length of In-Hospital Stay in Surgery
Nicole M. Santucci, Ayako Mayo, and Mariam C. Nikolin

7 Postoperative Patients Come to the Emergency Room because They Do Not Have Urgent Access to Surgical Clinics
Heather Lavoie and Teodoro Cleveland

8 Efficiency in the Operating Room: Get the Data, Make the Change
Melanie Morris, Irene Gabus, Bruce Ramshaw, and Timothy Zoph and Delaney W Simmons

9 Ensuring Access to Operating Room for Complex, Time-Sensitive Cases
Christopher L Skinner and Deborah Leyva, et al John

Building a Hospital-at-Home Program to Reduce Length of In-Hospital Stay in Surgery

6

NICOLE M. SANTUCCI, AYAKO MAYO, AND VAHAGN C. NIKOLIAN

Clinical Delivery Challenge

Nearly all modern-day healthcare systems are strained, with crowded emergency departments, diverted ambulances, full intensive care units, and booked operating room schedules that manifest as major limitations to in-patient capacity.[1,2] Higher patient acuity and volume all contribute to an overloaded system, negatively impacting healthcare delivery and patient outcomes, but a considerable proportion of hospital capacity is occupied by patients with a low burden of acute issues.[3] Patient length of stay (LOS) is often used as a metric to assess hospital management efficiency and is a significant contributor to hospital capacity strain.[4,5] LOS is complex and difficult to predict, with a patient's pre- and posthospital condition, available resources, insurance type, and provider preferences often resulting in a high degree of variation in hospitalization needs for patients undergoing similar procedures.[4] Evaluation of hospital-level data has determined that nearly a quarter of all hospitalizations may be defined as prolonged.[6] Innovative approaches to improving capacity and access to care are a primary focus of many systems and may be facilitated with modern communication and remote patient monitoring technologies. We explore the concept of expansion of in-patient services beyond the walls of the hospital—through Hospital-at-Home (HaH) and paramedicine programs.[7]

● WORKUP

Expanding hospital-level care beyond the physical walls of a hospital is not a new concept, yet studies on the feasibility of such an approach for surgical populations have been limited.[8,9] It has become clear that hospital capacity serves as a major barrier to access to timely and appropriate care. However, as telecommunication strategies, remote patient monitoring, and at-home testing have become more readily available, so too has the potential of extending the hospital beyond the traditional brick-and-mortar setting.[10–15] Developing an HaH program for surgical populations defines the next frontier in modern-day enhanced recovery after surgery (ERAS) programs.[16–18]

When developing an HaH program, a variety of factors must be considered and optimized to ensure successful implementation (see Key Steps in Change Management and Potential Pitfalls). Many systems have robust electronic medical record data related to perioperative outcomes and resource utilization. Defining low-acuity care and understanding the patient and service needs are important starting points for a program. Though the potential for the HaH program is high, strategic implementation with a vision for organic growth is both safe and advisable. Operational data evaluating current hospital bed and staffing shortages, assessing LOS, and understanding downstream care utilization and complication burden of various case types should be analyzed to determine the return on investment. Given the novelty of such an approach, surgical service lines and individuals who are most enthusiastic about such an approach should be enlisted as champions for programmatic growth.

An HaH program involves stakeholders in all phases of medical care. Patients, providers, institutional leadership, and paramedicine service lines must be considered.[19] The true list of stakeholders is essentially identical to the stakeholders that encompass traditional inpatient services in the brick-and-mortar setting. Forecasting and developing predictive models for hospital growth and care utilization can assist in defining

Table 6.1 Questions to Consider When Attempting to Expand Hospital Capacity

Domain of Interest	Considerations
Operational data	• Current bed shortage • Average LOS for specific operations • Strategies to safely reduce LOS (eg, ERAS)
Critical stakeholders	• Patients • Caretakers • Providers (nursing, physicians, consulting services) • Hospital administration • Ancillary services (laboratories, phlebotomy, diagnostic imaging)
Historical context and forecasting	• Accurate predictive modeling[19] • Innovation in strategies in care delivery • Hospital bed availability and utilization • High-surge hospital strain[45] (ie, COVID-19 pandemic, H1N1)
Equity	• Access to paramedical services • Traditional hospital catchment versus paramedicine catchment • Geographic accessibility • Resource and staffing availability

Abbreviations: LOS, length of stay; ERAS, enhanced recovery after surgery.

opportunities for program expansion to address hospital needs (Table 6.1). It is important to note that HaH can be a disruptive force, particularly in academic programs where perioperative management is not only an element of patient care but also a fundamental aspect of training future surgeons. As such, the integration of trainees into such a program should be considered. As we have seen with other innovations in modern-day patient care, the trainee experience is often overlooked despite trainee interest in being involved in new-age approaches to care.[20]

● DIFFERENTIAL DIAGNOSIS

Changes in patient population, hospital operations, and physical space can address the current strain on our hospital system. High-acuity and emergent patients often require lengthy and unpredictable inpatient hospitalizations, adding to hospital strain. Even when utilizing ERAS protocols to expedite postoperative recovery and reduce LOS,[16,18] there can be significant limitations related to admissions for various service lines. Improving hospital operations may take the form of care pathways, discharge protocols, audits to identify delays in LOS, admission planning checklists, and physician reminders.[21,22] Creating additional physical spaces to address hospital bed shortages would be the most direct, albeit cost-intensive, solution for inpatient capacity limitations. Planning, building, and running a hospital requires an enormous investment of human and financial capital. By expanding the potential for hospital-level care beyond the normal confines of a brick-and-mortar hospital, an HaH program has massive potential to increase access to care—importantly for the sickest patients who require postoperative hospitalization with a higher level of perioperative care.

● DIAGNOSIS AND TREATMENT

When physical space and resources are at a premium, we must be creative with existing spaces while maximizing expenditure to optimize healthcare delivery. The HaH system was envisioned in the 1990s at Johns

CHAPTER 6 • Building a Hospital-at-Home Program   35

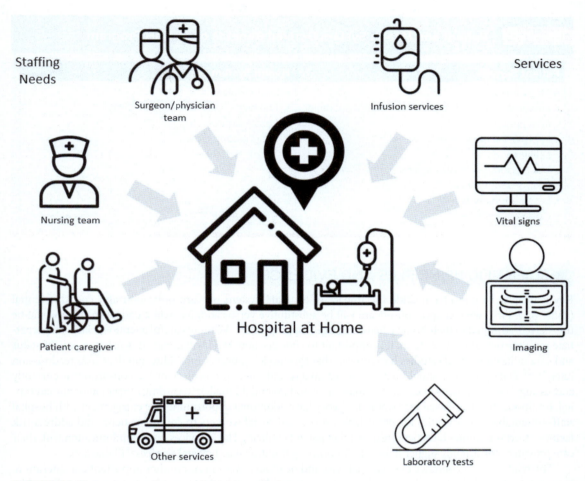

FIGURE 6.1 The network of support in HaH monitoring.

Hopkins Hospital as a solution to inpatient bed constraints, expensive hospital stays, and a loss of function seen in older adults following hospitalization.[23] The initial program focused on patients aged 65 and older with medical conditions including cellulitis, chronic heart failure, chronic obstructive airway disease, and community-acquired pneumonia (CAP). These patients receive care at home that is equivalent to an inpatient hospitalization,[9] including physician visits, nursing visits, vital sign monitoring, medication and intravenous fluid administration, basic laboratory and radiologic testing, and availability for transfer to traditional brick-and-mortar care, when appropriate (Figure 6.1). No additional physical space is needed to provide patients with appropriate care.

Since its inception, this model has been proven to be both feasible and effective, with approximately 30 successful HaH programs across the country,[24] including at Brigham and Women's Hospital, Massachusetts General Hospital, Mount Sinai Hospital, Oregon Health & Science University (OHSU), and several Veterans Health Administration hospitals.[25] In November 2020, the Centers for Medicare and Medicaid Services (CMS) expanded flexibility for hospitals to extend patient care outside of their walls in response to the COVID-19 pandemic.[26] The number of HaH programs has risen in response to the Hospital Without Walls and Acute Hospital Care at Home programs, with the pandemic providing further incentive to reduce in-hospital risks for patients, optimize inpatient availability, and maximize family and caregiver support.[24,26]

Table 6.2 Patient and Health System Derived Benefits of an HaH Program

Patient Benefit	Health System Benefit
• Shorter LOS[25,28,31]	• Cost savings[23,25,31,46]
• Fewer iatrogenic complications and nosocomial infections[25,28,31]	• Improves hospital bed availability[9]
• Improved caregiver and patient satisfaction[25,28,43,44]	• Less resource utilization[48]
• Decreased readmission rates[9,19,25,28,46]	• Patient-centric care[28,49]
• Decreased mortality[47]	
• Less sedentary time[48]	
• Cost savings[23,25,31,46]	

● SCIENTIFIC PRINCIPLES AND EVIDENCE

Key principles to consider include the impact of an HaH system on care utilization and cost differential (Table 6.2). First, what proportion of care will be substitutive versus additive; will a patient in the hospital be transferred/admitted to their home when discharge is appropriate?[27] Without careful attention, HaH can perpetuate resource overutilization. Next, it is important to consider how HaH will impact downstream patient status and care utilization. While studies have proven that this model improves morbidity and decreases readmission rates,[9,25,28] HaH programs should have standard quality and safety protocols, which a consortium is currently addressing[29] (see Key Steps in Change Management and Potential Pitfalls). Regarding utilization of human capital, traditional hospital-based care would in theory have additional opportunities for engagement with hospital staff—intangible opportunities for physicians, nurses, and social workers to counsel patients and address risk factors. However, studies have demonstrated that patients utilizing HaH services rate communication with their care providers consistently higher than patients utilizing traditional in-hospital services[28] (Table 6.2).

The relative cost difference between patients and healthcare systems is another important consideration. In countries including Australia, Canada, and the United Kingdom, HaH care has been integrated into the national payment models.[30] In the United States, HaH-specific payment was previously limited to Medicare Advantage and some commercial insurance plans. In 2017, the CMS introduced a pilot program that bundled HaH care within a 30-day postacute payment period, with a positive impact on patient outcomes.[28] The expansion of the CMS Hospital Without Walls program to include the Acute Hospital Care at Home program created the flexibility to provide inpatient care for patients in their own homes.[26] These initiatives have proven to be remarkably efficient in not only providing cost-effective care (up to 40% reduction in cost relative to comparable in-hospital care), but are associated with improved physical activity for patients while demonstrating no significant difference in quality, safety, or patient experiences.[23,25,31] A cross-sectional study looking at readmissions within 60 days of surgery found that nearly one-third of these readmissions met criteria for HaH, which would amount to millions of dollars in savings and thousands of bed days saved for medical systems. Currently, most hospital systems utilizing HaH programs will limit the distance that patients can be from the hospital to assure quality safety measures. As these programs evolve, catchments may be extended to allow for further support of patients who live long distances from the medical center. As the concept of remote patient monitoring continues to evolve, reimbursement patterns for HaH will likely follow patient and provider preferences and continue to benefit all stakeholders.

● IMPLEMENTING A SOLUTION

At the OHSU in Portland, Oregon, an HaH system was implemented in November 2021 at the main campus hospital with plans for expansion to a partner hospital.[32] Facing an increased demand for high-acuity

Table 6.3 Criteria for Establishing an HaH Program

	Criteria	Reasoning
Patients	• Safe home environment • Stable social support network • Geographically appropriate • Health-behavior congruent with at-home hospital care *See Table 6.4 for additional patient assessment criteria*	• Patients in safe and stable environments without risk factors for behavior incongruent with home-based care
Diagnosis	• Postoperative patients, nonoperative readmissions • Hemodynamically stable • Oxygen requirement <6 liters • No continuous infusions • Clinician agreement	• Maximize resource utilization in patients who are stable yet require hospital-level care
Resources	• Paramedicine staff • Remote patient monitoring system • Mobile laboratory • Mobile diagnostic imaging • IV infusions • Diet advancement • Pain management • Active staffing with in-hospital team • Drain management	• Services that are feasible to provide at home and allow for monitoring by care teams within the hospital system

admissions to the hospital, a shortage of inpatient beds, increased LOS, and discharge delays, the HaH system aimed to address capacity constraints at all three hospitals within the OHSU Health System. This system works when it is used for the right patient, with the right diagnosis, in the right physical space, and with stakeholder buy-in (Tables 6.3 and 6.4).

The successful HaH patient is an insured adult-aged patient that lives within a defined distance of the hospital providing care. OHSU uses an in-depth clinical and social stability screen to identify patients that are appropriate for HaH care (Table 6.4). Common medical diagnoses for an HaH patient include cellulitis, CAP, congestive heart failure, and urinary tract infection. In addition to these diagnoses, patients must be hemodynamically stable, not require any continuous infusions, have an oxygen requirement of less than 6 liters, and obtain clinician agreement and patient consent. HaH also has tremendous benefits for postoperative patients (Table 6.2),[33] particularly for case types associated with low acute complication burden (eg, minimally invasive ventral hernia repair, bariatric procedures, thyroidectomy, ileostomy reversal) who are generally observed for a short period of time using standardized postoperative pathways. Postoperative readmission issues including ileus, ileostomy dysfunction, surgical site infection, high-volume output after new ileostomy creation, and emesis/dehydration would also be favorable for hospital-level care received at the patient's home.[5]

Historically, utilization of HaH services appeared to be skewed toward higher socioeconomic status being associated with more opportunities for care—implying an opportunity to increase utilization in socioeconomically disadvantaged populations through strategic measures targeting patient awareness.[34] However, the COVID-19 pandemic has exposed many individuals to the concept of remote work, digital health care, and telemedicine, likely improving the potential for broader application of HaH services.

SECTION 2 • Efficiency of Inpatient Operations

Table 6.4	Assessing Patient Eligibility for HaH Care With Clinical Stability and Social Stability Screening

Clinical Stability Screen	Social Stability Screen
Does this patient have a negative COVID-19 status? Does this patient have a low diagnostic certainty that requires advanced diagnostics? *If yes, HAH services cannot be provided.* • Live telemetry monitoring • Advanced imaging (CT, MRI, nuclear stress) • Cardiac catheterization • Esophagogastroduodenoscopy/colonoscopy • Advanced lab monitor (troponin, labs > every 12 hours) Does this patient have high-acuity medical needs? *If yes, HAH services cannot be provided.* • Elevated intubation risks • New tracheostomy or need for mechanical ventilation • Unstable arrythmias • Elevated vasopressor risks • Home IV access limitations • Likely need for blood transfusions • Respiratory isolation/airborne precautions • Pain needs that required IV therapy Example services that cannot be provided in the home: • Surgical/IR procedures (significant wound debridement, thoracentesis, percutaneous nephrostomy tube placement, etc.)	Does the patient's fixed residence have reliable: • Electricity • Running water • Refrigerator (for medications) • Cell phone or internet access • Secure area for pets Is the patient: • Free from active recreational intravenous substance use • Able to perform activities of daily living without 24/7 support • Able to separate active smoker (by self or cohabitants) from oxygen source • Able to confirm they are not actively suicidal • Wiling to secure all firearms within the home Additional Home Needs Assessment: • Are there stairs to enter or within the home? • Does the patient live alone? • Does the patient have assistance at home? • Has the patient fallen within the last 6 months? • What is the patient's alcohol, tobacco, marijuana, and illegal drug use in the last year? • What is the patient's primary language?

Despite its proven benefits to patients, caretakers, and hospital systems, there are important considerations in equity when delivering care using an HaH model. Our HaH program requires patients to live within 25 miles of the hospital, which limits such options for a predominantly rural catchment area. One in five Americans lives in rural areas, which is associated with poor access to care, challenges with care coordination, and higher mortality rates.[35–37] Rural patients and clinicians overall have positive perceptions toward this modality of care and a Rural Home Hospital pilot program is working to implement an HaH program in Utah.[35,38] A similar pilot program is underway to establish an HaH program for Native American patients in rural areas in partnership with the Indian Health Service and First Nations.[38] Perceived challenges to establishing safe and sustainable rural HaH programs include poor cellular and internet access, poor health literacy, staffing availability, and challenging geographic accessibility.[35] Similar considerations in equity apply to individuals experiencing houselessness, with higher mortality,[39] attendance in emergency departments,[40] and postdischarge complications seen in this patient population.[39,41]

> ### Key Steps in Change Management and Potential Pitfalls
>
> **Key Steps in Change Management**
>
> 1. Identify key stakeholders to champion HaH care within departments.
> 2. Obtain operational data for inpatient bed utilization, LOS, and care utilization.
> 3. Establish qualifying criteria for patients.
> 4. Deliver high-quality care to patients outside the traditional four walls of the hospital.
> 5. Define a payment model for patients and hospitals.
> 6. Identify metrics for measuring effective and patient-reported outcomes with HaH care.
>
> **Potential Pitfalls**
>
> 1. Conflicting schools of thought on how the program should function.
> 2. Pushback from providers and staff to stray from the traditional model of care.
> 3. Difficult to model a variable and unpredictable process.
> 4. High-surge events are difficult to predict (ie, COVID-19 pandemic, natural disasters).
> 5. Risk of additive care.
> 6. Exacerbate existing disparities in access to care by strict qualifying criteria.
> 7. Existing staff shortage.
> 8. Availability of paramedicine resources.
> 9. Reluctant shift in patient and caregiver preferences toward traditional versus at-home hospital care.
> 10. Payment and reimbursement will vary based on the insurance type.
> 11. No current quality and safety standards.

● MEASURING OUTCOMES

Once an HaH system is in place, resource utilization and access, patient morbidity and mortality, and financial burden to both the patient and the healthcare system should be monitored as key outcome measures.[42] Important unintended consequences to consider are the utilization of downstream care following HaH. Prior studies have evaluated acute LOS, all-cause 30-day hospital readmissions and emergency department visits, skilled nursing facility admissions, and patient experiences with care as their primary measures of success for an HaH program.[28] Patient-reported outcomes are essential for assessing effectiveness, and in prior studies, patients self-selected receiving home care over traditional admission.[25,28,43,44]

● FOLLOW-UP AND MAINTENANCE

Optimizing opportunities for safe and effective patient care with an HaH model will allow patients and healthcare systems to reduce strain on the healthcare system and maximize outcomes. Similar to other patient-centered delivery modalities, including telemedicine, HaH provides numerous patient-derived benefits with positive health outcomes and lower in-hospital resource utilization. Improved access to patients outside of the traditional four walls of the hospital system with HaH programs will only provide more consistency among care at home and in the hospital.

REFERENCES

1. Schafermeyer RW, Asplin BR. Hospital and emergency department crowding in the United States. *Emerg Med (Fremantle)*. 2003;15(1):22–27.
2. Bazzoli GJ, Brewster LR, Liu G, Kuo S. Does U.S. hospital capacity need to be expanded? *Health Aff (Millwood)*. 2003;22(6):40–54.

3. Eriksson CO, Stoner RC, Eden KB, Newgard CD, Guise JM. The association between hospital capacity strain and inpatient outcomes in highly developed countries: a systematic review. *J Gen Intern Med*. 2017;32(6):686–696.
4. Baek H, Cho M, Kim S, Hwang H, Song M, Yoo S. Analysis of length of hospital stay using electronic health records: a statistical and data mining approach. *PLoS One*. 2018;13(4):e0195901.
5. Safavi KC, Ricciardi R, Heng M, et al. A different kind of perioperative surgical home: hospital at home after surgery. *Ann Surg*. 2020;271(2):227–229.
6. McDonagh MS, Smith DH, Goddard M. Measuring appropriate use of acute beds: a systematic review of methods and results. *Health Policy*. 2000;53(3):157–184.
7. Covinsky KE, Palmer RM, Fortinsky RH, et al. Loss of independence in activities of daily living in older adults hospitalized with medical illnesses: increased vulnerability with age. *J Am Geriatr Soc*. 2003;51(4):451–458.
8. Pajarón-Guerrero M, Fernández-Miera MF, Dueñas-Puebla JC, et al. Early discharge programme on hospital-at-home evaluation for patients with immediate postoperative course after laparoscopic colorectal surgery. *Eur Surg Res*. 2017;58(5–6):263–273.
9. Foley OW, Ferris TG, Thompson RW, et al. Potential impact of hospital at home on postoperative readmissions. *Am J Manag Care*. 2021;27(12):e420–e425.
10. Losorelli SD, Vendra V, Hildrew DM, Woodson EA, Brenner MJ, Sirjani DB. The future of telemedicine: revolutionizing health care or flash in the pan? *Otolaryngol Head Neck Surg*. 2021;165(2):239–243.
11. Nikolian VC, Williams AM, Jacobs BN, et al. Pilot study to evaluate the safety, feasibility, and financial implications of a postoperative telemedicine program. *Ann Surg*. 2018;268(4):700–707.
12. Liu X, Goldenthal S, Li M, Nassiri S, Steppe E, Ellimoottil C. Comparison of telemedicine versus in-person visits on impact of downstream utilization of care. *Telemed J E Health*. 2021;27(10):1099–1104.
13. Farias FAC, Dagostini CM, Bicca YA, Falavigna VF, Falavigna A. Remote patient monitoring: a systematic review. *Telemed J E Health*. 2020;26(5):576–583.
14. Mecklai K, Smith N, Stern AD, Kramer DB. Remote patient monitoring—overdue or overused? *N Engl J Med*. 2021;384(15):1384–1386.
15. Walker PP, Pompilio PP, Zanaboni P, et al. Telemonitoring in chronic obstructive pulmonary disease (CHROMED). A randomized clinical trial. *Am J Respir Crit Care Med*. 2018;198(5):620–628.
16. Forsmo HM, Pfeffer F, Rasdal A, Sintonen H, Körner H, Erichsen C. Pre- and postoperative stoma education and guidance within an enhanced recovery after surgery (ERAS) programme reduces length of hospital stay in colorectal surgery. *Int J Surg*. 2016;36(Pt A):121–126.
17. Ljungqvist O, Scott M, Fearon KC. Enhanced recovery after surgery: a review. *JAMA Surg*. 2017;152(3):292–298.
18. Smith TW, Jr., Wang X, Singer MA, Godellas CV, Vaince FT. Enhanced recovery after surgery: a clinical review of implementation across multiple surgical subspecialties. *Am J Surg*. 2020;219(3):530–534.
19. Buttigieg SC, Gauci D, Bezzina F, Dey PK. Post-surgery length of stay using multi-criteria decision-making tool. *J Health Organ Manag*. 2018;32(4):514–531.
20. Iqbal EJ, Sutton T, Akther MS, et al. Current surgical trainee perceptions and experiences in telehealth. *Telemed J E Health*. 2022;28(6):789–797. doi: 10.1089/tmj.2021.0237
21. Caminiti C, Meschi T, Braglia L, et al. Reducing unnecessary hospital days to improve quality of care through physician accountability: a cluster randomised trial. *BMC Health Serv Res*. 2013;13:14.
22. Topal B, Peeters G, Verbert A, Penninckx F. Outpatient laparoscopic cholecystectomy: clinical pathway implementation is efficient and cost effective and increases hospital bed capacity. *Surg Endosc*. 2007;21(7):1142–1146.
23. Leff B, Burton L, Guido S, Greenough WB, Steinwachs D, Burton JR. Home hospital program: a pilot study. *J Am Geriatr Soc*. 1999;47(6):697–702.
24. Weiner S. Interest in hospital-at-home programs explodes during COVID-19. https://www.aamc.org/news-insights/interest-hospital-home-programs-explodes-during-covid-19. Published 2020. Accessed February 8, 2022.
25. Leff B, Burton L, Mader SL, et al. Hospital at home: feasibility and outcomes of a program to provide hospital-level care at home for acutely ill older patients. *Ann Intern Med*. 2005;143(11):798–808.
26. CMS. CMS announces comprehensive strategy to enhance hospital capacity amid COVID-19 surge. https://www.cms.gov/newsroom/press-releases/cms-announces-comprehensive-strategy-enhance-hospital-capacity-amid-covid-19-surge. Published November 25, 2020. Accessed February 8, 2022.
27. Taylor SP, Golding L. Economic considerations for hospital at home programs: beyond the pandemic. *J Gen Intern Med*. 2021;36(12):3861–3864.
28. Federman AD, Soones T, DeCherrie LV, Leff B, Siu AL. Association of a bundled hospital-at-home and 30-day postacute transitional care program with clinical outcomes and patient experiences. *JAMA Intern Med*. 2018;178(8):1033–1040.

29. Hospital at Home Users Group. https://hahusersgroup.org/. Accessed February 15, 2022.
30. Montalto M. The 500-bed hospital that isn't there: the Victorian Department of Health review of the Hospital in the Home program. *Med J Aust*. 2010;193(10):598–601.
31. Cryer L, Shannon SB, Van Amsterdam M, Leff B. Costs for "hospital at home" patients were 19 percent lower, with equal or better outcomes compared to similar inpatients. *Health Aff (Millwood)*. 2012;31(6):1237–1243.
32. OHSU Health Hospital at Home. https://www.ohsu.edu/health/ohsu-health-hospital-home. Accessed February 1, 2022.
33. Shepperd S, Doll H, Angus RM, et al. Avoiding hospital admission through provision of hospital care at home: a systematic review and meta-analysis of individual patient data. *CMAJ*. 2009;180(2):175–182.
34. Fried TR, van Doorn C, O'Leary JR, Tinetti ME, Drickamer MA. Older person's preferences for home vs hospital care in the treatment of acute illness. *Arch Intern Med*. 2000;160(10):1501–1506.
35. Levine DM, Desai MP, Ross J, Como N, Anne Gill E. Rural perceptions of acute care at home: a qualitative analysis. *J Rural Health*. 2021;37(2):353–361.
36. Joynt KE, Harris Y, Orav EJ, Jha AK. Quality of care and patient outcomes in critical access rural hospitals. *JAMA*. 2011;306(1):45–52.
37. Garcia MC, Rossen LM, Bastian B, et al. Potentially excess deaths from the five leading causes of death in metropolitan and nonmetropolitan counties—United States, 2010–2017. *MMWR Surveill Summ*. 2019;68(10):1–11.
38. Rural Home Hospital. Adriane Labs. https://www.ariadnelabs.org/home-hospital/rural-home-hospital/. Accessed February 15, 2022.
39. Aldridge RW, Story A, Hwang SW, et al. Morbidity and mortality in homeless individuals, prisoners, sex workers, and individuals with substance use disorders in high-income countries: a systematic review and meta-analysis. *Lancet*. 2018;391(10117):241–250.
40. Gallagher TC, Andersen RM, Koegel P, Gelberg L. Determinants of regular source of care among homeless adults in Los Angeles. *Med Care*. 1997;35(8):814–830.
41. Davies A, Wood LJ. Homeless health care: meeting the challenges of providing primary care. *Med J Aust*. 2018;209(5):230–234.
42. Cai S, Intrator O, Chan C, et al. Association of costs and days at home with transfer hospital in home. *JAMA Netw Open*. 2021;4(6):e2114920.
43. Shepperd S, Iliffe S. Hospital at home versus in-patient hospital care. *Cochrane Database Syst Rev*. 2005(3):Cd000356.
44. Leff B, Burton L, Mader SL, et al. Comparison of stress experienced by family members of patients treated in hospital at home with that of those receiving traditional acute hospital care. *J Am Geriatr Soc*. 2008;56(1):117–123.
45. Rubinson L, Mutter R, Viboud C, et al. Impact of the fall 2009 influenza A(H1N1)pdm09 pandemic on US hospitals. *Med Care*. 2013;51(3):259–265.
46. Caplan GA, Sulaiman NS, Mangin DA, Aimonino Ricauda N, Wilson AD, Barclay L. A meta-analysis of "hospital in the home." *Med J Aust*. 2012;197(9):512–519.
47. Shepperd S, Gonçalves-Bradley DC, Straus SE, Wee B. Hospital at home: home-based end-of-life care. *Cochrane Database Syst Rev*. 2016;2(2):Cd009231.
48. Levine DM, Ouchi K, Blanchfield B, et al. Hospital-level care at home for acutely ill adults: a randomized controlled trial. *Ann Intern Med*. 2020;172(2):77–85.
49. Chua CMS, Ko SQ, Lai YF, Lim YW, Shorey S. Perceptions of hospital-at-home among stakeholders: a meta-synthesis. *J Gen Intern Med*. 2022;37(3):637–650.

Postoperative Patients Come to the Emergency Room Because They Do Not Have Urgent Access to Surgical Clinics

7

HEATHER L. EVANS AND LEEANNA CLEVENGER

Clinical Delivery Challenge

The evolution toward value-based surgical care has resulted in a dramatically decreased length of hospitalization and an increasing shift to outpatient procedures over the past 25 years. As a result, much of the burden of postoperative care has shifted to patients and their caregivers, whereas little has changed about standard postoperative care delivery. Between postoperative discharge to home and scheduled clinic follow-up visit, the surgical patient with a developing complication generally faces a lack of urgent surgical clinic access and overburdened emergency departments (EDs) with long wait times. Surgical site infections (SSIs) account for the majority of health care-associated infections and are the most common reason for readmission after surgery.[1] It is estimated that up to 5% of all surgical patients and up to 33% of patients undergoing abdominal surgery will develop SSI, costing USD$5–10 billion in excess healthcare expenditures.[2,3] About one-third of all postoperative complications and 87% of SSIs are diagnosed after hospital discharge.[4] Many patients with these problems present to the ED for care instead of the outpatient surgery clinic, contributing in part to the expenditure of billions of healthcare dollars.[5] In this chapter, we aim to address the challenge of providing personalized care delivery in the post-discharge period, acknowledging that the standard postoperative in-person clinic follow-up paradigm falls short for some patients, particularly those who have wound complications. To this end, we present 2 clinical scenarios to examine the current system barriers to early diagnosis and treatment of SSIs and to propose innovative care pathways to optimize access to postoperative care.

Case A: A 35-year-old woman with no past medical history presents to the ED 5 days after undergoing a laparoscopic appendectomy for acute perforated appendicitis.

Case B: A 72-year-old woman with obesity and diabetes mellitus is accompanied by her son when she presents to the ED 4 days following discharge from the hospital, after undergoing a laparoscopic converted to open appendectomy for acute perforated appendicitis.

● WORKUP

Factors leading to ED presentation for postoperative complications are multifaceted. With regard to SSI, when patients are discharged from the hospital, the responsibility for wound care and inspection usually shifts to the patients themselves. Patient education regarding wound management, expectations for the postoperative course, and feasibility for self-care are all factors to consider when preparing for hospital discharge. Additionally, postoperative complications usually arise during a time frame that is earlier than the scheduled postoperative clinic visit, leading patients to seek care elsewhere if they cannot make an urgent clinic appointment.[6] Patients often seek the nearest available care out of convenience or concern and may present at a different hospital emergency room from the facility in which they received surgical treatment, complicating care continuity and leading to underestimation of surgical complications.[3]

CHAPTER 7 • Postoperative Patients Come to the Emergency Room

It is important to identify all stakeholders and address their perspectives, challenges, concerns that may conflict with each other, and come to a solution that best addresses these in the existing system. Key stakeholders include not only the patients and their caregivers but also the healthcare providers who will help to take care of these postoperative complications, whether they are providers in the emergency setting or the surgical clinic staff. Others who might be affected by these outcomes include hospital administrators who are involved in allocating funding toward various clinic support systems.

● DIFFERENTIAL DIAGNOSIS

A recent qualitative study aimed to explore the barriers to post-discharge monitoring and patient–clinician communication.[7] By examining the content of interviews with over 30 patients and their families, as well as medical staff, including physicians, advanced care providers, nurses, and call center personnel, the authors highlighted patient and provider factors influencing post-discharge outcomes. Patient factors, such as education and perceived expectations, access to technology and healthcare literacy, resource and support availability, and communication preferences, were all found to be important determinants of post-discharge care. Several clinician-identified barriers were highlighted, including a shared notion that education is of paramount importance, in addition to easy access to the clinical team.[7]

Case A: The patient states that she first noticed redness around her wound on the third postoperative day. She was not sure what to expect regarding her wounds or the care of them. She attempted to call the surgeon's office clinic, but after not hearing back for a day, she decided to call the 24/7 nurse hotline. The nurse on call instructed her to "just go to the emergency department" if she was concerned. The patient decided to wait another day and attempted wound care by herself. On the fifth postoperative day, the peri-incisional redness and pain had again worsened, and she decided to go to the ED for care.

Case B: The patient states that she felt well on the day of discharge but felt like she had no energy when she returned home. On the second day at home, she noticed redness surrounding her wound. She was not sure what to expect, but she tried to dress the wound herself. She lives alone and had difficulty showering and keeping the wound clean. She called the surgical clinic to make an urgent visit, but there were no available appointments. On the fourth postoperative day, she developed fever, dizziness, and worsening redness surrounding her midline laparotomy incision. Her son decided to bring her to the ED. The patient is tachycardic and febrile, and there is purulent drainage coming from the incision.

● DIAGNOSIS AND TREATMENT

In both patient cases, there was a lack of education regarding expectations for the postoperative course, and there was no protocol in place to manage unplanned communications with the clinical team, or contingency plans for the emergence of worrisome postoperative symptoms before a scheduled follow-up clinic visit. The advice to seek care in the ED is the final common pathway for any worrisome symptoms in many surgical practices, dispensed routinely as an escalation option when urgent clinic appointments are unavailable. Consider the differences in cases, however, in that the patient in Case A may be able to perform better self-care and might have access to and familiarity with technology to allow additional modes of communication (eg, via mobile app or web-based patient portal). In the Case B scenario, this patient was unable to complete wound care by herself and was unable to be seen urgently in the surgical clinic.

● SCIENTIFIC PRINCIPLES AND EVIDENCE

Providing adequate education for patients regarding their postoperative course and information on wound care is essential. Surrounding the time of discharge, patients may have difficulty processing and retaining information due to pain, pain medications, or the large volume of information.[2] Even in the circumstance that they do receive an adequate education, they may not physically be able to follow wound care instructions. Insufficiencies in communication with the clinical team represent an area for potential improvement.

However, even when communication succeeds, there may be a lack of availability of urgent clinic appointments, perhaps due to existing high clinic volume or staffing problems. Deficits in wound care education, capacity for self-care, communication pitfalls, and limited time availability are the main factors leading to postoperative patients presenting to the ED instead of surgical clinics. Development and adoption of accurate risk-assessment prediction models can facilitate personalized follow-up intensity and timing. In elderly patients undergoing surgical procedures with high rates of postoperative complications, early follow-up with a primary care provider is associated with lower rates of readmission.[8] Other successful interventions include immediate post-discharge telephone communications with high-risk patients as part of a formal transitional care plan.[9] Use of a framework such as the "Ideal transition of care" model may help plan and implement processes to focus efforts across multiple domains, targeting patient, provider, and system stakeholder needs and limitations.[10]

● IMPLEMENTING A SOLUTION

To provide more adequate education and expectations for postoperative wound care, patients and their caregivers should be counseled both before and after surgery. For nonurgent operations, it is important to gauge a patient's ability to care for herself preoperatively. If there is a concern for a lack of home resources, it is a good idea to involve the patient's family or caretakers in their preoperative counseling. A preoperative questionnaire might help identify patients who are at risk for limited resources. Although guidance on wound care and providing warning signs for infection could improve patient confidence in their postoperative care,[11] it may not improve the reliability of diagnosis of infection. One randomized controlled trial found that detailed oral and visual instruction on local and systemic signs/symptoms of SSI actually resulted in patients overdiagnosing infections.[12]

An alternative approach to patient-initiated ad hoc post-discharge communications is remote patient monitoring, where patients submit serial symptom reports and vital data such as body temperature and wound photographs to aid in clinical decision-making and to personalize the timing of post-discharge follow-up. As patients alone may not be able to consistently recognize signs of early infection, a mobile phone application or other digital interfaces with the ability to upload patient-generated wound photographs may be helpful. A recent randomized controlled trial tested whether the use of a smartphone-based wound assessment tool resulted in earlier diagnosis and treatment of SSI after emergency general surgery.[13] The group of patients using the smartphone app had higher odds of SSI diagnosis within the first 7 postoperative days, and the incorporation of wound images offered an appreciable improvement in the specificity of correct SSI diagnosis. The smartphone group also showed better perceived quality of care and reduced rate of seeking urgent care elsewhere in the community. Another study showed an association between using mobile app platforms for postoperative surveillance with improved healthcare utilization. A randomized controlled trial in 2017 found that for one postoperative population, mobile app monitoring, including the daily upload of wound photos, was found to significantly decrease the number of in-person clinic visits.[14] This may alleviate some of the scheduling conflicts for patients who need to be seen in person on an urgent basis. Mobile apps also provide an avenue for entirely virtual postoperative visits.

Telehealth began to gain popularity before the COVID-19 pandemic, but with the mass closing of clinics and significantly decreased in-hospital resources for non–COVID-related illness, virtual visits became a mainstay for clinical communication. A recent randomized clinical trial found that for patients undergoing uncomplicated laparoscopic appendectomy or cholecystectomy, virtual visits were noninferior to in-person clinic visits, and they also provided shortened wait times and eliminated the need for travel.[15] One caveat to note in that study is the relatively young average age of the patients and their lack of comorbidities. This suggests that more research is needed to evaluate the efficacy of this mode of a clinic visit for the older, sicker population or for those who may not have access to the technology required to complete such a visit.

Shifting to virtual visits for routine follow-up care may allow for increased in-person clinic availability for urgent evaluations. Another possible way to optimize clinic utilization is to reexamine which patients need to be seen in the clinic after surgery—and when. Many institutions routinely schedule postoperative patients for their first clinic visit around 2 weeks after discharge. In a retrospective review evaluating the rates of 30-day outpatient follow-up and readmission for general or vascular surgical procedures, general surgery patients who were not readmitted were found to have an 88% follow-up rate at 2 weeks after discharge.[6] For those who were readmitted, half of them followed up before the first week after discharge. This suggests that the majority of 30-day readmissions occurred within 2 weeks of discharge before those patients could return for their scheduled return visit. Furthermore, the patients who came to their 2-week follow-up visit with compilations were already too advanced in their complications to avoid readmission. Earlier outpatient follow-up may prevent readmissions in select patients at higher risk for developing SSI. Identifying this group of patients was studied in a retrospective cohort design by Daneman and colleagues.[3] They found that increased procedure duration, American Society of Anesthesiology (ASA) class ≤ 3, breast and skin procedures, morbid obesity, diabetes or muscle disease, rural residence, and alcoholism contributed to postoperative SSI.

A patient's risk for developing SSI or other postoperative complications should be calculated around the time they are assessed for readiness for discharge. Ideally, case management would possess the resources and personnel to meet with each patient before discharge to identify what types of resources are available at home and next how best to interact with the clinical team—and when to make that appointment. A retrospective study found that the odds of returning to the emergency room within 30 days of surgery are 4.5 times higher if a patient is not case-managed compared to those who were evaluated by case managers.[16] It is important for the pre-discharge assessment to establish the patient's preferred mode of communication after hospital discharge, and for the clinical team to abide by it.

The patient in Case A might have been better suited to use a mobile monitoring app postoperatively. She could have uploaded pictures of her wound to allow the clinical team to act earlier in prescribing antibiotics.

Key Steps in Change Management

1. Enable clear communication with emergency providers in the surgical institution and in the community to identify areas for improvement. Ideally, emergency providers and primary care providers should have access to a communication system that would allow the surgeon to be notified anytime a patient is seen in the urgent or emergent setting. This would also eventually play a role in tracking progress.

2. Utilize case management and social workers to identify the needs of patients positioned for discharge *before* discharge. Patients should be screened to recognize who might need help with wound care, transportation, and communication with the surgical team. If a patient is deemed high risk for postoperative complications, they should be scheduled for a postoperative visit sooner than the typical 2-week follow-up visit. Conversely, patients may be deemed unnecessary for an in-person follow-up visit at all.

3. Provide adequate education regarding wound care before discharge. Education takes time, and this may prohibit the surgeon from being the sole provider of instructions and education. Utilize a discharge nurse to ensure patients feel comfortable with wound care before discharge. Educational pamphlets and videos may be of assistance.

4. Implement a telehealth system to allow patients to be closely monitored at home immediately following discharge. This system may include ways to easily and more rapidly communicate with the surgical team and it may help to identify problems (ie, SSI) sooner than the traditional 2-week follow-up visit. This may also present some patients with the opportunity to skip an in-person clinic visit if their procedure was routine and they do not show any signs of postoperative complications. Be aware that some patients may not feel comfortable using telemedicine or may not have the means necessary to do so.

5. Aim to reserve appointment space within surgical clinics for urgent visits. This may be more easily accomplished if the cohort of patients who do not need in-person follow-up actually follow up via telemedicine.

6. Identify a nurse navigator for after-hours communication access. This person should ideally be well versed in the care of surgical patients and potential complications. This person should be able to advise the patient on whether to actually seek emergent medical care or to wait for a clinic appointment within the next few days.

Instead, she sought care in the ED because she could not contact her surgical care team. A mobile app may not have been the most accessible mode of communication for the patient in Case B, however. This patient's risk for developing SSI was increased based on her comorbidities and the nature of her operation. She would have been better served with a thorough assessment by case management to ensure she had the means for adequate wound care, and a scheduled early postoperative clinic visit. Alternatively, preoperative engagement with her son who may have more facility with technology could provide improved surgical team connection and communication with a younger, more able caregiver.

Improving the problem of patients going to the ED instead of clinic visits and decreasing postoperative wound infections is not a one-size-fits-all solution; we must tailor each solution to the individual patients and their needs. Although remote patient monitoring shows promise in a select population, care must be taken to ensure that patients possess the equipment and education needed to successfully use the technology. This may even worsen health inequities for the underserved, rural, or geriatric populations without broadband access, and who are already at an increased risk for postoperative complications. Alternatively, telemedicine may help increase care for traditionally underserved populations, as 1 study found that telemedicine use actually increased in the Black population following the COVID-19 pandemic.[17]

FOLLOW-UP AND MAINTENANCE

In order to measure the effectiveness of the solution, key metrics, including patient satisfaction and clinical outcomes, should be assessed. Patients need to be able to communicate with the surgery team easily and quickly, and via their preferred method. The ability to schedule an urgent clinic appointment in a timely fashion must be improved. Patient satisfaction questionnaires may aid in discovering whether these communication interventions are effective. They may also help determine whether a patient felt confident with wound care before discharge. One example of an instrument used to measure care satisfaction in the surgical patient is the Consumer Assessment of Healthcare Providers and Systems, a recently validated tool used to determine which specific domains of operative care correlated most strongly with overall surgeon satisfaction to identify targets for quality improvement.[18]

In addition to patient satisfaction, clinical outcomes must be measured. The rate of SSI or wound complications should be closely followed, and individuals may compare their practice to data from the National Surgical Quality Improvement Program to evaluate overall performance in these areas.

Finally, healthcare utilization must be continually assessed. Communication with emergency providers and primary care providers in the community, in addition to chart review and careful tracking, may help delineate the number of unplanned visits within 30 days following discharge. Metrics to identify the number of preventable ED visits (eg, those that do not result in admission) should be developed and monitored so that future system changes can accommodate patient needs more effectively and efficiently. In addition, it will be important to evaluate whether there is ample time during a clinic period reserved for urgent visits. The number of in-person visits compared to virtual visits should be tracked to evaluate for efficiency of virtual visit care for the right population.

CONCLUSION

SSI are relatively common complications occurring in the postoperative period and account for a large majority of readmissions in this patient population. Tailoring discharge plans to the needs of patients may help identify and treat these complications more efficiently than applying a one-size-fits-all approach to routine postoperative follow-up. Utilizing new technology including mobile apps, as well as including dedicated personnel to help educate patients and their caregivers on the discharge plan and wound care instructions, may help prevent readmission or at least help identify complications earlier. Enabling a more direct line of communication between the patient and the surgical care team, and designating time during the clinic for unexpected, urgent visits may help reduce the burden of postoperative patients presenting to urgent care or ED settings.

REFERENCES

1. Woelber E, Schrick EJ, Gessner BD, Evans HL. Proportion of surgical site infections occurring after hospital discharge: a systematic review. *Surg Infect*. 2016;17(5):510–519.
2. Sanger PC, Hartzler A, Han SM, et al. Patient perspectives on post-discharge surgical site infections: towards a patient-centered mobile health solution. *PLoS ONE*. 2014;9(12):e114016.
3. Daneman N, Lu H, Redelmeier DA. Discharge after discharge: predicting surgical site infections after patients leave hospital. *J Hosp Infect*. 2010;75(3):188–194.
4. Hart A, Furkert C, Clifford K, Woodfield JC. Impact of incisional surgical site infections on quality of life and patient satisfaction after general surgery: a case controlled study. *Surg Infect*. 2021;22(10):1039–1046.
5. Kocher KE, Nallamothu BK, Birkmeyer JD, Dimick JB. Emergency department visits after surgery are common for Medicare patients, suggesting opportunities to improve care. *Health Aff (Millwood)*. 2013;32(9):1600–1607.
6. Saunders RS, Fernandes-Taylor S, Rathouz PJ, et al. Outpatient follow-up versus 30-day readmission among general and vascular surgery patients: a case for redesigning transitional care. *Surgery*. 2014;156(4):949–956.
7. Brajcich BC, Shallcross ML, Johnson JK, et al. Barriers to post-discharge monitoring and patient-clinician communication: a qualitative study. *J Surg Res*. 2021;268:1–8.
8. Brooke BS, Stone DH, Cronenwett JL, et al. Early primary care provider follow-up and readmission after high-risk surgery. *JAMA Surg*. 2014;149(8):821–828.
9. Medina D, Zil-E-Ali A, Daoud D, Brooke J, Lee Chester-Paul K, Aziz F. Implementation of transitional care planning is associated with reduced readmission rates in patients undergoing lower extremity bypass surgery for peripheral arterial disease. *Ann Vasc Surg*. 2022;84:28–39.
10. Burke RE, Kripalani S, Vasilevskis EE, Schnipper JL. Moving beyond readmission penalties: creating an ideal process to improve transitional care. *J Hosp Med Off Publ Soc Hosp Med*. 2013;8(2):102–109.
11. Tanner J, Padley W, Davey S, Murphy K, Brown B. Patient narratives of surgical site infection: implications for practice. *J Hosp Infect*. 2013;83(1):41–45.
12. Whitby M, McLaws ML, Doidge S, Collopy B. Post-discharge surgical site surveillance: does patient education improve reliability of diagnosis? *J Hosp Infect*. 2007;66(3):237–242.
13. McLean KA, Mountain KE, Shaw CA, et al; TWIST Collaborators. Remote diagnosis of surgical-site infection using a mobile digital intervention: a randomised controlled trial in emergency surgery patients. *NPJ Digit Med*. 2021;4(1):160.
14. Armstrong KA, Coyte PC, Brown M, Beber B, Semple JL. Effect of home monitoring via mobile app on the number of in-person visits following ambulatory surgery: a randomized clinical trial. *JAMA Surg*. 2017;152(7):622–627.
15. Harkey K, Kaiser N, Zhao J, et al. Postdischarge virtual visits for low-risk surgeries: a randomized noninferiority clinical trial. *JAMA Surg*. 2021;156(3):221–228.
16. Kelly EA, Keller CC, Sax MR, Rossi RA. Emergency department utilization of case-managed patients following benign gynecologic surgery. *Int J Emerg Med*. 2020;13(1):34.
17. Eruchalu CN, Bergmark RW, Smink DS, et al. Demographic disparity in use of telemedicine for ambulatory general surgical consultation during the COVID-19 pandemic: analysis of the initial public health emergency and second phase periods. *J Am Coll Surg*. 2022;234(2):191–202.
18. Schmocker RK, Cherney Stafford LM, Siy AB, et al. Understanding the determinants of patient satisfaction with surgical care using the CAHPS Surgical Care Survey (S-CAHPS). *Surgery*. 2015;158(6):1724–1733.

Efficiency in the Operating Room: Get the Data, Make the Change

8

MELANIE S. MORRIS, BRENDA CARLISLE, BROOKE REEVES VINING, JIMMIE LOATS, AND JEFFREY W. SIMMONS

Clinical Delivery Challenge

Operating rooms are frequently the most precious resource in a healthcare system and running them efficiently is vital to the health and well-being of patients, staff, surgeons, anesthesiologists, and the financial success of the organization. To run efficiently, operating rooms must have a strong collaborative leadership and perioperative governance structure, accurate data with shared definitions, transparent policies, and appropriate staffing levels.

● WORKUP

Obtaining and reporting accurate data are necessary to determine the efficiency of the operating rooms and identify areas to target improvement. Key operational metrics should include at a minimum the following: day of surgery cancellation rate, first case on-time starts, turnaround time (TAT), and the rate of cases running over the allocated time in the schedule. Definitions of some of our key operational metrics are shown in Table 8.1. To collect these data, you need team members, including information technology and data analytics to automate data collection based on your electronic medical record (EMR). This includes an identified sole source repository for data capture combination, automation, and data integrity logic control. For example, we have Cerner EMR, but we do not use the Cerner Anesthesia package, which made data extraction from the anesthesia record more challenging. An operational team including perioperative nursing, anesthesia, surgeons, and data decision support staff should review these data regularly to ensure accuracy and identify trends.

● DIFFERENTIAL DIAGNOSIS

In our organization, we currently have both block scheduling (at our main university hospital, North Pavilion) and operating rooms that are allocated as "first come, first served" (at our smaller hospital, Highlands, which provides less complex care). Additionally, cardiovascular, neurosurgery, vascular, acute care surgery, orthopedic trauma and transplant services all have an allocated number of daily safe, reserved rooms. Our surgeons can operate at both locations. We must measure efficiency differently based on the scheduling model. Our main university hospital blocks are allocated from 7 am to 5 pm and are staffed accordingly. Our smaller hospital is staffed from 7 am to 3 pm. Both facilities regularly incur block overrun or extended days to facilitate our surgical acuity, level 1 traumas, and case volume growth over the past 7 years. Additionally, we accommodate 25+ urgent and emergent add-on cases daily. To understand which model will work more effectively for your institution, you need to understand the proportion of cases that are elective and those which are urgent or emergent. We view "elective" as a scheduling term and find that most of our cases are more complex "essential" surgeries. You should also examine the balance of outpatient cases to those which will require an inpatient stay.

CHAPTER 8 • Efficiency in the Operating Room: Get the Data, Make the Change

Table 8.1 — Key Operational Metric Definitions

Metric	Definition	Best Practice
Prime-time room utilization	The sum of the time duration to perform each surgical procedure ("OR In" to "OR Out") plus the total turn-over time, divided by the prime time available UAB Main (7 am–5 pm; 8 am–5 pm Tuesdays); Highlands (7 am–3 pm; 8 am–3 pm Tuesdays). Note: No. of rooms available will decrease on holidays and weekends.	80%
Block utilization	The sum of the time duration to perform each surgical procedure (including preparation of the patient in the OR, anesthesia induction, and emergence) plus the total turnover time, divided by the block time available	75%–80%
Block run-over utilization	The sum of the time duration of surgical procedure performed in 2-hour increments after the assigned block [North Pavilion (5 pm–7 pm; 7 pm–9 pm); Highlands (3 pm–5 pm; 5 pm–7 pm)] divided by the hours available based on scheduled rooms during those time increments	
First case on-time starts	Percentage of first cases scheduled as of 6 am the day of surgery with an in-room start time (wheels in) that is either early or not more than 5 minutes after the scheduled start time with a cutoff time of 7:30 am	90% 5 minutes 95% within 15 minutes
Case TAT	The time (in minutes) that elapsed between the prior patient exiting the room and the succeeding patient entering the room	25–30 minutes

● DIAGNOSIS AND TREATMENT

Approximately 20% of the daily cases in our main hospital with 43 operating rooms are add-on urgent or emergent cases. We needed a shared language to prioritize the most time-sensitive add-on cases. To facilitate this, we developed a case-leveling system (Table 8.2). Our anesthesiologist and certified registered nurse anesthetist along with OR nursing leadership use this case leveling to manipulate the schedule to accommodate urgent and emergent add-on cases. If a room is open, a level 1 emergent case will be placed in it. However, if a room is not available, the case will bump other scheduled cases with priority to bumping the same surgeon or service line that is performing the level 1 case.

We allow surgeons to decide their start time of 7 am, 7:15 am, or 7:30 am. Any requested start time after 07:30 am is considered a to-follow (TF) case and has the potential to start later based on total first-start case volumes. Additionally, we are working to optimize these start times across all anesthetizing locations. The nursing staff transparently document the intended start time, actual start time, and reason for the delay that is attributed to the surgeon, anesthesia staff, operating room, or patient with names attached. This is shared with all surgical faculty and staff daily in an automated email. As shown in Figure 8.1, our first case on-time start ranges from 70% to 75%, with a stretch goal of 90%. We use these data to look for trends in our first case start time delays and make changes to improve our first case on-time starts.

Table 8.2 Case Triage Levels and Definitions

- **Level 1**
  - **Definition:** Immediate threat to life, as determined by the attending surgeon.
  - Takes priority over all other elective cases and levels 2–4.
  - The surgeon MUST be immediately available.
  - Requires a phone call by the OR desk to the anesthesia attending coordinator immediately after the case is posted.
- **Level 2**
  - **Definition:** Life or limb-threatening condition that requires operative intervention within 1–2 hours as determined by the attending surgeon.
  - Requires a phone call by the OR desk to the anesthesia attending coordinator immediately after the case is posted.
  - The surgeon must be immediately available.
  - Takes priority over routine/level 5 and levels 3 and 4 add-on cases.
- **Level 2T (transplant cases)**
  - If 3 or greater kidney transplants or kidney–pancreas + kidney transplants are posted for 1 weekend day, a page is sent to the weekend charge nurse running the desk, anesthesia attending running the board, transplant surgery attending on call, and the attending of the service being considered for "bumping."
- **Level 3**
  - **Definition:** Substantial risks to the patient that requires operative intervention within 6 hours of case posting.
  - Takes priority over level 4 cases and level 5/Routine cases.
  - The surgeon must be available within 60 minutes of being informed of the projected OR availability.
  - If surgeon has other cases scheduled, the level 3 add-on case will take priority over the Routine/level 5 cases.
  - If surgeon is not available to start the case within 60 minutes, OR will be given to the next case on the triage list.
  - Level 3 cases not accommodated within 6 hours will be redesignated to level 2 cases and will be offered the next available OR.
  - Cases will not be given higher priority in the leveling system if the surgeon was not available on the prior 2 notifications.
- **Level 4**
  - **Definition:** Cases deemed to be medically necessary, OR.
  - **Definition:** Add-on cases so as not to extend the length of stay for inpatients, require operative intervention within 24 hours of case posting.
  - Level 4 cases not started within 24 hours will be prioritized for the next available OR.
  - The surgeon must be available within 60 minutes of being informed of the projected OR availability.
  - If surgeon is not available to start case within 60 minutes, OR will be given to the next case on the triage list.
  - If surgeon is not available to start the case within 60 minutes of the second notice, the case will be moved to the end of the triage list.
- **Level 5/Routine**
  - Cases posted for next day or future.

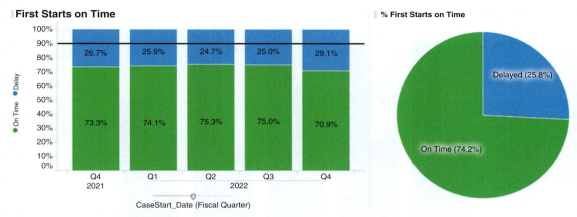

FIGURE 8.1 Percentage of first case on-time starts.

We all know surgeons who routinely over- or underestimate the time it will take them to perform certain surgical procedures. Collecting historical data on operative times by surgeons for specific procedures will allow accurate estimation of future procedure lengths. Accurate case postings are required for both historical data and future predictions. Inaccurate case postings or bad historical data will lead to either unutilized operating rooms or operating rooms running later than the staffing model planned. Of course, unanticipated events can happen during surgical procedures, but estimating case length is important for estimating staffing levels for our operating rooms.

● SCIENTIFIC PRINCIPLES AND EVIDENCE

In order to minimize our day of surgery delays or cancellations, we developed a robust Preoperative Assessment, Consultation, and Treatment (PACT) clinic. These 2 geographically separated clinics (1 at each hospital) are staffed by 1 anesthesiologist and 10 nurse practitioners (NPs) with a goal of evaluating all patients with an electively scheduled surgery either in person or by phone. Staffing levels for a similar clinic should be based on anticipated volume and adjusted as needed. An inpatient preoperative evaluation team consisting of 9 NPs performs daily add-on case evaluations, trauma/ER evaluations, and staff high-volume procedural areas such as endoscopy and interventional labs. The patients are evaluated for preoperative medical conditions that could affect their postoperative outcome such as diabetes, smoking, malnutrition, and delirium. The patients are also risk assessed for postoperative cardiac or pulmonary complications. We have standardized the laboratory values checked preoperatively and standardized perioperative anticoagulation management.

We now successfully screen 73% of our patients in the PACT clinic which has led to a sustained day-of-surgery cancellation rate of 6% at the main hospital and 5% at our smaller hospital as shown in Figure 8.2. One key to communicating pertinent findings from our PACT clinic, such as a history of malignant hyperthermia, is the use of flags within our Anesthesia Dashboard. Flags communicate missing elements of operative readiness and pertinent history and physical findings that guide the patient's course throughout the perioperative continuum.

We continually measure TAT at both our hospitals. As a large academic medical center, a 30-minute TAT was a stretch goal; however, we thought it was important to ensure continued focus for improvement. Our TATs have decreased from an average of 77 minutes 7 years ago to a more consistent 38–45 minutes. Our cases are primarily large complex cases at North Pavilion and mostly orthopedic cases at Highland Hospital, both of which require more extensive setup times. Over the past

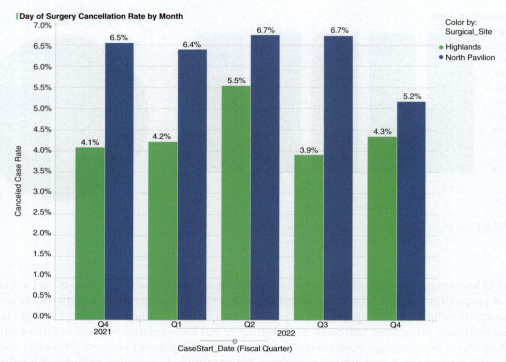

FIGURE 8.2 Day of surgery cancellation rate by month.

4 years, we have moved out to ambulatory surgery centers with over 8,000 outpatient and less complex cases from both of our campuses. Those cases transitioned to ambulatory centers averaged TATs of 27–30 minutes. Since this case transition, we are successfully sustaining TATs of 41–45 minutes, which we feel is likely a best practice for large academic hospitals. These TATs for both hospitals are shown in Figure 8.3.

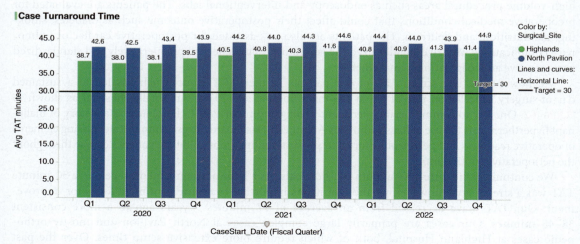

FIGURE 8.3 Case TAT in minutes.

CHAPTER 8 • Efficiency in the Operating Room: Get the Data, Make the Change

● IMPLEMENTING A SOLUTION

Centralized scheduling and empowering our schedulers to manipulate the OR schedule with guidance from our policies and support from our OR leadership allows our operating rooms to be more efficient. For example, we have 1 operating room dedicated to cystoscopy. If urology has booked enough cystoscopy cases to fill the day, then no cases are added. If, however, urology has not booked cystoscopy cases, then the schedulers can move other appropriate cases such as anorectal cases into the room with surgeon approval. This optimization of the surgery schedule happens the day before surgery around midday as the scheduling team huddles.

Our assistant nurse managers, lead CRNA, and nursing team leaders huddle twice a day at 05:30 and noon to ensure optimization of the schedule for the day of and the next day's operative schedule. In this huddle, they look for opportunities to fill unanticipated holes in the OR schedule with creative strategies of case placement focused on throughput and guided by our case leveling system. Case movement at the noon huddle often requires phone calls to surgeons and patients to adjust arrival times for the following day, which has been key to optimizing the surgery schedule relative to preventing block overruns whenever possible.

Key Steps in Change Management and Potential Pitfalls

Key Steps in Change Management

1. Identify key operational metrics to track and target for improving efficiency in the operating rooms.
2. Understand the types and volume of surgical cases your organization performs to inform your policies and procedures for routine block scheduling and urgent case additions.
3. Empower and support your frontline staff (centralized surgery schedulers, nursing team leaders, etc.) to make real-time decisions based on your policies.
4. Standardize and hard-wire as many processes as possible.
5. Pilot test any new process or intervention prior to widespread implementation and be flexible with changing the process to fit your institution's unique needs.

Potential Pitfalls

1. Lack of accurate, robust data and transparent definitions will lead to surgeon mistrust.
2. Lack of an OR governance structure with visible engagement from surgical, anesthesia, and nursing leaders.
3. Constant turnover of staff leads to a lack of institutional memory of policies and procedures, so continuous education is necessary.

● MEASURING OUTCOMES

Our OR Executive Committee meets monthly to review the percentage of all operating room minutes used out of the total operating room minutes that are available. A national best practice is using 85% of the total minutes available. This allows some flexibility in the schedule to accommodate both staffing challenges and urgent or emergent cases. We also review monthly the block time utilization of each surgical division or department. If a division or department is not utilizing (75%) its available block time over a 3-month period, it will be notified that it may have its block time taken away. If it is not utilized, then they lose that block time. By ensuring relatively predictable volumes, understanding our add-on case rate, and tracking our block overrun time, we can staff the operating rooms appropriately. Additionally, all monthly perioperative reports are shared transparently with Surgical Department Chairs, OR Executive Committee, and hospital Senior Leadership.

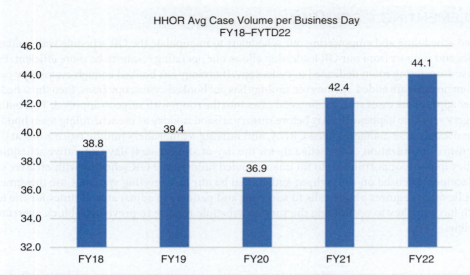

FIGURE 8.4 Highland Hospital average case volume by day.

Measuring the data and making appropriate changes have allowed us to increase our surgical volumes year over year, with the exception of the COVID-19 pandemic restrictions. In fiscal year 2012, we performed 30,592 cases at both our hospitals. In fiscal year 2021, we performed 37,973 cases and in 2022, we are projected to perform 39,466 cases. By utilizing the first come, first served model at Highlands Hospital, we have increased our daily case volumes significantly as shown in Figure 8.4. This model increases access for surgeons who do not have allocated block time, or who are able to operate more frequently than their assigned block time.

● FOLLOW-UP AND MAINTENANCE

Maintaining efficiency and optimal throughput in the operating room requires constant attention and engagement from the OR leadership. It also requires continuous investing in the education of new staff and trainees to ensure everyone understands our policies, key performance indicators, and goals. In addition to continuous education, we standardize and hard-wire processes as much as possible to try to neutralize the effects of staff turnover. We constantly balance meeting the needs of our healthcare system (providing surgical care as safely and efficiently as possible) with the needs of our staff, anesthesiologists, and surgeons. Finding this right balance will lead to healthier and happier healthcare systems, patients, providers, and staff to ensure the future success of our mission.

Ensuring Access to Operating Room for Complex Time-Sensitive Cases

9

CHRISTOPHER L. CRAMER AND VICTOR M. ZAYDFUDIM

Clinical Delivery Challenge

In the spring of 2020, the world faced a crisis. A novel coronavirus, COVID-19, spread quickly to become a global pandemic. Hospital systems were flooded with patients, rapidly overtaking available acute care beds, ICU beds, ventilators, materials, and healthcare worker resources. Urgent operations were streamlined; elective operations either slowed or came to a halt at many medical centers. Ensuring access to complex time-sensitive cases became a priority for many surgeons not involved in direct critical care of COVID-19 patients. Most healthcare systems needed an ability to stratify elective care needs to help prioritize patient needs and allocate surgical care.

Mass casualties, natural disasters, and infectious disease outbreaks are just some examples of unexpected events that incite an enormous logistical burden on a healthcare system. Such large-scale events tax available resources including consumable resources, human staff (nurses, patient care technicians, respiratory therapists, environmental services personnel, physicians, just to name a few), bed space, and operating room (OR) space and personnel. As surgeons, this strain on resources can limit our ability to offer and perform elective operations for time-sensitive cases.

The first surge of COVID-19 pandemic is a recent model example of unprecedented strain on our healthcare system demanding restriction, and in some cases, near complete cessation of elective operations. The unanticipated lack of human resources and available hospital bed space in many hospitals necessitated urgent development of triage systems for performing time-sensitive operations while postponing operations that could be safely delayed.

● WORKUP

While elective surgical volumes can be estimated with relative precision based on historical data, system strain arising from a disaster management condition is more challenging to estimate. Relatively short-term system limitations, such as those resulting from a mass casualty, can typically be resolved to accommodate access for time-sensitive cases without significant delay. Resources needed to treat patients and manage healthcare system strain associated with global pandemic, however, are more challenging to predict, and a vast pool of data with complex forecasting are needed to estimate the quantity of elective surgical cases a healthcare system would be able to provide. A substantial body of questions and changes in prediction models manifested during the first and second waves of the COVID-19 pandemic, as such forecasting evolved using an iterative process of data collection, data review, and prediction generation to maximize the number of time-sensitive elective cases performed.

Developing streamlined methods for efficiently collecting these data requires multidisciplinary collaboration of key stakeholders and leadership across the healthcare system. Essential perioperative data include historical operative volumes, new surgical outpatient clinic visits, planned volume of daily elective cases, operations and operative indications, predicted level of postoperative care required (acute care, intermediate care, intensive care), and estimated length of stay. During the acute phases of COVID-19 surge, planning also required a hospital's operational data, including available beds, planned discharges, number of available nursing (and in some cases physician) staff, as well as an estimated number of non-COVID- and COVID-related admissions. Ultimately, these data allowed for estimating the volume of elective cases our system could accommodate after allocating hospital beds and resources toward the care of COVID-19 patients and other higher priority patients.[1]

Resource management is critical to maximize care and minimize the number of delayed elective cases. We can borrow several ideas from disaster preparation principles discussed more heavily in the trauma and emergency medicine literature. Key principles of resource utilization include the following[2]:

1. Preparation—This step involves maintaining stocks of supplies and working equipment for situations that tax the system beyond typical levels. Part of preparedness includes planning for disaster situations and stockpiling critical supplies such as equipment needed for managing airways.
2. Conservation—Critical resources should be conserved to accommodate the critical situation at hand. In our example, these important resources include physical bed space and personal protective equipment needed for the care of patients with COVID. Resource conservation could involve limiting elective operations to maximize supplies of the aforementioned resources.
3. Substitution—This principle involves using functionally equivalent or near equivalent resources to minimize the consumption of other resources. An example might be substituting medical therapy for surgical therapy in a young fit patient with uncomplicated appendicitis to limit the volume of elective operations and thus conserve hospital beds.
4. Adaptation—Typically, adaptation involves using devices safely for purposes they were not intended. On a broader scale in the COVID example, adaptation would involve assigning critically ill COVID-positive patients to hospital beds in the procedural ICUs.
5. Reallocation—Critical resources may need to be reallocated to patients in greater need after extensive risk–benefit analysis. During the peak of the COVID pandemic, given the space and personnel constraints, the number of elective operations offered was limited to those in greatest need.

● DIFFERENTIAL DIAGNOSIS

The following is just a fraction of the factors that may contribute to an inadequate ability to perform all needed elective operations during a crisis, such as a natural disaster, mass casualty, or pandemic:

- Insufficient equipment including bed availability or ventilators
- Insufficient personal protective equipment
- Insufficient hospital staff
- Influx of inpatient admissions or patients seeking emergent evaluations
- Delayed hospital discharges
- Volume of needed elective surgical cases and procedures
- Financial constraints, which may impact other factors

● DIAGNOSIS AND TREATMENT

All the items on the differential contribute directly to capacity level and hospital occupancy rate. Although all these contributing factors need to be addressed to create a highly functional healthcare system, for the purpose of this chapter, we will focus on elective surgical case volume as a contributor to limited bed space in the setting of the acute phase of the COVID pandemic.

During the peak of the pandemic, as patients with COVID occupied greater than 25–50% of hospital beds (or greater) in many healthcare systems, and hospitals' physical and employee resources stretched thin, delays and cancellations of elective cases were inevitable. A multidisciplinary approach to triage was needed. For the triage system to be successful, key stakeholders including cross-specialty surgeons and proceduralists composed a tier-based triage system for elective operations requiring hospital admission. Multidisciplinary consensus is paramount to ensure individual specialty buy-in and implementation of the triage system.

Operative cases that need to be performed urgently and those that could be delayed several months with minimal or no associated morbidity are typically easy to differentiate; however, there is a large group of patients that are in the gray zone between these 2 groups. To help address triage needs, operative cases are classified into 3 tiers using a standardized criterion. Procedures and operations that need to be done urgently or emergently are the highest tier, whereas cases that can be safely delayed without a direct short-term negative effect on a patient are in the lowest tier.[1] It is also critical to establish a real-time daily communication system to discuss atypical cases that do not neatly fit into one of the triage tiers. When possible, optimal active medical management is used in patients in the lower tier groups until the operation can be performed.

● SCIENTIFIC PRINCIPLES AND EVIDENCE

Surgical triage is the foundational principle used for deciding how to ensure OR access to those in greatest need during the time of crisis (eg, COVID pandemic).[3]

Traditionally, in the United States, urgent or emergent procedures (life or limb saving) are established as offering the greatest amount of benefit during a disaster situation. Under more dire circumstances, the goals of triage can change to give priority to those who stand to gain the greatest number of quality life years from intervention.

Next, it is important to consider reasonable alternatives to surgery that may help preserve more scarce resources. Examples of a reasonable alternative to surgery include the use of antibiotics for appropriate cases of uncomplicated appendicitis. In cancer patients, the use of a neoadjuvant approach or prolonging the use of neoadjuvant therapy can be safe and effective in select malignancies until operative management is pursued. Decision-making in cancer care is complex and requires individualized review by a multidisciplinary team for each patient. Cancer operations that cannot be delayed should be pursued to avoid negative life-limiting consequences. For smaller hospital systems or those that are overwhelmed by the emergent condition, the transfer of elective patients who are in need of time-sensitive elective operations should be considered and pursued.[4]

While some procedures can be delayed indefinitely (eg, cosmetic surgery), most elective operations are performed for progressive diseases, disease processes that risk acute exacerbation, or diseases associated with disability and/or pain. Expected gains in life expectancy and quality of life from intervention must be weighed against the potential for worsened morbidity, long-term harm, and disease progression from postponing surgery. Other considerations to the triage process include prioritizing procedures that can be performed without the need for admission, those with short hospital stays, low likelihood of complications, and the lowest likelihood of requiring critical care. Resource utilization required for operations such as organ transplantation or extensive oncologic operations must be judiciously allocated as these operations can consume large amounts of consumable and human resources.

Given the complexity of these problems, systems have been proposed to help make equitable decisions that involve daily real-time management with discussion in a multidisciplinary team including key stakeholders such as physicians, administrators, other providers, and hospital leadership.[5] Input from multidisciplinary surgeon team and strong surgical leadership is particularly prudent to emphasize camaraderie and joint decision-making. Diagnoses that are either prioritized or de-prioritized should be reviewed with department and hospital leadership to assure the alignment of resources and the best available patient care. It is also imperative for surgeons to have a thorough discussion with each patient whose operation is to be delayed ensuring patient engagement, understanding of both decision-making and disease process, proposed short-term alternative treatment, projected time-course for postponed operation, and expected outcomes of alternatively proposed treatment with clear methods for communication should alternative

58   SECTION 2 • Efficiency of Inpatient Operations

treatment require change or re-consideration for operative management. Patients must be aware of indications to contact the surgeon in the setting of delayed intervention.

● IMPLEMENTING A SOLUTION

The following tier-based patient triage stratification system was developed for patients requiring elective operations. Importantly, the tier system and individual components were developed in a multidisciplinary setting, including collaboration between all surgical specialties and key administrative stakeholders, and were rooted in guidance from the American College of Surgeons who released recommendations for triage systems along with procedure-specific guidelines across various surgical specialties.[6,7]

- Tier 1: Purely elective—case can be scheduled at any time without risk to the patient (eg, aesthetic or cataract surgery).
- Tier 2: Medically necessary, time-sensitive—case delay will lead to a decrement in patient outcome (eg, in the case of progressive deterioration of a joint or nerve condition, delay will lead to a poor outcome, increased pain, or further disability).
- Tier 3: Critical—Case delay will lead to imminent harm (eg, malignancy, impending neurologic deterioration, need for coronary artery bypass).
  (Tier 2 and Tier 3 involve a delay in treatment that may lead to patient harm.)

To improve efficiency, the tier system is implemented directly into the case request process for each patient. Additional comments are encouraged, particularly for Tier 2 patients, as individual case review might be required to optimize resource allocation for sub-prioritization of the Tier 2 patient group. Based on predictive modeling for admissions, discharges, and bed availability, the number of elective cases that can be performed is estimated giving priority to Tier 3 cases and working on less urgent cases as resources allow. When bed utilization is the primary limiting factor, Tier 3 operations are prioritized as first-start cases allowing later-day cases to be flexed dependent on daily discharges and bed availability.

Key Steps in Change Management and Potential Pitfalls

Key Steps in Change Management

1. Data collection to allow for guided and precise resource management.
2. Multidisciplinary approach to the development of a triage system involving key stakeholders including surgeons from all specialties.
3. New data should be reviewed regularly to ensure the maximal number of elective cases are being performed to minimize disease progression and risk from case delays.
4. Thorough communication with patients discussing the rationale for the delay along with the alternative therapy and clear indications for reevaluation (eg, acutely worsening symptoms).

Potential Pitfalls

1. Failing to prepare for the potential moral distress and staff burnout associated with crisis situations.
2. Lacking a system to discuss atypical cases that do not fall cleanly within the triage criteria.
3. Not addressing other areas that could save resources (or gain resources) to allow for more elective operations (eg, performing all possible operations safely in an outpatient setting).
4. Lack of a backup plan for when resources are depleted (eg, a system for transferring patients who need urgent/timely care to a different facility with available resources that is capable of caring for the specific patient).

MEASURING OUTCOMES

In a setting such as the COVID pandemic, resources needed to be conserved and reallocated to allow for the care of COVID patients requiring hospitalization; this situation demanded the delay and triaging of elective operations. The goal of our change management was to ensure timely access to the OR for time-sensitive elective cases as resources allowed using a 3-tiered system. Success was measured by maintaining the capacity and resources needed to care for COVID-19 patients while maximizing the number of elective cases performed. Unintended consequences of delaying elective cases included possible worsening morbidity, disease progression, and acute exacerbation of the disease. Patients with adverse outcomes from surgical delay were dealt with on a case-by-case basis, while addressing each patient's specific needs and reevaluating continued postponing of the case groups.

FOLLOW-UP AND MAINTENANCE

The 3-tier-based triage system successfully stratifies patients into the urgency of operative intervention among elective surgical patients. Healthcare system and departmental leadership regularly reassess the ability to expand elective services amid the pandemic. Active reevaluation of data improves prediction models to regularly ensure accommodation of elective cases based on available resources. It is important to remember that as resources become more available, the volume of cases will be greater, and patients may have more advanced disease, possible associated comorbid conditions, and potential for greater complications, greater resources needed, and possible prolonged hospitalizations.

Acute rehabilitation and skilled nursing discharge facility destinations continue to experience high volumes of patients and ongoing staff shortages. The process of expanding elective surgical services after a large-scale crisis, such as the COVID pandemic, involves careful planning, frequent reevaluation, and continued awareness of the potentially ongoing crisis. A significant backlog of patients whose operations were delayed and who still require surgical intervention can continue to tax a system long after the crisis has peaked. It is crucial to anticipate and prepare for an increased volume and complexity of cases with more advanced diseases as well as the rise of urgent/emergent operations from delayed and unmet population needs.

REFERENCES

1. Babidge WJ, Tivey DR, Kovoor JG, et al. Surgery triage during the COVID-19 pandemic. *ANZ J Surg.* 2020;90(9):1558–1565. doi: 10.1111/ans.16196
2. Hick JL, Hanfling D, Cantrill SV. Allocating scarce resources in disasters: emergency department principles. *Ann Emerg Med.* 2012;59(3):177–187. doi: 10.1016/j.annemergmed.2011.06.012
3. Rathnayake D, Clarke M. The effectiveness of different patient referral systems to shorten waiting times for elective surgeries: systematic review. *BMC Health Serv Res.* 2021;21(1):155. doi: 10.1186/s12913-021-06140-w
4. Brindle ME, Doherty G, Lillemoe K, Gawande A. Approaching surgical triage during the COVID-19 pandemic. *Ann Surg.* 2020;272(2):e40–e42. doi: 10.1097/SLA.0000000000003992
5. Qadan M, Hong TS, Tanabe KK, Ryan DP, Lillemoe KD. A multidisciplinary team approach for triage of elective cancer surgery at the Massachusetts General Hospital during the novel coronavirus COVID-19 outbreak. *Ann Surg.* 2020;272(1):e20–e21. doi: 10.1097/SLA.0000000000003963
6. COVID-19: Elective Case Triage Guidelines for Surgical Care. ACS. Accessed July 1, 2022. https://www.facs.org/for-medical-professionals/covid-19/clinical-guidance/elective-case/
7. COVID-19: Guidance for Triage of Non-Emergent Surgical Procedures. ACS. Accessed July 1, 2022. https://www.facs.org/for-medical-professionals/covid-19/clinical-guidance/triage/

SECTION 3

Site of Care Optimization

10 **"Right Case, Right Place": High Number of Outpatient Cases at an Inpatient Facility**
Pratyusha Yalamanchi, Sapan N. Ambani, Amir A. Ghaferi, and Kelly Michelle Malloy

11 **Avoiding Life-Threatening Complications at an Ambulatory Surgery Center**
Pratyusha Yalamanchi and Andrew J. Rosko

12 **Low Acuity Inpatient Cases at High Acuity Hospital**
Nabeel R. Obeid and Dana A. Telem

13 **Home Monitoring for Surgical Home Hospital**
Biqi Zhang, Jayson S. Marwaha, Kavya Pathak, Malcolm K. Robinson, and Thomas C. Tsai

14 **Service Line With Low Operating Room Utilization at Ambulatory Surgery Center**
Andrew M. Ibrahim, Geoffrey E. Hespe, and Amir A. Ghaferi

"Right Case, Right Place": High Number of Outpatient Cases at an Inpatient Facility

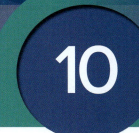

PRATYUSHA YALAMANCHI, SAPAN N. AMBANI,
AMIR A. GHAFERI, AND KELLY MICHELLE MALLOY

Clinical Delivery Challenge

Despite significant unused ambulatory surgery center (ASC) capacity (Figure 10.1), the majority of cases performed at an academic tertiary care center inpatient facility in the fiscal year 2019 (FY 2019) were outpatient procedures. Given that the inpatient facility operated at full capacity, this resulted in limited availability for urgent or emergent inpatient operative procedures. Safe and timely surgical care for acutely ill patients was often delayed, resulting in an increased risk of complication. As 1 patient noted, "A procedure that is rather common got delayed and rescheduled to the point where it became a life-threatening procedure with painful side effects. I arrived at the emergency department with appendicitis and ended up in the operating room nearly 40 hours later with a ruptured appendix."

Optimization of operative block time, defined as time available for specific surgical services to schedule procedures, across the inpatient and outpatient facilities became an urgent clinical delivery challenge to ensure the availability of inpatient operating rooms (ORs) for urgent and emergent procedures.

The rise in ASCs in the last 2 decades has been driven by efforts to reduce perioperative care costs while delivering equivalent patient outcomes and improved patient satisfaction.[1] Despite the increased capacity of ASCs and hospital outpatient departments (HOPDs) over time, there remains wide variation in the utilization of these sites for the delivery of outpatient surgical care.

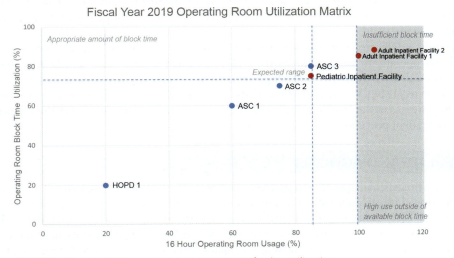

FIGURE 10.1 FY 2019 inpatient and outpatient facility utilization.

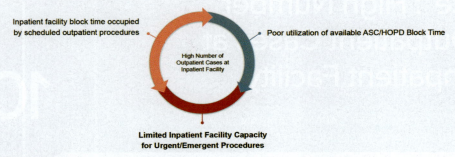

FIGURE 10.2 Clinical delivery challenge.

Here we present the clinical delivery challenge of insufficient inpatient OR capacity for urgent and emergent cases due to overscheduling of routine outpatient cases within an inpatient facility (Figure 10.2). The workup and management of this case study are discussed. We then review the available literature and present change management solutions and continuous process improvement strategies for addressing a high number of outpatient cases within an inpatient facility.

● WORKUP

Workup first involves a review of operational data by facility leadership. Institution-specific operational metrics include commonly tracked key performance indicators that offer insight into business efficiencies such as case turnover time, block scheduling, and cancellation rates, as well as operative outcomes and complications that can be reviewed to inform additional primary data collection.

In our case study, surgeon leadership and operations analysts reviewed FY 2019 OR block time utilization, scheduling delays, and OR usage at the inpatient facility, ASCs, and HOPDs. This resulted in the identification of an additional capacity need of 4 16-hour ORs per week at the inpatient facility to ensure timely access for urgent (defined as within 6 hours of booking) and emergent (defined as within 1 hour of booking) procedures.

Having identified the scope of the problem, inpatient facility leadership proceeded to identify surgical services in need of urgent and emergent inpatient facility operative block time such as acute care and trauma surgery, plastic surgery, and orthopedic surgery. Additionally, the surgical leadership team characterized lower acuity outpatient procedures performed at the inpatient facility that may be candidates for ASC/HOPD care. These included cases from surgical services such as orthopedics, otolaryngology, general surgery, and urology.

Subsequently, a dedicated multidisciplinary work group was established with key stakeholders including clinical and operations team members from each inpatient facility, ASC, and HOPD sites, surgical service faculty, and anesthesiology leadership. This group defined key operational metrics for operative site optimization as (1) block time utilization at ASCs/HOPD, (2) time from booking to the procedure for urgent/emergent cases at the inpatient facility, and (3) percent of cases performed at the inpatient facility which were outpatient procedures.

● DIFFERENTIAL DIAGNOSIS

Addressing the clinical challenge of operative case and operative site mismatch, defined as a high number of outpatient procedures in an inpatient facility in our case study, requires systematic root cause analyses. Returning to our case scenario, primary qualitative data from key stakeholders identified 3 barriers to outpatient case movement to alternative sites that were not evident from the operational data review alone. These included (1) availability of equipment at ambulatory facilities, (2) concern for patient eligibility for care at ASC/HOPDs based on comorbidities, and (3) surgeon preferences.

Based on these findings, the multidisciplinary working group identified a core principle for reframing outpatient case scheduling: *outpatient procedures should occur at outpatient facilities (ASCs/HOPD)*. While ASCs/HOPDs had been open with available OR block time for a few years, surgeons and anesthesiologists alike expressed efficiency and patient safety concerns for transitioning outpatient procedures from the inpatient facility to ambulatory centers. Ensuring accurate patient risk stratification and ASC/HOPD preparedness were identified as critical to ensuring that outpatient procedures would occur at the inpatient facility *only* for patient-specific clinical needs.

DIAGNOSIS AND TREATMENT

Based on the previously described workup, the highest leverage areas for addressing operative case and site mismatch in our case study included (1) moving operative block time for surgical services from the inpatient facility to outpatient facilities for low-acuity, outpatient procedures in a one-to-one fashion and (2) obtaining needed equipment and staff training at outpatient facilities to ensure efficient, safe outpatient procedures.

Through this process, the multidisciplinary working group was able to identify 4 surgical services which would "relinquish" a portion of their inpatient facility OR block time in exchange for ASC/HOPD OR time. As shown in Figure 10.3, this resulted in creating an additional capacity of 14 16-hour rooms per month at the inpatient facility for emergent and urgent cases.

SCIENTIFIC PRINCIPLES AND EVIDENCE

Outpatient procedures performed at an ambulatory center compared to inpatient setting have repeatedly been shown to offer significant cost savings and equivalent or improved 30-day outcomes in appropriately selected patients.[1,2] Appropriate patient selection is critical to ASC success, and current literature has identified both patient and procedural factors associated with perioperative complication and safety of surgery in an ambulatory setting. Studies have demonstrated that patients with age greater than 80 years, body mass index > 25 kg/m^2, chronic obstructive pulmonary disease, history of transient ischemic attack or stroke, moderate to severe obstructive sleep apnea, and/or previous cardiac surgery are at increased risk of perioperative complications and may benefit from outpatient surgical management in a hospital setting.[3-5]

Given the increasing interest in the allocation of limited healthcare resources, procedure specialization within ASCs has also contributed to efficiencies in OR turnover and perioperative time. The economic logic of specialization supports the trend toward dedicated ambulatory surgery care environments given the increasing Centers for Medicare and Medicaid Services interest in value-based reimbursement systems such as bundled payments and reduced site-neutral payments.[6]

IMPLEMENTING A SOLUTION

A data-driven, multidisciplinary problem-solving approach is critical to ensuring that the "right case occurs in the right place." In our case study, decision-making involved (1) facilitating improved patient selection and scheduling of cases at ASCs, (2) ensuring appropriate equipment availability at ambulatory care centers,

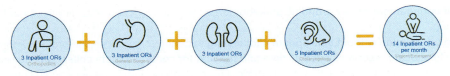

FIGURE 10.3 Inpatient facility OR capacity obtained by block time transfer to ASC.

and (3) gaining surgeon buy-in for transfer of site of care delivery from the inpatient facility to an outpatient setting by enhancing the physician experience at ASCs.

Specifically, facilitating improved patient selection involved regular meetings of the multidisciplinary work group of anesthesia and ambulatory and inpatient facility leaders. This group spearheaded the development of a readmission risk assessment tool based on FY 2019 data to advise surgeons on patient candidacy for surgical care at an outpatient facility and to offer a comparison with longitudinal patient outcomes. After the development of this tool, a 2-month pilot program with 2 surgical services, Urology and Surgical Oncology, was designed to track patient perioperative outcomes and better understand the surgeon experience at ASCs and perioperative care at these facilities.

Choice architecture such as a best practice alert (BPA) within the electronic medical record to support scheduling of outpatient procedures in outpatient facilities was designed as shown in Figure 10.4. The resulting data informed the awareness of day-to-day barriers to case movement to ambulatory care centers.

Based on the BPA data, the multidisciplinary working group performed frequent assessments of operative equipment and instrumentation at the ASCs/HOPDs and ensured staff preparedness for equipment utilization within cases. Further enhancement of the surgeon experience at ASCs was also ensured through the development of a formal onboarding process.

Key Steps in Change Management and Potential Pitfalls

Key Steps in Change Management

1. **Define the problem:** *There is an additional capacity need of 4 16-hour ORs per week at the inpatient facility, to ensure timely access to urgent and emergent procedures.*
2. **Understand the process:** *Surgical services in need of urgent and emergent inpatient facility operative block time and lower acuity outpatient procedures performed at the inpatient facility are identified.*
3. **Engage key stakeholders:** *A dedicated multidisciplinary work group including clinical and operations team members from each inpatient facility and ASC sites, surgical service faculty, and anesthesiology leadership is established.*
4. **Define key operational metrics:** *Measurable outcomes are identified including (1) block time utilization at the inpatient and ambulatory surgery facilities, (2) time from booking to procedure for urgent/emergent cases at the inpatient facility, and (3) percent of cases performed at the inpatient facility which are outpatient procedures.*
5. **Introduce and implement possible solutions:** *At least 4 surgical services that "relinquish" a portion of their inpatient facility OR block time for ASC operative time are identified. Feedback and barriers to implementation are identified by key stakeholders. Consistent communication across surgical services, departments, schedulers, and sites is critical toward implementing this "Right Case, Right Place" solution.*
6. **Continuous process improvement:** *Continuous data collection, including monthly postoperative admission rates, rates of outpatient procedures at inpatient facilities, and block time utilization at inpatient and outpatient facilities, is critical to driving durable change aimed at reducing the number of outpatient cases performed at an inpatient facility.*

Potential Pitfalls

1. **Lack of engagement of key, frontline stakeholders** at the inpatient and ASC facilities prior to piloting a solution.
2. **Scaling the solution without appropriate pilot testing** to generate feedback and process improvement.
3. **Failure to allocate resources such as time and funding for continued data collection** and review after solution implementation, which is critical to (1) identify unintentional consequences and (2) prevent reversion to the pre-intervention state after changes have been implemented.

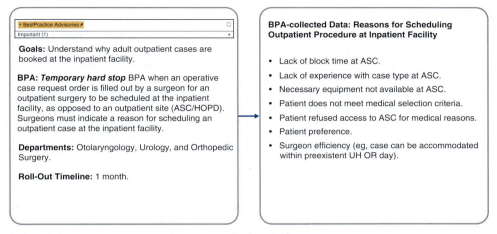

FIGURE 10.4 BPA within the electronic medical record.

● MEASURING OUTCOMES

Development of a monthly standard review process of block time utilization for all sites by senior leadership should be performed, with in-depth analyses of utilization by each OR and day to assess turnover times, case length, and availability of necessary operative equipment and training. Success within the continuous process improvement effort requires implementation of Plan-Do-Check-Act (PDCA) cycles to measure and improve outcome metrics such as movement of outpatient cases from the inpatient facility, rate of perioperative complications and unplanned hospital admissions, and time from booking to procedure for urgent/emergent cases at the inpatient facility.[7]

In our case study, the multidisciplinary working group found that consistent communication across surgical services, departments, schedulers, and sites was critical toward implementing "Right Case, Right Place," specifically reframing the provider mindset to performing outpatient procedures at the inpatient facility only for patient-specific or unique procedure-specific clinical needs. The work group continued to meet monthly for over a year to monitor the movement of cases out of the inpatient facility and ensure that 14 OR days per month remained available for urgent/emergent procedures. By FY 2021, surgeon leaders reported not only satisfaction with their ASC/HOPD experience but also preference for ambulatory surgical sites over the inpatient facility for available operative block time due to perioperative efficiency and patient preference. Moreover, acute care surgeons reported increased access and flexibility for scheduling time-sensitive inpatient surgeries beyond the measurement of time from booking to OR.

● FOLLOW-UP AND MAINTENANCE

Continuous data collection, including monthly postoperative admission rates, rates of outpatient procedures at inpatient facilities, and block time utilization at ASCs, is critical to driving durable change aimed at reducing the number of outpatient cases performed at an inpatient facility. While our case study demonstrated the need to address operative case and site mismatch to improve inpatient OR access for urgent and emergent care, there is an increasing pressure across health systems to lower healthcare delivery costs while providing excellent patient outcomes. Appropriate patient selection is critical to ensuring the safety of outpatient procedures performed in an ambulatory setting. Ultimately, optimal utilization of lower-cost, specialized centers such as ASCs/HOPDs is an important component of cost-effective surgical care delivery.

The use of continuous process improvement strategies can lead to iterative improvements in care delivery over time.[7] Potential pitfalls include failure to allocate resources such as time and funding for continued data collection and review, which remain critical to prevent reversion to the pre-intervention state after changes have been implemented.

REFERENCES

1. Makanji HS, Bilolikar VK, Goyal DK, Kurd MF. Ambulatory surgery center payment models: current trends and future directions. *J Spine Surg.* 2019;5(Suppl 2):S191.
2. Friedlander DF, Krimphove MJ, Cole AP, et al. Where is the value in ambulatory versus inpatient surgery? *Ann Surg.* 2021;273(5):909–916.
3. Mathis MR, Naughton NN, Shanks A, et al. Patient selection for day case-eligible surgery: identifying those at high risk for major complications. *Anesthesiology.* 2013;119(6):1310–1321.
4. Kent C, Metzner J, Bollag L. An analysis of risk factors and adverse events in ambulatory surgery. *Ambul Anesth.* 2014;1:3–10. https://doi.org/10.2147/AA.S53280. doi: https://doi.org/10.2147/AA.S53280.
5. Fortier J, Chung F, Su J. Unanticipated admission after ambulatory surgery—a prospective study. *Can J Anaesth.* 1998;45(7):612–619.
6. Carey K, Mitchell JM. Specialization and production cost efficiency: evidence from ambulatory surgery centers. *Int J Health Econ Manag.* 2018;18(1):83–98. https://doi-org.proxy.lib.umich.edu/10.1007/s10754-017-9225-9.
7. Knudsen SV, Laursen HVB, Johnsen SP, Bartels PD, Ehlers LH, Mainz J. Can quality improvement improve the quality of care? A systematic review of reported effects and methodological rigor in plan-do-study-act projects. *BMC Health Serv Res.* 2019;19(1):683. doi: 10.1186/s12913-019-4482-6.

Avoiding Life-Threatening Complications at an Ambulatory Surgery Center

11

PRATYUSHA YALAMANCHI AND ANDREW J. ROSKO

Clinical Delivery Challenge

A high-volume thyroid surgeon is determining which of her patients are candidates for thyroidectomy at a new ASC versus tertiary care hospital where she has admitting privileges. While thyroidectomy is historically an inpatient procedure due to the potential life-threatening complication of airway obstruction related to postoperative neck hematoma, this surgeon has increasingly been discharging patients undergoing hemithyroidectomy on the same day of surgery with low complication rates and high anecdotal patient satisfaction. She is also increasingly encouraged by her departmental leadership to transition outpatient surgical procedures to the new ASC given lower associated costs, and possible decreased patient exposure to multidrug-resistant organisms and other nosocomial infections.[1,2] In addition, this would offer additional hospital-based operating room (OR) time for her surgical colleagues performing inpatient procedures.

In order to avoid significant complications at the stand-alone ASC, she seeks to understand the likelihood of major morbidity and mortality at an ASC and risk stratify her own patients to better identify who may be a safe candidate for outpatient surgery at the new outpatient surgery center.

Life-threatening complications at ambulatory surgery centers (ASCs) are fortunately rare events. Still, management of these events can be challenging due to limited on-site resources and poses life-altering consequences to both patient and provider, in addition to potential legal and financial loss to health systems. Therefore, clinical preparedness involves both (1) prevention of complications through accurate preoperative risk stratification and assessment of patient candidacy for outpatient surgery and (2) readiness for management of complications with timely patient stabilization and activation of appropriate, higher acuity care with rapid transport to the nearest hospital's emergency department (ED).

Here we present a case study of the assessment of candidacy for outpatient thyroidectomy to investigate the workup and management of this clinical delivery challenge. We then review the available literature and present change management solutions and continuous process improvement strategies for avoiding life-threatening complications at an ASC.

● WORKUP

Approximately 1% of patients in ASCs develop severe complications that require transfer to a hospital after a procedure.[3] Institution-specific operational data regarding case volume, rates of complications requiring hospital transfer as well as associated patient and procedural factors, and provider staffing are critical to understanding the current state and mitigating the risk of avoidable complications. Given the variability in mandatory quality reporting practices for ASCs across states, some of this data may be unavailable and need to be collected in a prospective fashion.

Key stakeholders for obtaining institution-specific ASC operations data include the ASC medical director and operations manager, who likely have access to collected data such as case volume, outcomes, and financial data related to the day-to-day management of the ASC. These administrative leaders are tasked with reviewing key performance indicators (KPIs) which are operational metrics that keep track of business efficiencies such as case turnover time, block scheduling, and cancellation rates, as well as operative

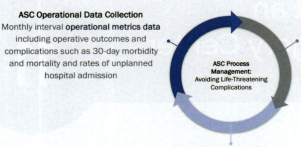

FIGURE 11.1 ASC process management—key metrics and process tools framework for avoiding life-threatening complications.

outcomes and complications. Each ASC complication, defined as any event posing morbidity or risk of mortality, should trigger a root cause analysis to identify contributory factors and relevant process tools that can be used to identify areas for improvement such as resource allocation (Figure 11.1). Comparisons with national databases such as the ACS National Surgical Quality Improvement Program (NSQIP) and closed claims analysis can offer further benchmark data.

Returning to our case study, our surgeon completed her own "workup" by obtaining data from her ASC leadership regarding rates of unplanned hospital admissions and factors associated with life-threatening complications after outpatient surgery. The ASC's rate of unplanned admissions was 1.5% over the course of a year with 5% of these admissions associated with major cardiopulmonary events and 1% due to significant procedure-related bleeding requiring further intervention. There were no mortality events. The indications for unplanned hospital admission were 45% surgical, 45% anesthetic, and 10% social. Multivariate logistic regression analyses identified longer case length, ASA class 4, age > 85 years, and body mass index (BMI) > 30 as associated with complications at the ASC requiring hospital transfer and admission. She then proceeded to compare this with existing literature as well as guidelines from the American Thyroid Association (ATA) to determine candidacy in her patient panel for outpatient thyroidectomy at the ASC.

● DIFFERENTIAL DIAGNOSIS

The rare nature of life-threatening complications at ASCs makes these events challenging to study. Institutional-specific outcome metrics as outlined above and data from national databases described below can inform root causes of potential life-threatening complications and establish effective preventative and management measures. Preventative measures involve accurate risk stratification of preoperative patients to assess candidacy for ASC-based procedures based on patient age, BMI, comorbidities such as obstructive sleep apnea or need for chronic anticoagulation, and other procedure-specific factors such as length of procedure, risk of complication, and likelihood of the need for postoperative monitoring. Other patient-specific factors such as patient distance from the hospital and adequate social support such as available transportation and caregivers in the setting of anesthetic recovery are additional considerations.

Preparedness with the goal of avoidance of life-threatening ASC complications is the primary goal. Regular training for staff regarding the management of potential complications is also an important consideration often identified during process improvement efforts. These may range from awareness of emergency crash cart locations and contents, as well as identifying other skilled on-site providers such as additional anesthesiologists who may assist with airway or acute cardiopulmonary management.

CHAPTER 11 • Avoiding Life-Threatening Complications at an Ambulatory Surgery Center

● DIAGNOSIS AND TREATMENT

Based on the workup described previously, the highest leverage areas for improvement are (1) prevention of complications through accurate preoperative risk stratification and assessment of patient candidacy for outpatient surgery at ASCs and (2) readiness for management of complications with timely patient stabilization and activation of appropriate, higher acuity care when needed.

Solutions include the exclusion of patients with clinical and social factors associated with unplanned hospital admission and risk of serious complication from ASC care. Individual patient candidacy for ASC care should be assessed by multiple providers including an initial screening by the surgeon at the time of case request, subsequent necessary preoperative medical clearance, and finally by the anesthesiology team at the ASC prior to scheduling surgery. Establishment of institution-specific patient clinical and social factor criteria as well as procedure-related considerations by a multidisciplinary team involved in ASC and hospital management can offer standardization in ASC candidacy and allow surgeons to educate patients regarding their likely site of care delivery at the time of consultation.

Additionally, regular training for the management of possible complications offers preparation and prevention of significant morbidity and mortality at ASCs. Emergency crash carts are present and available in all OR settings, and biannual training among all OR faculty and staff in this equipment can ensure that carts are appropriately stocked and can be used efficiently if needed. Team-based simulation of possible code events during these training events can further ensure smooth delivery of care. Additionally, protocols establishing ease of contacting 911, facilitating urgent transfer to the closest ED, and communicating with providers at the higher acuity care center regarding impending transfer are all additional means of ensuring preparedness.

Ultimately, continuous process improvement as described in Figure 11.1 is required to assess complication rates and the effectiveness of preventative interventions.

● SCIENTIFIC PRINCIPLES AND EVIDENCE

Existing literature has identified both patient and procedural factors associated with surgical complications and the need for unplanned hospital admission. A prospective Canadian study, among a study population of 15,172 patients, identified a 1.4% hospital admission rate after ambulatory surgery. The most common types of adverse events were associated with temporary morbidities such as poorly controlled nausea and vomiting, poorly controlled pain, and procedure-related bleeding requiring treatment or observation. The indications for admission were surgical in 38% of cases, anesthetic in 25%, social in 20%, and medical in 17%. Five percent of admissions or 1 in every 1400 were a life-threatening complication such as a major cardiopulmonary event.[4] A similar case–control study in Canada found factors associated with unplanned admission on multivariate logistic regression included length of surgery greater than 3 hours (OR 4.26), American Society of Anesthesiologists (ASA) class 3 or (OR 4.60 and 6.51, respectively), age $\geq$ 80 years (OR 5.41), and BMI > 30 (OR 2.81).[5]

Similarly, a 2013 study of 250,000 subjects within the NSQIP database identified a postoperative mortality rate of 0.009% within 72 hours of surgery, a major morbidity rate of 0.1%, and an unplanned admission rate of 1.1%. Factors associated with perioperative morbidity and mortality included patient comorbidities such as chronic obstructive pulmonary disease, history of cerebrovascular accident or transient ischemic attack, hypertension, BMI > 30, as well as prolonged operative time. The procedures associated most frequently with adverse outcomes were laparoscopic cholecystectomy and inguinal or abdominal wall hernia repair.[6] Studies of pediatric ambulatory surgery have identified an increased risk of apnea in former preterm infants as well as patient age, severity of OSA, history of Down syndrome or craniofacial disorders, and distance from the hospital as predictive of airway morbidity, particularly in children undergoing tonsillectomy and adenotonsillectomy.[7]

Returning to our case study, the surgeon made herself aware of this existing body of literature as well as the ATA guidelines on candidacy for outpatient thyroidectomy, which highlight patient clinical and social factors as well as procedural considerations that merit postoperative admission given the risk of significant complication (Figure 11.2).

Clinical
- Cardiac or respiratory disease
- Dialysis for renal failure
- Anticoagulation
- Anxiety or seizure disorder
- Obstructive sleep apnea
- Mental or sensory impairment
- Pregnancy

Social
- Excessive distance from skilled facility
- Living alone with lack of transportation
- Patient preference
- Communication barrier

Procedural
- Massive and/or substernal goiter
- Locally advanced cancer
- Challenging hemostasis
- Difficult thyroidectomy with Hashimoto's thyroiditis or Graves' disease

FIGURE 11.2 Relative contraindications to outpatient thyroidectomy (adapted from American Thyroid Association).[2]

● IMPLEMENTING A SOLUTION

Approaching the problem of avoiding rare, life-threatening complications at an ASC requires a data-driven, multidisciplinary problem-solving approach with thoughtful consideration as to prevention, preparedness, and process improvement. As highlighted in Figure 11.1, the use of continuous process improvement strategies described in the quality improvement literature can lead to adaptive changes that facilitate iterative improvements in care delivery over time.[8]

A multidisciplinary team of key stakeholders including ASC leadership such as the ASC medical director, operations manager, anesthesiologists, nursing leaders, as well as surgeons operating at both the ASC and the admitting hospital should be assembled for review of collected outcomes and adverse event data. Based on the available institution-specific data as well as national benchmark data, institutional criteria for patient candidacy for ASC surgery and Postanesthesia Care Unit (PACU) criteria for safe discharge should be established with the goal of avoiding life-threatening complications. Regular monthly or quarterly meetings of this group are critical to ensuring the appropriate rigor of implementing these guidelines and subsequent review of resulting operating outcomes and complications to facilitate iterative improvement. Additionally, this group can be tasked with facilitating simulation-based training to ensure preparedness for the management of complications such as utilization of emergency crash carts and activating patient transport and access to higher acuity care.

Regarding our case study, our surgeon joined a multidisciplinary team of key ASC stakeholders at her own institution to define criteria for ASC surgical candidacy based on patient factors and procedure type, as well as requirements for safe discharge from PACU for nursing and anesthesia providers to follow. The latter included (1) adequate oxygenation, vital signs, and blood pressure control, (2) appropriate pain control and ability to tolerate PO, (3) return to baseline neurologic status, and (4) adequate social support with transportation home.[9,10] In this process, she identified her patients that were candidates for hemithyroidectomy at the ASC and clarified who would benefit from admission with standardized criteria. These were ultimately guiding principles and she felt that it was important to treat each patient individually as well given the danger of a one-size-fits-all approach (see Figure 11.3).

● MEASURING OUTCOMES

Success in this continuous process improvement effort requires thorough root cause analysis of complications and implementation of Plan-Do-Study-Act (PDSA) cycles to measure and improve various outcome metrics such as rate of postoperative adverse events and unplanned hospital admissions, as well as process metrics such as time to transport of the patient with complication to the nearest hospital. Process measures can offer proxy measurements to assess designed interventions given the rare nature of the primary

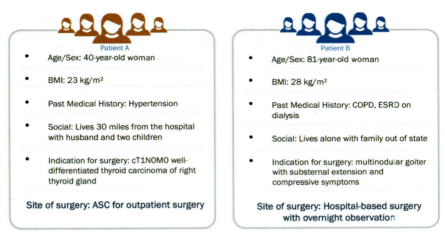

FIGURE 11.3 Avoiding ASC complications through preoperative risk stratification for determination of site of surgery.

outcome of life-threatening complications after ambulatory surgery. The multidisciplinary group should also continue to evaluate the previously outlined KPIs such as case turnover time, block scheduling, and cancellation rates, which may demonstrate unintended consequences of designed interventions.

● FOLLOW-UP AND MAINTENANCE

Avoiding rare, significant life-threatening complications at an ASC does require significant, continuous investment in leadership, expertise, and resources for change. Potential pitfalls include failure to allocate resources to prevent reversion to the prior state after changes have been implemented to reduce complication rates. "Project postmortems" as described in the business world are regular analyses of changes made to assess their success. If implementation was ultimately a failure, a "postmortem" analysis can offer insights and lessons for future change efforts. The process tools framework outlined in Figure 11.1 can be used to continuously collect data to drive change to achieve and maintain desired patient outcomes.

Returning to our thyroid surgeon, she continued to attend quarterly ASC stakeholder meetings where case outcomes and complication data were reviewed. This group also worked to design biannual preparedness simulations for the staff to ensure efficient, appropriate responses to complications, which ranged from emergency crash cart access to trialing the protocol for calling 911 and alerting the nearest hospital of an impending patient transfer. Continued time and labor allocation to this multidisciplinary working group ultimately facilitated continuous process improvement of care delivered at the ASC.

REFERENCES

1. Terris DJ, Moister B, Seybt MW, et al. Outpatient thyroid surgery is safe and desirable. *Otolaryngol Head Neck Surg*. 2007;136(4):556–559.
2. Terris DJ, Snyder S, Carneiro-Pla D, et al. American Thyroid Association statement on outpatient thyroidectomy. *Thyroid*. 2013;23(10):1193–1202.
3. Boodman S. Popularity of outpatient surgery centers leads to questions about safety. *Medpage Today*. 2014. Accessed May 5, 2023, https://www.medpagetoday.com/publichealthpolicy/publichealth/49213
4. Fortier J, Chung F, Su J. Unanticipated admission after ambulatory surgery—a prospective study. *Can J Anaesth*. 1998;45(7):612–619.
5. Whippey A, Kostandoff G, Paul J, Ma J, Thabane L, Ma HK. Predictors of unanticipated admission following ambulatory surgery: a retrospective case-control study. *Can J Anaesth*. 2013;60(7):675–683.
6. Mathis MR, Naughton NN, Shanks A, et al. Patient selection for day case-eligible surgery: identifying those at high risk for major complications. *Anesthesiology*. 2013;119(6):1310–1321.

SECTION 3 • Site of Care Optimization

7. Kent C, Metzner J, Bollag L. An analysis of risk factors and adverse events in ambulatory surgery. *Ambul Anesth.* 2014;1:3–10. doi: https://doi.org/10.2147/AA.S53280
8. Knudsen SV, Laursen HVB, Johnsen SP, Bartels PD, Ehlers LH, Mainz J. Can quality improvement improve the quality of care? A systematic review of reported effects and methodological rigor in plan-do-study-act projects. *BMC Health Serv Res.* 2019;19(1):683. doi: 10.1186/s12913-019-4482-6
9. Fortier J, Chung F, Su J. Unanticipated admission after ambulatory surgery—a prospective study. *Can J Anaesth.* 1998;45(7):612–619.
10. Clarkson E, Jung E, Lin S. How to avoid life-threatening complications associated with implant surgery. *Dent Clin North Am.* 2021;65(1):33–41. doi: 10.1016/j.cden.2020.09.002

Low Acuity Inpatient Cases at High Acuity Hospital

12

NABEEL R. OBEID AND DANA A. TELEM

Clinical Delivery Challenge

Your health system's strategic priorities include decentralization of care delivery and have acquired a local community hospital with strong market shares. A top clinical priority is the regional expansion of the bariatric surgery program. Currently, all bariatric surgeries are performed at the high acuity, quaternary care hospital in the system with specialty-trained bariatric surgeons. To effectively expand the clinical program, there will need to be processes implemented to optimize the site of care and align with levels of acuity.

One of the key principles of health system operations is the alignment of appropriate patients and procedures to the appropriate site for clinical delivery. Site of care optimization is critical to operations and resource allocation while maintaining safety and quality. According to the American Hospital Association, 84% of hospitals in the United States are community hospitals, of which 68% are affiliated with health systems.[1] For such multihospital systems containing hospitals of varying acuity, it is essential to identify less complex cases and lower acuity patients to be cared for at lower acuity facilities. This chapter explores this concept on a deeper level, providing practical examples and potential solutions for optimizing and aligning the level of acuity to the site of care.

● WORKUP

The most important first step in tackling operational decisions is gaining a deeper understanding of the current state. When considering a shift of a proportion of operative cases to a lower acuity facility, current annual case volume and procedure case mix are important data points. The raw data can be obtained from electronic health record reports, which are then often refined by department administrators. It is also important to understand the number of surgeons involved and their respective percentage of effort dedicated to clinical care. With that information, it will be possible to identify opportunities for restructuring a clinical program, including the distribution of cases across sites.

Understanding what types of procedures to perform and patients to care for in a safe and effective way at a lower acuity center requires a thorough understanding of available resources. Specific hospital information to gather should include number of hospital beds and capacity, intensive care capabilities, specialty-specific structural elements and equipment needs, subspecialty consultants, and available ancillary care services. Much of this information can be gathered from discussions with hospital leadership/administrators (Chief Executive Officer, Chief Medical Officer), department chairs, and medical directors.

With the above information, one can begin to quantify the proportion of low acuity cases that are being performed at a higher acuity facility which may highlight an opportunity for better alignment. This becomes the key operational metric: maximizing low acuity patients and cases to low acuity facilities. In turn, this will result in better resource utilization and increased capacity at higher acuity hospitals for higher levels of care.

SECTION 3 • Site of Care Optimization

> Which bariatric procedures would be appropriate to perform at a lower acuity facility? How will you identify patients who can be cared for safely in a community hospital setting? How will this affect the current clinical practice for you and your team?

● DIFFERENTIAL DIAGNOSIS

There is great variability in the makeup of American health systems. Systems that consist primarily of a single inpatient facility naturally have less opportunity for distribution of cases, particularly nonambulatory surgery. In contrast, multihospital systems have a prime opportunity to leverage the numerous sites of care to optimize acuity alignment. Despite this innate advantage, though, not all multihospital systems are successful in achieving this metric. Reasons are usually multifactorial and may include conflicting high-level strategic priorities, difficulty with operationalization, or resistance to change from affected personnel or groups. The challenge of site of care optimization becomes even more pronounced when a hospital is newly acquired by a system given the added pressures to leverage that opportunity and the countless unknowns of a new partnership.

● DIAGNOSIS AND TREATMENT

Once the key information and data are obtained, efforts should then turn to identification of the most impactful opportunities for improvement. As explained above, the highest leverage area should be the movement of low acuity surgical cases to a lower acuity facility. This should be accomplished in a step-wise manner with input from key stakeholders at all facilities involved, including surgeons, administrators, clinical program coordinators, and staff.

Case acuity is predominantly defined by the complexity of the technical aspects of an operation and/or the complexity of the patient's medical and comorbid conditions and the resultant likelihood of requiring inpatient subspecialty services. Facility resources, capabilities, and infrastructure largely dictate what is considered inclusion versus exclusion criteria and can help serve as guardrails by which to abide. In addition, there may be health system-specific considerations for shifting of cases across the enterprise. These factors will aid in the development of protocols or triage points to allocate the appropriate patients and cases to the intended facility based on core principles of site of care optimization. Society-sponsored consensus statements or accreditation standards are frequently published and serve as invaluable references.

> You have determined that primary bariatric surgery, including Roux-en-Y gastric bypass and sleeve gastrectomy, is appropriate to perform at the low acuity hospital given the available equipment and surgical team expertise. However, the Metabolic and Bariatric Surgery Accreditation and Quality Improvement Program (MBSAQIP) standards have strict criteria against the performance of revisional bariatric surgery at low acuity hospitals. In addition, your team has concluded that patients with end-organ dysfunction or the need for subspecialty consultative services not available at the intended facility should be excluded.

● SCIENTIFIC PRINCIPLES AND EVIDENCE

Decentralization has been shown to improve quality and safety metrics in specific healthcare delivery settings.[2] Considerations should include case and patient complexity, volume projections, necessary resources and expertise, and appropriate infrastructure for system-based practice. The successful implementation of decentralization relies on an environment in which relevant stakeholders are included, innovation is encouraged, and post-implementation outcomes are closely monitored.[3]

Site of care optimization is an increasingly important priority for health system leaders to improve hospital capacity, increase efficiency in care delivery, and enhance the patient experience. Data from market analyses project a significant shift of patient volumes from the inpatient hospital setting to hospital outpatient departments and ambulatory surgery centers in the years ahead.[4] Developing a sound strategy for shifting surgical care to various practice settings will allow systems to effectively adjust to the changing landscape and create future opportunities for growth.

> You have estimated that 40% of your annual primary bariatric surgical volume could be considered low acuity. Working with department and hospital administrators, bariatric surgery team, and perioperative staff, you have developed a method for identifying such eligible patients and preferentially scheduling them for surgery at the low acuity center under the newly acquired operating room block time for your surgeons. The MBSAQIP standards manual was referenced for criteria appropriate for low acuity center designation, which aligns well with your lower acuity hospital resources and prepares your program for future accreditation of the secondary site.[5] In doing so, your program will still maintain the volumes necessary for program accreditation at both health system sites while improving patient access and increasing hospital capacity at the quaternary care hospital.

● IMPLEMENTING A SOLUTION

When developing a comprehensive plan for addressing the realignment of surgical cases based on acuity, it is critical to have a practical approach. No singular solution is likely to fully address all the priorities, but the strategy should be to influence as much positive change to achieve the greatest effect. For example, it is highly unlikely that a process developed to optimize the site of care will result in complete alignment of acuity but having a mechanism in place to allow for shifting is invaluable. Starting with realistic, achievable goals and expectations is important and can serve as a building block for further change.

Key Steps in Change Management and Potential Pitfalls

Key Steps in Change Management

1. Clearly identify the problem and greatest opportunities for improvement.
2. Develop a deep understanding of the processes and workflows involved in case assignment and designation of acuity level.
3. Identify relevant data sources (eg, electronic medical record synopsis, case request, OR activity reports) that illustrate the gap in the alignment of acuity with facility.
4. Articulate the problem and discuss potential solutions with key stakeholders to evaluate the feasibility and unintended consequences and solicit feedback to refine the proposed solution.
5. Begin with a pilot implementation with a subset of surgeons and very low acuity patients for the initial rollout at the lower acuity facility and adjust based on regular feedback prior to expanding.
6. Continually track measurable outcomes as previously identified (eg, better alignment of acuity, increased access, and quality/safety metrics).

Potential Pitfalls

1. Rushing to reach a conclusion about the root cause without fully investigating all aspects from multiple perspectives.
2. Not engaging key stakeholders (surgeons, schedulers, program staff) when designing the new scheduling process.
3. Approaching the solution/change with a fixed or rigid mindset.
4. Broad implementation of the solution (low acuity cases scheduled at low acuity centers) across all bariatric surgeon practices without piloting or considering potential barriers to successful implementation (other surgeon commitments, case mix).
5. Not developing a reliable method for the review of progress or outcomes.

Significant change is often met with the greatest resistance, but with a gradual and inclusive approach, the outcome is likely to be favorable. When engaging stakeholders most affected by the change (surgeons being asked to relocate a portion of their surgical volume), it is imperative to clearly articulate why the acuity misalignment is problematic and why change is necessary. This will result in greater understanding and flexibility. As the leader orchestrating the change, it is essential to have a deep understanding of the processes involved from multiple perspectives. Prior to full implementation, pilot the case shifting with a few surgeons and proper patient selection with the lowest acuity to maximize the chance of initial success. Finally, ensure that there is a reliable mechanism for periodic review of outcomes and solicitation of feedback in order to refine the process accordingly.

● MEASURING OUTCOMES

Once the proposed solution or set of solutions has been implemented, continuous reassessment of key metrics is vital for process improvement. Specifically, one should monitor the volume of low acuity cases as a percentage of total eligible patients as a marker for the site of care optimization. Annual volume and projections are important for a hospital's financial viability, given that approximately half of a hospital's budget may be allocated to supporting perioperative services.[6] Additionally, the rate at which acuity exclusion criteria are not properly applied (error rate) should be measured periodically and efforts made to understand the root causes behind such errors, as errors will decrease process efficiency and delay care unnecessarily. When a new service line is introduced (even among low acuity patients), the clinical practice may be susceptible to deviation from usual or expected outcomes until care pathways and nuanced management are normalized. Therefore, one must implement a continual quality improvement process to ensure that high standards for quality and safety are maintained.

● FOLLOW-UP AND MAINTENANCE

Over time, there may be opportunities to broaden low acuity criteria and increase the pool of eligible patients and procedure types. This may occur as a result of increased resources or enhanced infrastructure at the lower acuity hospital, a relaxation of originally restrictive exclusion criteria, or a change to society guidelines. Following key strategies such as continuous process improvement and monitoring quality and safety metrics will ensure long-term success.

REFERENCES

1. American Hospital Association. *Fast Facts on U.S. Hospitals, 2022.* https://www.aha.org/infographics/2020-07-24-fast-facts-infographics
2. Iverson KR, Svensson E, Sonderman K, et al. Decentralization and regionalization of surgical care: a review of evidence for the optimal distribution of surgical services in low- and middle-income countries. *Int J Health Policy Manag.* 2019;8(9):521–537.
3. Liwanag HJ, Wyss K. What conditions enable decentralization to improve the health system? Qualitative analysis of perspectives on decision space after 25 years of devolution in the Philippines. *PLoS One.* 2018;13(11):e0206809.
4. American Hospital Association. *3 Ways to Prepare for Coming Shifts in Care Delivery Sites, 2021.* https://www.aha.org/aha-center-health-innovation-market-scan/2021-06-15-3-ways-prepare-coming-shifts-care-delivery
5. Metabolic and Bariatric Surgery Accreditation and Quality Improvement Program. *Optimal Resources for Metabolic and Bariatric Surgery, 2019 Standards.* https://www.facs.org/media/fguhte1t/2019_mbsaqip_standards_manual.pdf
6. Healthcare Financial Management Association. *Integrating Care to Improve Surgical Outcomes and Reduce Costs, 2018.* https://www.hfma.org/topics/hfm/2018/august/61399.html

Home Monitoring for Surgical Home Hospital

13

BIQI ZHANG, JAYSON S. MARWAHA, KAVYA PATHAK, MALCOLM K. ROBINSON, AND THOMAS C. TSAI

Clinical Delivery Challenge

Ms. H is a 27-year-old woman with a history notable for obesity (BMI = 42), gastroesophageal reflux disease, polycystic ovarian syndrome, and no abdominal surgeries who presented to the bariatric surgery clinic for evaluation prior to planned laparoscopic sleeve gastrectomy. Much to her dismay, her surgery had been postponed numerous times due to the COVID-19 pandemic and associated state-mandated deferments in all elective procedures, specifically those that involved postoperative hospital admissions.

The COVID-19 pandemic placed significant strain on hospitals around the nation, highlighting that few institutions had adequate surge capacity. Many states canceled—and deferred indefinitely—all surgeries save for those that were urgent or emergent. This created year-long backlogs of elective cases, which, while not urgent, were still time-sensitive and left patients such as Ms. H waiting for elective inpatient surgery to resume. Nearly a year into the COVID-19 pandemic, recognizing both the need to address these backlogs and to maintain future bedspace as COVID-19 uncertainty persisted, the U.S. Centers for Medicare and Medicaid Services (CMS) announced the Acute Hospital Care at Home waiver, an innovative payment and delivery system reform that focused on Home Hospital (HH) care models.[1] Providing hospital-level care in a patient's home was recognized as an opportunity to accelerate the conversion of inpatient to HH surgeries and increase surgical throughput. This was thought to enable hospitals to reschedule elective surgeries and maximize the use of in-house bedspace to care for higher-risk patients. The possible benefits of HH were further underscored by our nation's continued focus on value-based care. To date, U.S. health system reform has focused primarily on reducing utilization through population health reform; *shifting* utilization of care and optimizing the site of care had not yet been emphasized. With CMS' November 2020 announcement, the promise of HH came to the forefront. Studies on HH conducted in the United States since as early as the 1980s and more recently in Europe and Australia revealed that perhaps the greatest reductions in inpatient length of stay, 30-day readmissions, and harms related to hospital stays (ie, iatrogenic infections, delirium, post-hospital syndrome) could be realized by adopting HH models of care.

● WORKUP

The bariatric HH program was the pilot for the broader surgical HH initiative in our health system. We obtained data on the types of procedures with lengths of stay typically in the 1–3-day period, which would benefit the most from the HH model. Additionally, we identified the volume of procedures with patients from within a 10-mile radius of the hospital, which was specified as part of our HH protocol in order to allow for expeditious transfer back to the hospital should a higher level of care or additional interventional procedures be needed in the acute postoperative period.

The development of a successful HH program necessitates multi-stakeholder consensus regarding which components of care to implement during the various phases of care as well as which quality metrics to measure. A sample of care components, quality metrics, and primary stakeholders needed to implement a perioperative HH program is outlined in Table 13.1.

Table 13.1 Development of a Successful Home Health Program

Phase of Care	Components	Quality Metrics	Stakeholders
Preoperative	• Preoperative home safety evaluation • Surgical prehabilitation and biometric assessment • Multimodal pain and PONV premedication and management • Medication management (eg, anticoagulation)	• Adherence to prehabilitation regimen • Equity-focused metrics of access	• Patients, families and health care providers
Operating room	• Multimodal pain management and prophylaxis of PONV	• Use of totally intravenous and opioid-free anesthesia • Use of antiemetics	• Health care providers
PACU	• Observation in PACU • Assessment of nausea and pain control	• Time until discharge to HH from PACU • Nausea and pain medication requirements	• Patients and families • Hospital system • Payer
Recovery	• Daily visit by surgeon remotely and/or surgicalist/advanced practice clinician • Twice and as-needed visits by nursing or paramedicine, wound care, physical/occupational, and respiratory therapists • Point-of-care postoperative laboratory tests and imaging • Administration of intravenous fluids and medications • Continuous biometric monitoring	• Rate of complications • Rate of safety events, including falls • Escalation of care to inpatient hospitals • Failure to rescue/unanticipated mortality • Steps taken and time spent laying down	• Patients and families • Health care providers • Hospital system • Payer
Discharge	• Discharge to normal postoperative follow-up	• 30-day post-discharge mortality and readmission • Patient satisfaction and experience	• Patients and families • Health care providers • Hospital system • Payer

Abbreviations: PONV, postoperative nausea and vomiting; PACU, Postanesthesia Care Unit.

Adapted with permission from Bryan et al.[2] Copyright © 2021 American Medical Association.

The 3 levers by which to guide implementation, and around which operational data must be gathered to understand the environment in which one is building an HH model, are the following: patient safety and care quality, patient satisfaction, and cost. While the possible benefits of HH are numerous, there are key strategic operational metrics by which to drive momentum in early implementation phases. For instance, the HH model has been shown to improve patient safety, including by reducing iatrogenic harms such as postoperative infections especially those by resistant organisms, delirium, sedentariness, and post-hospital syndrome.[3] As HH seeks to replace inpatient admission, safety metrics also must be tracked to ensure

CHAPTER 13 • Home Monitoring for Surgical Home Hospital

that nosocomial complications, time to provider response, ability to rescue or transfer/escalate care, and mortality outcomes do not suffer.

In response to patient needs such as those of Ms. H, our Metabolic and Bariatric Surgery group implemented HH for short-stay elective surgical patients. A randomized controlled trial to evaluate the effectiveness of HH for sleeve gastrectomy patients was launched. At Ms. H's preoperative evaluation, she met the criteria for enrollment in the trial. She was randomized to the study arm: instead of usual care consisting of an overnight hospital stay, she would be transported home from the post-anesthesia care unit with continuous biometric monitoring.

● DIFFERENTIAL DIAGNOSIS

Perhaps the newest and thus most challenging component of implementing HH is integrating home monitoring technology into the clinical workflow. What is most apparently lost in transitioning care from an inpatient to an outpatient setting is a provider's ability to see and physically examine the patient. The greatest challenge to overcome is, therefore, the integration of secure, HIPAA-compliant, easy-to-use, reliable, in-home, and noninvasive biomonitoring. Such technologies as well as the ability to communicate with patients via phone, photo-sharing, and/or videoconferencing can enable surgeons to engage, assess, and escalate care quickly with the rest of the care team and the patient in the home. The adoption of these new technologies, with the various stakeholders as well as an institution's existing care platforms (ie, electronic health records), will likely be expensive and time-consuming. It will require troubleshooting and iterative feedback cycles to configure evidence-based pathways to address both best- and worst-case scenarios.

Ms. H underwent an uncomplicated laparoscopic sleeve gastrectomy. She was recovered in the PACU and deemed clinically stable for transfer to HH. A BioVitals patch was applied and ensured in working order prior to arranging transportation home. Her PACU RN gave a direct report to the HH RN who, along with an HH hospitalist, met the patient and the patient's partner at Ms. H's home for intake. A physical exam was performed, and the plan for symptom management and reaching the HH team was reviewed with the patient and her partner.

● DIAGNOSIS AND TREATMENT

Crucial components of HH implementation include allocating clinical personnel and supplies and establishing protocols to deliver appropriate care to patients in the home. Personnel, such as deployable nurses (for phlebotomy, IV fluids, lab draws) and paramedics for in-home visits during intake and as needed, must be recruited to administer HH care. Surgery physician assistants and attendings must be available to communicate with patients via telehealth as needed and routinely prior to discharge from HH. Patients in HH may also need specialty care from other services, necessitating methods of integrating consulting teams into surgical HH care. Designing processes to deliver medical supplies, medications, and special foods (protein shakes and specialized diets) will also be essential. In addition to personnel and supply allocation, HH programs must have robust workflows to integrate HH care into hospital care delivery. Establishing new methods of rounding on patients as well as integrating residents and fellows into HH will be critical.

Another important part of HH implementation is the selection and integration of home-based technologies into the HH program. At Brigham and Women's Hospital, usage of the Biofourmis platform has integrated data from multiple remote monitoring devices, including real-time telemetry, blood pressure, and temperature, as well as a secure telehealth platform for virtual visits. As health systems implement HH, choosing technologies that allow for data integration with a hospital's electronic medical records is crucial to ensure success.

SCIENTIFIC PRINCIPLES AND EVIDENCE

A key principle underlying HH is the establishment of care around where patients ought to be, rather than where their clinicians are most conveniently—and currently—located. HH may prove to be a natural extension of Enhanced Recovery After Surgery (ERAS) protocols, which have dramatically accelerated patients' postoperative recovery times. By learning from existing HH frameworks, most of which were initially developed in nonsurgical patient populations but could be adopted into surgery, it is possible to strive for a new ERAS metric such as conversion to same-day surgeries.

The majority of research and protocol development in HH has centered around medical patients. The Hospital at Home Users Group is an academic collaborative that disseminates best practices for medical HH patients and gathers academic literature in the field of HH.[4] Johns Hopkins has created an HH toolkit with both adoption and implementation tools that health systems can use to start HH programs.[5] Prior studies of medical HH have demonstrated that this care model is both safe and feasible in the medical setting. A study measuring the effectiveness of HH in caring for COPD patients found decreased rates of 6-month readmission and higher quality of life scores.[6] Further medical HH studies have shown decreased utilization of diagnostic testing and increased physical activity in HH patients.[3] While the potential cost savings of HH programs are still being understood, 1 study found savings of 19% compared to a traditional inpatient stay.[7]

While the majority of HH studies have been conducted in medical patients, there is an emerging body of evidence on surgical HH. Small studies of surgical hospital-at-home programs have reported the safety of this care model, with no deaths during HH and resolution of complications that required readmission.[8,9] These studies focused on low to medium complexity, primarily minimally invasive cases. As surgical leaders look to expand HH to more patients, innovations from medical HH programs can be used to develop surgical HH programs.

> Four hours after Ms. H arrived home, the biomonitoring patch stopped recording. A paramedic was sent to replace this patch. A concurrent health check was performed: she was sinus tachycardic up to the 110s–130s and reported more incisional abdominal pain. She was treated with IV Toradol on top of available PO Tylenol and oxycodone. The surgery attending was notified of all these events. A basic metabolic panel and comprehensive blood count were drawn, and she was given a 1-liter bolus of lactated ringers, which improved her tachycardia.

IMPLEMENTING A SOLUTION

As an initial step toward implementing hospital-at-home program for surgical patients, the team at Brigham and Women's Hospital first began by carving out a discrete and manageable set of clinical conditions and procedures for which the program could be practically deployed, iterated upon, and learn from, and then scaled from there if it successfully manages to demonstrate impact. The "lowest hanging fruit" that could be used to demonstrate the value of HH was identified to be procedures in which the standard of care was to keep patients for just 1 day in the hospital postoperatively, as these postoperative inpatient stays could practically be translated to the home. While not an entirely risk-free endeavor, caring for these lower acuity patients affords opportunities to learn what works and what does not, smooth out the small but critical wrinkles in the execution of the HH program, and plan for the program's future direction as its care team and patient capacity scales.

Implementation of the program required constant anticipation and evaluation of its potential effects on payors, providers, and patients. While CMS has begun to signal early support for such programs, a clear pathway to reimbursement among commercial insurers remains less clear[1]; further research on its potential for value creation and partnerships with health systems are likely needed before commercial payers begin to embrace this form of care delivery and incorporate it into their plans. For providers such as large health systems, HH is currently a financially viable way of delivering care, and will remain viable if CMS's Acute Hospital Care at Home waiver remains in place or is expanded. However, scaling a successful

Key Steps in Change Management and Potential Pitfalls

Key Steps in Change Management

1. Select a narrow, specific use case that can be used to initially demonstrate the value of HH. In our case, we began with sleeve gastrectomy procedures.
2. Constant evaluation of upsides and downsides for payors, providers, and patients:
   a. Payors: CMS is supportive but commercial plans to be determined, warrants research, partnerships.
   b. Providers: Can remain profitable if waiver remains in place. But, there are significant costs associated with scaling HH's success.
   c. Patients: Care quality, outcomes, and safety will ultimately determine value.

Potential Pitfalls

1. Preventing failure to rescue events when patients experience postsurgical complications such as pulmonary embolus, stroke, and myocardial infarction.
2. Maintaining surgical team involvement for high-caliber care in HH patients.
3. Ensuring equity and social determinants of health are kept in mind in how patients are selected and managed via HH.

HH program requires significant upfront investment and potential costs in the form of new processes and tools for billing, patient monitoring, clinical documentation, care delivery partnerships with nursing and paramedical organizations, and more.[10] Finally, for patients, the quality of care, outcomes, and safety of this mode of care delivery will ultimately dictate its value. Essential to the process of evaluating HH's impact on patient care will be taking advantage of new opportunities to digitally phenotype the trajectory of postsurgical patients, collect and study patient-reported outcomes, and more.

Many important potential pitfalls must be kept in mind throughout the implementation process for an HH program—among the most important ones are avoiding failure to rescue, anticipating the need for surgical reevaluation, and ensuring the program serves to reduce—and not widen—disparities in access to quality care. Failure to rescue is an important metric to monitor in these programs as many rare but potentially catastrophic postsurgical complications exist including stroke, pulmonary embolus, myocardial infarction, and sepsis; HH programs must have the infrastructure to promptly detect and act upon these events. It is also important to ensure that the training and expertise of the care team matches what a patient would receive if they were in the hospital. Ongoing involvement and monitoring by the surgical team that operated on the patient can help ensure that the HH team is qualified to make appropriate care decisions for the patient in the home. Finally, while HH programs undoubtedly have the potential to improve access to quality postsurgical care in the home, It is important to recognize its potential unintended consequence of widening disparities for patients who do not have sufficient resources (eg, housing and social support in the home) required for HH care to be delivered safely. For these types of patients, it is important to recognize that alternative postsurgical care plans and discharge options should be considered.

● MEASURING OUTCOMES

To appropriately measure the value that HH programs add to the current care delivery landscape, appropriate evaluation metrics should be selected that align well with its intended purpose of improving patient satisfaction and reducing inpatient resource utilization, all while not adversely impacting the recovery of postsurgical patients. Patient experience is a primary outcome of our HH program and is measured using validated patient-reported outcomes, such as the Body-Q score and captures patient satisfaction with the information they received, with the provider, and with the entire care team.[11] Secondary outcomes measured in our program include presentation to the ED or readmissions within 30 days of surgery, cost of care, morphine milligram equivalents consumed after surgery, length of stay, postoperative pain scores, and postoperative complication rates; the goal of capturing these metrics is to demonstrate that HH-based care is noninferior to standard brick-and-mortar inpatient hospital care.

In addition to tracking HH performance as it relates to patient satisfaction and quality of care, we also measure its impact on clinical processes and operations including inpatient bed-days saved, time to resuming a stage 2 bariatric diet (ie, a full liquid diet), and patient's ability to stay out of bed for at least 6 hours on the first postoperative day. Cases are also treated just like all other surgical patients: our program involves the primary surgical team throughout the patient's postoperative course, includes HH cases in weekly Morbidity and Mortality conferences alongside other surgical patients, and includes representation from our institution's diversity, equity, and inclusion office to ensure care is equitable and accessible.

A few hours later, Ms. H continued to endorse abdominal pain and new bilateral shoulder pain; her earlier labs resulted and were notable for hemoglobin drop to 11.1 from 13.8 preoperatively and creatinine elevation to 1.5 from a baseline of 0.65. The paramedic made a second overnight visit to provide a second-liter bolus of intravenous fluids and start her on maintenance fluids at 100 milliliters per hour. Given persistent abdominal pain and her concerning labs, it was decided with the surgery attending to transfer the patient back to the hospital for a timely CT angiography of her abdomen/pelvis to rule out intraabdominal hemorrhage.

● FOLLOW-UP AND MAINTENANCE

Patient's CT scan revealed intraabdominal hematoma. Repeat CBC upon transfer back to the hospital revealed another drop in her hematocrit. She was taken urgently to the operating room for a washout, which she tolerated well. She recovered well after this washout and the remainder of her postoperative recovery was uneventful.

Numerous studies as well as our own experiences highlight the feasibility, opportunities, and challenges of the surgical HH model. The COVID-19 pandemic has accelerated national interest in the HH model, with nearly 100 hospitals receiving the US Centers for Medicare and Medicaid Services Acute Hospital Care at Home waiver. To ensure the long-term viability, desirability, and feasibility of the surgical HH model, several issues must be addressed. First, there must be a clear pathway toward long-term financial sustainability of this model; 1 pathway might be getting most commercial payers to recognize the value of HH and offer coverage for it. Another largely unanswered question is what role emerging technologies should play in HH programs. Remote patient monitoring, ambient sensing, and artificial intelligence are all rapidly evolving fields that may help to optimally select and manage HH patients if they are incorporated into these programs strategically. As these programs scale and evolve, equity must always remain a priority so that the HH model of care always serves to eliminate and never exacerbate disparities in access to quality surgical care. In conclusion, appropriate patient monitoring with strong clinical oversight can allow HH programs to provide patients with the same level of care as inpatient services.

REFERENCES

1. CMS announces participants in new value-based bundled payment Model. https://www.cms.gov/newsroom/press-releases/cms-announces-participants-new-value-based-bundled-payment-model
2. Bryan AF, Levine DM, Tsai TC. Home hospital for surgery. *JAMA Surg.* 2021;156(7):679–680.
3. Levine DM, Ouchi K, Blanchfield B, et al. Hospital-level care at home for acutely ill adults: a randomized controlled trial. *Ann Intern Med.* 2020;172(2):77–85.
4. Hospital-level care for adult patients where they live. *Hospital-level care for adult patients where they live | Hospital at Home* https://www.hahusersgroup.org/ (2020).
5. Toolkit. https://www.hospitalathome.org/develop-your-program/toolkit.php
6. Aimonino Ricauda N et al. Substitutive "hospital at home" versus inpatient care for elderly patients with exacerbations of chronic obstructive pulmonary disease: a prospective randomized, controlled trial. *J Am Geriatr Soc.* 2008;56:493–500.

7. Cryer L, Shannon SB, Van Amsterdam M, Leff B. Costs for "hospital at home" patients were 19 percent lower, with equal or better outcomes compared to similar inpatients. *Health Aff.* 2012;31(6):1237–1243.
8. Safavi KC, Frendl D, Ellis D, et al. Hospital at home for surgical patients: a case series from a pioneer program at a large academic medical center. *Ann Surg.* 2022;275(1):e275–e277.
9. Pajarón-Guerrero M, Fernández-Miera MF, Dueñas-Puebla JC, et al. Early discharge programme on hospital-at-home evaluation for patients with immediate postoperative course after laparoscopic colorectal surgery. *Eur Surg Res.* 2017;58(5–6):263–273.
10. Brody AA, Arbaje AI, DeCherrie LV, Federman AD, Leff B, Siu AL. Starting up a hospital at home program: facilitators and barriers to implementation. *J Am Geriatr Soc.* 2019;67(3):588–595.
11. Klassen AF, Cano SJ, Alderman A, et al. The BODY-Q: a patient-reported outcome instrument for weight loss and body contouring treatments. *Plast Reconstr Surg Glob Open.* 2016;4(4):e679.

Service Line With Low Operating Room Utilization at Ambulatory Surgery Center

14

ANDREW M. IBRAHIM, GEOFFREY E. HESPE, AND AMIR A. GHAFERI

Clinical Delivery Challenge

Each year Michigan Medicine performs approximately 18,000 surgical procedures at our ambulatory surgery centers across seven different surgical service lines. The typical process for a patient involves the patient being referred to a specialty clinic, evaluation by a surgeon, possible additional workup, and then scheduling for the appropriate surgery. Like many institutions, ambulatory operating room (OR) block time is at an all-time premium and watched quite closely by hospital administrators. In the summer of 2020, it became clear that at Michigan Medicine, there was suboptimal utilization of operative block time at our ambulatory surgery centers. As would be discovered (and discussed in detail below), we observed that along with *unused block time*, there was a frustratingly long waitlist of *patients waiting to be scheduled*. The timing of this evaluation coincided with the first and second waves of COVID, which would underscore even more the need to optimize our OR capacity at multiple sites of care to improve patient access to care.

● WORKUP

To understand why ambulatory OR block time was underutilized, we first had to ask the question, "What are all the processes and steps that need to happen for a patient get from clinic to an OR?" To do so, we created a "journey map" or "process map" subdivided into three phases: prior to clinic, clinic to OR scheduling, and OR scheduling to actual OR (Figure 14.1).

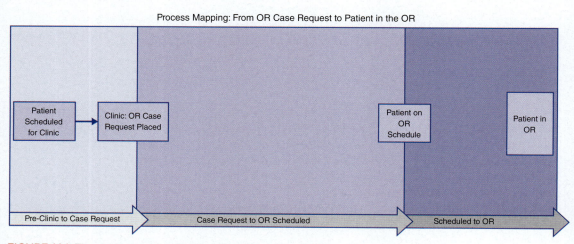

FIGURE 14.1 Three phases of patient journey from clinic to OR.

CHAPTER 14 • Service Line With Low Operating Room Utilization   87

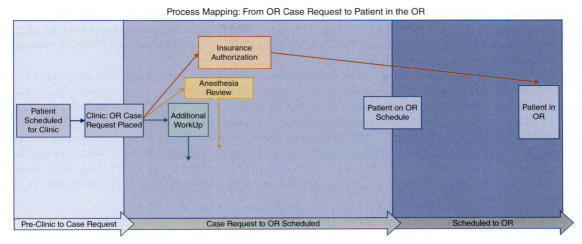

FIGURE 14.2 Processes initiated after a case request is created.

We focused our attention on bettering our understanding of the process from the time a case request is placed to the patient arriving in the OR. We discovered at least three separate streams of approval are initiated at our institution including insurance approval, anesthesia review, and medical workup (Figure 14.2).

Once the anesthesia review is performed (to ensure a case is appropriate for the ambulatory setting) and additional preoperative medical workup is completed, the patient can now enter the scheduling pathway. Scheduling involves multiple steps including the availability of patient, surgeon, consulting surgeon (if applicable), and facility (Figure 14.3). Once an OR date is set, the patient is scheduled for a Pre-Op clinic visit and COVID testing before the OR. Sometimes Pre-Op clinic identifies the need for additional workup, and the patient may need to return to additional workup prior to their procedure (dashed red line in Figure 14.3).

With our conceptual model in place for a patient's journey from clinic to OR, we then needed data to help identify where the bottleneck(s) may be occurring. Gathering these data came from three sources:

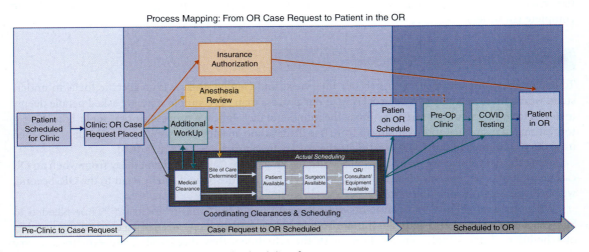

FIGURE 14.3 Coordinating clearances and scheduling for surgery.

1. *Electronic Medical Record (EMR)*—Because many of the key processes along the journey had a date stamp associated with them in the EMR (eg, clinic date, when OR case requests order was placed, etc.), we used our internal analysts to pull this data from the EMR. In doing so, we could start to estimate the average time needed for each phase.
2. *Interviews with Key Stakeholders*—As we developed our process map, we realized there were many key stakeholders involved, including residents, advanced practice providers, surgeons, schedulers, clinical supervisors, OR managers, and patients. We iteratively improved our process map with their input and asked for hypotheses about what might be leading to underutilization of our ambulatory ORs.
3. *Gemba Walks*—"Gemba Walks" (discussed more below) refers to the process of immersing where the key processes occur. For us, that meant spending time in a clinic, sitting at a desk alongside schedulers, and visiting our ambulatory ORs. This overlapped with our stakeholder interviews, but allowed for much more organic exchanges and frontline exposure closer to potential sources of the problem.

It is worth noting that no one source of data told the whole story, and we often had to cycle through the data sources over time to help understand the process. Additionally, each immersion unearthed new questions worth exploring in order to gain the most complete understanding of this process possible.

● DIFFERENTIAL DIAGNOSIS

With our process map in place (Figure 14.3), we were then able to develop a robust differential diagnosis for potential causes for underutilization of ambulatory ORs by following any of the arrows. Possible sources of underutilization included the following:

- Delays due to insurance authorizations
- Delays due to anesthesia approval
- Additional or unforeseen medical workup
- Misalignment of patient and surgeon schedules
- Inadequate number of patients seen in a clinic
- Inadequate number of schedulers to process OR case requests
- Lack of availability of preoperative clinic or COVID testing sites

It is worth mentioning here that some of these sources of possible underutilization are related to each other (occur in series), and some are independent (occur in parallel). For example, insurance authorization happens almost entirely independently from medical workup (in parallel). In contrast, the schedulers choosing an OR date is entirely dependent on prior steps (eg, anesthesia review) being complete (in series).

● DIAGNOSIS AND TREATMENT

To explore our differential, we revisited our interviews and Gemba walks with a specific focus to understand where these delays might be occurring in our process map. As a simple start, we asked people deeply involved in these streams of care to estimate the number of days for each process. For example, administrators estimated insurance approval ranged from 0 to 28 days and anesthesia review from 1 to 2 days. We then used the timestamps in our EMR to estimate the days between each phase (Figure 14.4).

Using the data above, we made a few observations. First, there was a significant delay from when an OR case request for a patient was placed until a date was chosen and the patient finally went to the OR. Second, we observed a significant wide variation across service lines.

With our data (Figure 14.4) in hand, we narrowed our differential to focus on "Time Needed to Schedule" (light blue bars) with the initial thought being that we likely needed to expand the number of schedulers. Interestingly, when talking with the schedulers they disagreed. They explained a very different problem. When an OR scheduler opens their list of OR case requests, all requests appear

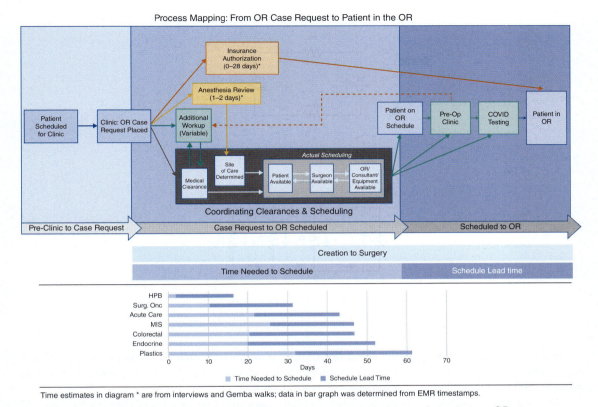

FIGURE 14.4 Using quantitative data to identify bottlenecks in patient journey from clinic to OR.

the same even though not all patients may be ready to schedule. Thus, surgery schedulers have no way of determining which patients are ready to schedule now, which still need more workup, or which of them were there as "placeholders" should the patient want surgery later. As such, the schedulers exerted a significant amount of time going through these patients' charts trying to sort out those details, rather than actually scheduling patients for surgery. One of them described the process as a recurring scene from Groundhog Day, and they had started to memorize the patient names at the top of the list each morning who were still awaiting clearances to get scheduled. This was clearly an area of wasted time and resources that needed to be addressed.

Cycling through our EMR data, interviews, and Gemba walks, we learned that a potential solution to improving OR utilization was clarity in the OR case request. Specifically, schedulers needed an efficient way to identify who was ready to schedule, and who was awaiting additional workup or clearance.

● SCIENTIFIC PRINCIPLES AND EVIDENCE

Our clinical delivery challenge was founded on three important management principles: processing mapping, Gemba walks, and LEAN thinking. We discuss these in further detail.

Process mapping is a common approach used in business and large organizations to understand delays or bottlenecks along a process.[1,2] Essential to an accurate process map is distinguishing which processes occur in series versus in parallel (Figure 14.5).

Process in Series—Processes that occur in series are ones where the second step cannot occur until the first one is complete. In our example above, a patient cannot be scheduled for a COVID test until an OR date is chosen. And an OR date cannot be chosen until a patient has clear medical clearance and anesthesia review.

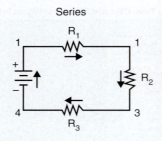

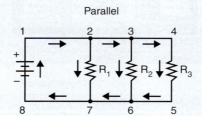

FIGURE 14.5 Processes in series or in parallel.

Process in Parallel—Processes that occur in parallel are ones where each step is independent and can occur simultaneously with the others. For example, in our scenario above, insurance authorization can occur at the same time the patient is undergoing medical workup.

Once you have developed your process map, you can assign times for each leg of the process. This will allow you to determine bottlenecks that slow down your process. Improving inefficiencies at bottlenecks decreases the time needed to complete a task and thus increases the effectiveness of the entire process. It should be noted that improving one bottleneck will lead to the emergence of a new bottleneck that may or may not need to be addressed depending on overall goals.

The other important principle relevant to this clinical challenge is the value of Gemba walks.[3] The term originates from the Japanese word "Gemba," which means "the actual place." As was seen multiple times in this example, while our data told one story, being on the front line with providers ("in their place" of work) provided new insight. Our management principle is in line with "no data without stories, and no stories without data." In fact, the ultimate source of OR underutilization was not even on our initial differential until we went back to schedulers with our proposed ideas.

We also utilized the principles of LEAN thinking during this project. LEAN principles look to reduce inefficiency and waste in order to improve value for a system based on the consumer input. This line of theory was originally indoctrinated by Toyota as the Toyota Production System but has been since adopted by many other companies and sectors. In health care, these principles also exist as we strive to make medicine more patient centered to reduce costs and improve outcomes. Underutilization of ambulatory ORs delays patients' care and as a result their interest in our healthcare system. By determining inefficiencies that result in increased delays, we are able to improve the experience and value to our patients.

● IMPLEMENTING A SOLUTION

At this point, it became clear that to improve ambulatory OR utilization, we needed to improve our OR request process. We first evaluated the existing case request form within our EMR and made two important observations. First, there were a lot of optional questions that were added over time that are no longer relevant to most cases. Second, there was no opportunity to identify if the patient was "ready to schedule."

Key Steps in Change Management and Potential Pitfalls

Key Steps in Change Management

1. Identify a clear problem with a measurable outcome of ambulatory OR utilization.
2. Understand the process and steps leading up to patients getting their procedure.
3. Spend time on the front line (eg, Gemba Walks) with key stakeholders involved including residents, APPs, surgeons, schedulers, administrators, and patients.
4. Identify sources of quantitative data (eg, EMR timestamps) to bring measurable outcomes to understand your potential sources of OR underutilization.
5. Introduce possible solutions to key stakeholders to test face validity (ie, do they think that is actually the problem?) and refine based on feedback.
6. Pilot the potential solution (eg, new OR case request) in a high-yield area and have regular opportunities to solicit feedback. Make sure you can track a measurable outcome (ideally what you identified in #1).

Potentially Pitfalls

1. Jumping straight to a solution (eg, we need more schedulers) without exploring alternatives.
2. Lack of a clear conceptual model for the process from clinic to OR.
3. Not engaging enough of the correct stakeholders and spending time with them, in their space, while their work is in action.
4. Forgetting to monitor for unintended consequences of your solution. Correcting one bottleneck will almost certainly identify another, especially in a complex process.
5. Broadly implementing your solution (eg, new OR case request) across the whole department, without pilot testing it within one division or section first.

We reviewed the case requests with a broad range of stakeholders who frequently engage it including residents, APPs, surgeons, and schedules. To support any changes we made to the current case request form, we utilized once again our internal analysts to collect data on how frequently each field was filled in. Based on these discussions and data, we considered several options and ultimately decided to remove questions that are rarely used and add one:

Is the patient ready to be scheduled for surgery now? Yes/No.

We then worked with our EMR Team so that any case request that was labeled "Yes" for this question could be readily identified in the schedulers list as well as sortable. If the requester responded "No," it gives options to provide what additional medical workup is required or to provide other reasons for why the patient is not ready to schedule.

While the problem existed across all of our service lines, we decided to implement this change in only one service line at first. As such, we could measure if it achieved our desired result as well as if it had any unintended consequences before disseminating it to other services. A summary of our key steps and potential pitfalls are summarized below.

● MEASURING OUTCOMES

The original challenge identified was underutilization of our ambulatory ORs. As such, the percent utilization of ORs became our initial outcome to measure the success of our implemented solution. However, it also became clear that the lengthy delays from case requests to scheduling should also be prioritized as a patient-centered measure of improvement. As such, we created an automated dashboard that pulled this information from our EMR and allowed us to track desired metrics in real time. As a committee, we meet once a month to review interval changes.

● FOLLOW-UP AND MAINTENANCE

Since its introduction in our plastic surgery division, we have now disseminated this new OR case request to other divisions in a step-wise fashion. In addition to monitoring the outcomes mentioned above (OR utilization and delays in scheduling), we also needed to monitor unintended consequences. Specifically, as we created a system to quickly identify which patients were ready to do "now," we needed to make sure the other patients were not lost to follow-up. As such, we now measure those patients separately to make sure this new OR case request has not paradoxically worsened their experience or timeliness of care.

As described above, OR scheduling is a very complicated process that entails many different stakeholders and steps in order to get the patient from the clinic to the OR. Improving schedulers' efficiency as described above was a key aspect of the process but during our interviews and Gemba walks, other areas for improvement were identified. As mentioned above, improving the efficiency of one bottleneck will lead to the emergence of others. In our scenario, this included patient–scheduler correspondence and the back-and-forth that occurs due to a centralized phone system at our institution. We found in interviewing schedulers that if they call a patient and leave a message to schedule a surgery, when the patient calls back, they have to go through the call center first. The call center then transfers the patient to the scheduler but if they are busy or on the phone with another patient there is a limit for how long the patient can wait before having to call back. This can result in multiple attempts by bother parties before being able to connect to schedule a surgery. Future work looks to improve this, and multiple possible solutions have been brainstormed (eg, ability to directly communicate through the portal, providing schedules with a secure way to text patients, and a possible digital scheduling platform where patients can select the date from available dates via the patient portal). The overall goal of this process is to improve our patient-centered approach to delivering health care.

REFERENCES

1. Antonacci G, Reed JE, Lennox L, Barlow J. The use of process mapping in healthcare quality improvement projects. *Health Serv Manage Res*. 2018;31(2):74–84. doi: 10.1177/0951484818770411. Epub 2018 Apr 30.
2. DeGirolamo K, D'Souza K, Hall W, et al. Process mapping as a framework for performance improvement in emergency general surgery. *Can J Surg*. 2018;61(1):13–18. doi: 10.1503/cjs.004417. Epub 2017 Dec 1.
3. Markovitz D. Go to where the actual work is being done. *Harv Bus Rev*. March 31, 2014. https://hbr.org/2014/03/go-to-where-the-actual-work-is-being-done.

SECTION 4

Building Regional Networks

15 Hospital Losing Market Share: Is Joining a Hospital Network the Answer?
Andrew Shin and Cynthia Lewis Kavanagh

16 Low-Volume Surgery Within One Site of a Hospital Network
Kyle H. Sheetz and Hari Nathan

17 Disseminating Quality Standards Across a Hospital Network
Caroline E. Reinke and Michael Barringer

18 Ensuring Quality while Exporting Brand to New Network Affiliates
Ronald B. Hirschl

19 Outreach and Referral Building at New Network Affiliates
Brent D. Matthews

20 Coordinating Care and Referrals Across Affiliates
Ryan A. J. Campagna and Andrew C. Chang

21 Investing in Health Outside the Hospital: Public and Community Infrastructure
Pooja Chandrashekar and Sachin H. Jain

22 Working With Employers to Build Destination Programs for Complex Surgery
Caitlin Halbert

Hospital Losing Market Share: Is Joining a Hospital Network the Answer?

15

ANDREW SHIN AND CYNTHIA LEWIS KAVANAGH

Clinical Delivery Challenge

St. Elmo's Hospital is an independent, 200-bed community hospital in a suburban setting. Over the years, in no small part due to a reputation for high-quality care, St. Elmo's resisted numerous acquisitions and/or merger attempts from other hospitals/health systems and even private equity firms. Many clinicians cite their choice to practice at St. Elmo's over their larger and better-resourced competitors in the local market, due to the unique culture that supports the "heart of medicine" over profits and growth. However, after decades of stable operations and critical investments to maintain infrastructure and adopt an electronic medical record and other technology investments, the hospital was on the verge of its third quarter in a row of missing its operating income target. If this trend continued, then St. Elmo's would need to tap their balance sheet reserves, putting the hospital at risk of a credit downgrade and likely layoffs.

Today, many hospitals in the United States face a similar challenge: St. Elmo's was losing market share to competing hospitals and free-standing facilities. Though St. Elmo's maintained patient volume at near maximum capacity, revenue was down, especially in surgical services, which were most responsible for positive contribution and operating margin. The challenge for St. Elmo's leadership would be to understand why they were losing market share and how they could best reverse that trend while preserving their unique culture as an independent community hospital for decades to come.

Hospital markets are increasingly becoming more competitive. As a result, many hospitals find themselves tracking their market share. What happens when a hospital loses market share? What are the consequences? And what are the options to improve? This chapter considers a theoretical hospital (St. Elmo) that has lost market share and considering joining a hospital network as a strategy to improve.

● WORKUP

To better understand sources of losing market share, we conducted both an external analysis and an internal analysis. Both provide different types of data, that together inform the source of the problem.

Initial External Analysis

When faced with the prospect of losing market share, it is critical to start with an external analysis to understand both the opportunities, and in this case threats, that could be contributing to changes in volume and/or position in the local market. In many cases, there are multiple drivers, necessitating the broadest lens possible. Starting with an internal analysis can often foreclose possibilities, especially if we lack the access and/or experience with relevant data to uncover the root cause(s). To quickly assess market threats and opportunities, we focused on five key elements of our healthcare market and degree of change: population, purchasers (employers and payers), regulatory, competitors, and clinical/therapeutic innovations. For each area, we conducted secondary research leveraging data available to the public or to healthcare providers.

Table 15.1 · External Analysis Process to Understand Changes in Hospital Market Share

Measures		Data Source
Demographic/Population Changes	• Suburban market, moderate size, and growth	• Census data and/or Claritas
Economic/Payer Coverage Changes	• Increasing push toward value-based care from both public and commercial payers	• Industry report
Regulatory	• CMS elimination of the inpatient-only list triggering a downshift of high-growth, high-margin services • Certificate of Need (CON) state	• CMS, consulting report • Department of health
Competition/New Entrants	• One large academic health system • Several for-profit owned community hospitals • Growing number of independent, single-specialty ASCs	• Local business journal • State/local hospital associations • Public Health Department website • All-claims databases
Clinical/Therapeutic	• American Society of Anesthesiologists' Relative Value Guide (ASA RVG)	• ASA RVG • Peer-reviewed journals/conferences

Using hospital volume data from our state hospital association, we could see that total market inpatient and outpatient volumes for all hospitals had been trending downward over the last few quarters which ran counter to our market's demographic trends, which were modestly positive. Industry reports indicated similar trends nationally.

Using our external analysis process (Table 15.1), we found market share remained fairly stable as most hospitals experienced a similar degree of volume declines. However, financial impact appeared to vary across hospitals in the region. The analysis did not sufficiently explain the magnitude or likely cause of the revenue deficit or the specific conditions that seemed to be shifting somewhere, as the market share data did not include service-specific data.

Although the external analysis was helpful, it did not explain the market force changes. Although our market share seemed to be stable, we could see that volume was going down overall, but the volume decrease did not seem to be explained by factors that usually drive market share changes. However, we realized that local hospital volume trends collected by our state hospital association were an incomplete picture, as some providers, especially those owned by private equity firms and some for-profit entities tend not to participate in voluntary state-wide surveys.

Additional Internal Analysis

To either test hypotheses or develop de novo ones when the external data is not compelling, an internal analysis can be a very effective tool (Table 15.2). Department-specific data can help determine whether all or select services are experiencing volume and revenue decline. Physician and patient interviews can reveal potential nuances that higher-level data can mask. See below for summarized findings from St Elmo's internal analysis.

Table 15.2	Components of an Internal Analysis to Understand Hospital Market Share
Department-level data	Review of internal department volume and revenue indicated growth in medical cases and decline in surgical cases and revenue, most notably orthopedic. Review of consult-to-surgery ratios indicated a lower conversion rate than in prior years, particularly for outpatient orthopedic surgeries.
Physician interviews	Most physicians indicated concern regarding volume decline. Few commented that private surgical centers recruit surgeons with a promise of equity share.
Patient follow-up and interviews	Patients indicate concern regarding out-of-pocket costs and/or cited lower-cost option within the marketplace.

● DIFFERENTIAL DIAGNOSIS

With our external and internal analysis complete, we identified a differential diagnosis for three likely causes for St. Elmo's decline in surgical volume, most notably orthopedics. Most likely causes included the following:

1. New Entrant Ambulatory Surgery Centers (ASCs) majority or wholly owned by private and/or for-profit entities
2. Referral shift as payor and/or employer/provider steer patients to lower-cost hospitals, free-standing ASC, or participate in a bundle/destination program out of state
3. Patients delaying care

These hypotheses would not necessarily be evident on a surface-level view of market share metrics, because as discussed above, the sources of market share shifts are not always reported through standard channels and with new competitors.

● DIAGNOSIS AND TREATMENT

To explore this differential, we revisited our analyses and discussions with physicians to understand which of our hypotheses were contributing the most to our volume decrease in surgical volume, particularly orthopedic procedures. Decline in surgical volume and reduced conversion rate from consult to surgery suggest patients are either delaying care or seeking alternatives. Follow-up calls with orthopedic patients who did not elect to proceed with recommended procedures at St Elmo's indicate that patients are seeking alternatives due to concern regarding undergoing surgery or cost of care.

While most patients refrained from naming where they received care, several mentioned a surgical center in the neighboring town. Physician interviews confirmed a national for-profit group had recruited local surgeons to the new surgical center and offered them an equity stake in the venture. We conducted a "secret shopper" field trip to the new surgical center which confirmed a current offering focused on orthopedics; however, research on the national chain indicated they were starting to enter other markets in bariatrics and publishing thought leadership on the future of cardiac care.

To effectively compete with this national chain and others in our market who would likely soon follow suit, we believed a multispecialty ASC approach would be the most effective way to leverage our clinical capabilities and compete for market share, especially in the future.

● SCIENTIFIC PRINCIPLES AND EVIDENCE

Our approach to this challenge started within the overall context of hospital consolidation. Retention or growth of market share represents one potential objective of consolidation, but recent evidence provides a serious reevaluation of when and why a multi-hospital network can be a viable solution. In less than a decade, hospital consolidation has resulted in the top 10 U.S. health systems controlling 24% of total market share and revenue growth at twice the rate of the rest of the market.[1]

While there is evidence that most mergers fail to improve clinical and financial performance or patient experience,[2] there is also significant data that demonstrates that with adequate clinical–operational integration, mergers into multi-hospital networks can result in lower costs and improved quality outcomes.[3] Thus, scale may be *an approach* to solving a market share challenge for a hospital, but shifts in "where we care" and lack of transparency among new entrants likely necessitate a broader lens.

Many hospitals only consistently track (due to data transparency limitations) inpatient market share, yet nationally between 2011 and 2018, hospital outpatient revenue outpaced inpatient annual revenue growth (9% versus 6%), nearly matching inpatient as a share of total revenue for hospitals.[4] ASCs, virtual, and the home represent a growing share of the care delivery modalities that will adversely affect hospital volume and profitability, but are not often measured and reported in the same way inpatient market share is.

The ambulatory arena in particular has long been an analytic blind spot, partly because of the service volume and coding complexity found in this setting. Unlike traditional inpatient diagnosis-related groups, the International Classification of Disease, Current Procedural Terminology, Healthcare Common Procedure Coding System, and revenue codes that comprise ambulatory claims activity lack a common, straightforward, and meaningful grouping schema, especially one that functions across sites of care. Thus, the root cause for changes in volume and/or market share is not immediately evident, requiring analysis of another layer or two deeper. This is where local knowledge may be more helpful than sophisticated data analytics because the frontline primary care practices, local payors, and purchasers are likely more aware of what is happening on the ground.

● IMPLEMENTING A SOLUTION

To effectively compete for market share with these ASC entrants, we had to determine what procedures to focus on, how we would go about standing up an ASC to recapture volume, and perhaps most importantly, how to get the internal buy-in to be successful. Current data and a "secret shopper" field trip to the new surgical center indicated that orthopedic procedures have already begun to shift to the ASC setting. Industry reports and national ASC trends indicate additional specialties beginning to shift to outpatient, spurred by changes in the CMS inpatient-only list.

Interviews with physicians indicated cardiologists were interested in expanding diagnostic capabilities in the community setting to increase reach and prevention efforts, whereas orthopedic surgeons were interested in increased OR time and turnover efficiency of an orthopedic-focused OR. Physician input suggested exploring options to build a freestanding clinic with diagnostic and ORs for multispecialty use. Patient interviews and surveys indicated an emphasis on the need for convenient "one-stop shopping" for both preventive and procedural care with less preference for how close the site would be relative to St. Elmo's hospital campus, but a higher preference for a location not subject to "rush hour" traffic congestion to and from the downtown area. Finally, a conversation with the head of the payer contracting team indicated that in recent negotiation, the health plan noted St. Elmo's high HOPD rates and countered with rate increases far below inpatient rates.

CHAPTER 15 • Hospital Losing Market Share: Is Joining a Hospital Network the Answer?

Key Steps in Change Management and Potential Pitfalls

Key Steps in Change Management

1. Analyze unmet needs to determine whether the local market can support ASC expansion.
2. Focus on one or a few specialties that drive margin and volume.
3. Select partners carefully. When purchasing an existing ASC, a re-syndication of surgeon shares may be needed to make sure the right specialties and surgeons are being selected.
4. *Align economics* to ensure adequate volume and surgeon participation in facility management through joint ventures and other shared equity models.
5. Embrace *new operational models and metrics* that over-index toward efficiency and patient experience.

Potential Pitfalls

1. Reactive ambulatory surgery strategy that does not advance system goals or match the market's service demands.
2. Unclear service distribution plan that optimizes sites of care and scope of license.
3. Ineffective business and operational alignment with key partners.
4. Inefficient operations and poor throughput, including fragmented referral volume.
5. Missing the mark on consumer experience that drives convenience and differentiated access.

To implement the multispecialty approach, we decided that we would need to find the right match of services our target market needed and providers who were enthusiastic about the opportunity to practice in a different model.

● MEASURING OUTCOMES

Although losing market share was our original challenge and that was most evident in inpatient volume, it was only through further analysis that the true root cause was evident. Macro trends shifting care from the inpatient to the outpatient setting combined with local market competitors/new entrants were putting downward pressure on our ability to maintain surgery volume. Keeping abreast of procedures that were more likely to shift to ASCs in the future is critical to determine when/where to build ASCs.

● FOLLOW-UP AND MAINTENANCE

With the emergence of national for-profits, private equity firms, and other new entrants into our local market, St. Elmo's (along with other local nonprofit hospitals) has had to develop new processes that go a layer deeper than the normal market share analysis between "traditional" competitors. This is critical to evaluate local market dynamics and opportunities for growth with new lower-cost and improved experience models. This includes new sources of data, such as proactively seeking intelligence and feedback from surgeons, patients, and purchasers/payers. It also means purchasing new analytic tools from solutions companies that can more comprehensively assess volume shifts to the outpatient setting, beyond voluntary and self-reported surveys.

Finally, as we look toward growth and not just market share protection, it is incumbent on us to be more aggressive about opportunities to innovate around new models of care that improve experience and efficiency. This may involve partnerships with new entrants who bring ASC operational expertise, but likely also requires internal stakeholder change-management to realign our financial models toward value-based care and to rely less on the traditional inpatient acute care that has fueled our core mission for nearly our entire history.

REFERENCES

1. Traci P, Ion S, Wendy G, and Debanshu M. The potential for rapid consolidation of health systems. Deloitte Insights, 2020. Retrieved from https://www2.deloitte.com/us/en/insights/industry/health-care/hospital-mergers-acquisition-trends.html
2. Martin G, Adam S, Raffaella S, Chad S, and Shruthi V. The Anatomy of a Hospital System Merger: The Patient Did Not Respond Well to Treatment (December 2021). CEPR Discussion Paper No. DP16787. Available at SSRN: https://ssrn.com/abstract=4026652
3. Erwin W, Sonia A, Simon J, et al. Quality and safety outcomes of a hospital merger following a full integration at a safety net hospital. *JAMA Netw Open.* 2022;5(1):e2142382. doi: 10.1001/jamanetworkopen.2021.42382
4. Wendy G and Ankit A. Hospital revenue trends. Deloitte Insights, 2020. https://www2.deloitte.com/us/en/insights/industry/health-care/outpatient-virtual-health-care-trends.html

Low-Volume Surgery Within One Site of a Hospital Network

16

KYLE H. SHEETZ AND HARI NATHAN

Clinical Delivery Challenge

There is robust evidence that higher procedural volumes are associated with improved outcomes for complex surgery.[1,2] The mechanisms by which volume impacts quality are likely varied. Higher volumes can lead to more familiarity with complex procedures for nurses, anesthesiologists, and surgeons.[3] Surgical decision-making (including whether to operate) improves with institutional experience. Rescue from complications can be improved due to early recognition of complications at high-volume hospitals as well as ready access to services such as surgical intensive care units, interventional radiology, and advanced endoscopy.[3] While not all procedures exhibit strong volume–outcome relationships, complex cardiovascular procedures (eg, aortic or mitral valve repair) and complex cancer procedures (eg, pancreatectomy, esophagectomy, pneumonectomy) have consistently shown strong associations between volume and mortality in numerous studies.[4]

With the known volume–outcome relationship or complex procedures in mind, how then should we approach low-volume surgery at 1 site of care within a network?

There has been a strong and ongoing trend in the U.S. healthcare system of hospitals consolidating into regional delivery networks. Rates of hospital consolidation have doubled since 2009.[5] This trend has broad consequences for how health care is delivered, including how hospitals and their networks organize their surgical services. It has also created unique opportunities to reorganize care delivery due to the availability of multiple sites of care within the network. One potential benefit of hospital consolidation is the ability to concentrate procedural volume for high-risk surgery and avoid the potentially unsafe practice of low-volume complex surgery. This chapter explores the scenario of a low-volume hospital within a newly formed hospital network.

● WORKUP

As we begin to think about low-volume sites of care, it is important to gather more information about that site of care to better inform a solution.

Procedure Case-Mix and Volume

First, and perhaps, most importantly, what procedures are being performed. If the operations are common, low-risk procedures (eg, inguinal hernia repair), then care may be appropriate there at lower volume. However, if the procedures are more complex (eg, pancreatectomy) and are performed at low volume, then there is concern that the volume–outcome relationship is not being optimized.

In the United States, the Leapfrog Group reports whether hospitals meet modest volume thresholds for complex surgery, but there are few regulatory requirements to prevent hospitals from performing low-volume complex surgery.[6] One exception is the modest minimum volume requirements for heart, intestine, liver, lung, and kidney transplants established by the Centers for Medicare & Medicaid Services. However, mandatory standards have been implemented in other countries. For example, a volume requirement of 20 pancreaticoduodenectomies per year was implemented in 2013 for hospitals in the Netherlands, with consequent improvements in resection rates and survival for pancreatic cancer patients.[7] In the Netherlands, pancreatic surgery is now concentrated in 16 centers. In the absence of such requirements in the United States, hospital networks may be uniquely positioned to implement such volume concentration on their own.

Hospital Capabilities

Next, it is important to understand what capabilities each hospital has available and how they align with the procedures being performed. For many common procedures (eg, endoscopy, laparoscopic cholecystectomy), the capabilities needed are usually specific to the procedure itself (eg, endoscopy tower, laparoscopic instruments.) For more complex operations, additional resources are needed after the procedure is complete. For example, for sites of care performing pancreatectomy, it would be important to have interventional radiology and intensive care unit available.

Mission and Service

Finally, in some contexts, a low-volume hospital may be needed because it ensures access to surgical care. For example, Critical Access Hospitals receive federal subsidies because they are more than 35 miles away from any other source of care. In the United States, these small rural hospitals are the predominant source of care for more than 80 million Americans. Although they may be acceptable as a low-volume provider for common low-risk procedures, they likely should avoid more complex operations.

● DIFFERENTIAL DIAGNOSIS

Individual hospitals have limited options to increase their procedural volume, as this market share generally must come from competitors. Hospital networks, on the other hand, may both increase their aggregate volume and consolidate volume among hospitals within their networks. The impact of hospital network formation is perhaps best understood as a balance between various competing priorities. For example, a newly formed hospital network may choose to consolidate certain high-risk procedures in a single tertiary care hospital or "hub." In exchange, they maximize safety and quality by restricting care to the surgeons and teams with the most experience. On the other hand, this decision may have an impact on access for patients seeking care at other lower-volume affiliated hospitals farther away from the hub. Similar tensions exist with respect to potential revenue. Consolidating certain (potentially lucrative) service lines at particular hospitals within a network may present problems for smaller (and presumably low-volume) hospitals losing that revenue because of network affiliation.

● DIAGNOSIS AND TREATMENT

What should be done about a low-volume hospital within a network? Is it acceptable? Should the service line be redesigned to consolidate procedures elsewhere in the network?

One common framework for how hospital networks arrange surgical services is based on the overall complexity of care.[8] It proposes that hospital networks centralize high-risk, complex procedures (eg, major liver resection), standardize care pathways for moderate-risk surgeries (eg, colon cancer surgery), and decentralize low-risk surgeries (eg, inguinal hernia repair) (Figure 16.1). This framework attempts to balance some of the tensions discussed above to maximize safety, access, and shared revenue from surgical care within a hospital network. The remaining barriers to this strategy include surgeon reluctance to refer to a colleague as well as patient travel. Many patients prefer to have surgery locally even when informed that travel to a regional center could result in lower mortality risk.[9] However, more recent data

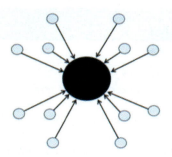 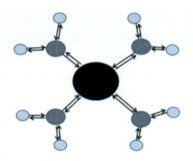

Centralize More Complex Procedures   **Decentralize Less Complex Procedures**

FIGURE 16.1 Conceptual model for how hospital networks can organize surgical services. Used with permission of Massachusetts Medical Society from Ibrahim and Dimick.[10] Permission conveyed through Copyright Clearance Center, Inc.

suggest that many patients can be motivated to travel for complex surgery, especially if financial support is available.[11]

● SCIENTIFIC PRINCIPLES AND EVIDENCE

The current best evidence suggests that the relationship between hospital network formation and clinical quality is mixed.[12-15] In other words, it remains unclear whether the quality of care improves as hospitals affiliate with existing hospital networks. For surgical care, 1 recent study of patients undergoing a range of general, cardiac, vascular, or orthopedic operations found that hospital network participation was not associated with improvement in rates of postoperative complications.[16] Moreover, time-in-network as a surrogate for the potential development of network strategies, reorganization of care delivery, and accrual of network benefits were also not associated with improvement in outcomes. Most hospital networks exhibit substantial variation in complication rates and spending across affiliated hospitals, suggesting that standardization of care and appropriate consolidation of volume have not taken place in many networks.[17,18] Another study compared the surgical outcomes of hub hospitals and their affiliates among the networks ranked highest by the U.S. News and World Report.[19] While rates of failure to rescue were lower at the hub (U.S. News Honor Roll) hospitals compared to affiliates, complication rates were higher at hub hospitals and the overall rates of complications varied widely within each network.

On the other hand, networks that have consolidated complex surgery do achieve better overall outcomes, including both complications and mortality, even in networks with low volumes.[20] While it is possible that networks that consolidate volume take other steps to improve the quality of care, it is likely that volume concentration itself exerts direct effects as described above. Taken together, the evidence suggests that consolidation of complex procedures within networks can lead to improvements in outcomes, although these benefits remain largely unrealized because networks have not adequately developed these internal referral strategies.

● IMPLEMENTATION OF A SOLUTION

Several real-world examples of within-network consolidation have been reported that provide important insight into how surgical service lines may be overoptimized within a hospital network. Providence St. Joseph Health (PSJH) system operated 21 cardiac surgery programs in 2016, of which two were in the state of Oregon.[21] These hospitals were only 9 miles apart but together accounted for 35–40% of the

Key Steps to Change Management and Potential Pitfalls

Key Steps in Change Management
1. Recognize the potential risk of low-volume sites of care for complex operations.
2. Identifying referral patterns within the network can be optimized to take advantage of known volume–outcome relationships.
3. Separate phases of care to identify which parts can be safely done locally (eg, outpatient preoperative workup) and which should be centralized (eg, pancreatectomy procedure).
4. Develop measures and safeguards that take into account trade-offs of centralization, including possible increased travel burden on patients.

Potential Pitfalls
1. Assuming that good outcomes at low-volume sites of care are measuring true quality as opposed to statistical noise.
2. Centralizing procedures without taking into account potential access trade-offs.

local cardiac surgical market share. In 2016, network leaders decided to close the Portland program with lower volumes and inferior outcomes over the course of 6 months, consolidating the system's local cardiac surgical volume at the remaining Portland PSJH program. Overall PSJH cardiac surgical volume was maintained, and outcomes at the remaining higher-volume center remained consistent with its favorable historical outcomes, even as it absorbed the additional volume. The Willis-Knighton Health System in Louisiana has used a hub-and-spoke model for 30 years, whereby patients needing complex services are referred to referral centers.[22] Travel support can be provided by the network. This approach has yielded efficiencies in avoiding duplication of resource-intensive services and has resulted in superior quality by concentrating volume at hospitals with the most experienced teams and the most comprehensive resources for service lines such as cardiovascular surgery.

In our opinion, several elements are necessary to successfully implement a strategy to avoid low-volume surgery in a healthcare network. First, network and hospital leadership must recognize the drawbacks of low-volume surgery and the benefits of volume concentration. They must, in turn, achieve buy-in or at least compliance from surgeons across the network. Second, an efficient referral system must be devised. Depending on various network characteristics, including the availability of imaging technology at outlying hospitals and geographic dispersion of the hospitals in the network, the referral system may take different forms. Patients may be immediately referred for all remaining diagnostic workup and therapy once the diagnosis is suspected. When the capability exists, some of the diagnostic workup may be completed locally. For cancer patients, remote review of clinical data by a central tumor board may alleviate some of the need for travel, especially for patients who either are not surgical candidates or require some type of preoperative optimization (eg, prehabilitation) or therapy (eg, neoadjuvant chemotherapy), prior to surgery. Third, attention must be paid to travel burden and equitable access to ensure that all populations served by the network can access expert high-volume care. Finally, hospital and network leadership can think strategically about how patients access the expertise needed to provide quality care. This means leveraging technology, where possible, to limit the physical displacement of patients or providers.

● MEASURING OUTCOMES

There are several important measures relevant to optimizing care within a network. These include important clinical outcomes such as 30-day mortality, failure to rescue, and complications. It is equally important to track patient-centered outcomes. For example, 1 drawback of centralizing surgery across a network would be great patient travel burden. As such, these centralization efforts likely come with inherent trade-offs that need to be measured and constantly reevaluated.

● FOLLOW-UP AND MAINTENANCE

It is ultimately the responsibility of the health system and surgical leadership to recognize the opportunities and potential pitfalls that come with hospital network formation. However, regulators, healthcare policymakers, and the broader public should also take note of whether new affiliations, mergers, and acquisitions make good on their promise to improve care quality and decrease costs. Low-volume surgery, in certain contexts, is unsafe and should be avoided. Hospital networks may possess a unique opportunity to implement selective referrals to consolidate volume while avoiding the loss of revenue that might stymie such referrals between rival hospitals. However, this takes planning and deliberate strategy but might be viewed as a hospital network quality measure, as a surrogate for a broader, intentional care optimization effort. At present it remains unclear whether hospital networks are collectively recognizing this opportunity to address the quality and safety concerns associated with low-volume care that have long been a neglected priority for surgical care.

REFERENCES

1. Birkmeyer JD, Siewers AE, Finlayson EV, et al. Hospital volume and surgical mortality in the United States. *N Engl J Med*. 2002;346(15):1128–1137. doi: 10.1056/NEJMsa012337
2. Finks JF, Osborne NH, Birkmeyer JD. Trends in hospital volume and operative mortality for high-risk surgery. *N Engl J Med*. 2011;364(22):2128–2137. doi: 10.1056/NEJMsa1010705
3. Birkmeyer JD, Stukel TA, Siewers AE, Goodney PP, Wennberg DE, Lucas FL. Surgeon volume and operative mortality in the United States. *N Engl J Med*. 2003;349(22):2117–2127. doi: 10.1056/NEJMsa035205
4. Hata T, Motoi F, Ishida M, et al. Effect of hospital volume on surgical outcomes after pancreaticoduodenectomy: a systematic review and meta-analysis. *Ann Surg*. 2016;263(4):664–672. doi: 10.1097/SLA.0000000000001437
5. Dafny L. Hospital industry consolidation—still more to come? *N Engl J Med*. 2014;370(3):198–199. doi: 10.1056/NEJMp1313948
6. Sheetz KH, Chhabra KR, Smith ME, Dimick JB, Nathan, H. Association of discretionary hospital volume standards for high-risk cancer surgery with patient outcomes and access, 2005–2016. *JAMA Surg*. 2019;154(11):1005–1012. doi: 10.1001/jamasurg.2019.3017
7. Latenstein AEJ, Mackay TM, van der Geest LGM, et al. Effect of centralization and regionalization of pancreatic surgery on resection rates and survival. *Br J Surg*. 2021;108(7):826–833. doi: 10.1093/bjs/znaa146
8. Ibrahim AM, Sheetz KH, Dimick JB. Improving the delivery of surgical care within regional hospital networks. *Ann Surg*. 2019;269(6):1016–1017. doi: 10.1097/SLA.0000000000003182
9. Finlayson SR, Birkmeyer JD, Tosteson AN, Nease RF, Jr. Patient preferences for location of care: implications for regionalization. *Med Care*. 1999;37(2):204–209. doi: 10.1097/00005650-199902000-00010
10. Ibrahim AM, Dimick JB. Redesigning the delivery of specialty care within newly formed hospital networks. *NEJM Catalyst*; 2017. doi: 10.1056/CAT.17.0503
11. Resio BJ, Chiu AS, Hoag JR, et al. Motivators, barriers, and facilitators to traveling to the safest hospitals in the United States for complex cancer surgery. *JAMA Netw Open*. 2018;1(7):e184595. doi: 10.1001/jamanetworkopen.2018.4595
12. Beaulieu ND, Dafny LS, Landon BE, Dalton JB, Kuye I, McWilliams JM. Changes in quality of care after hospital mergers and acquisitions. *N Engl J Med*. 2020;382(1):51–59. doi: 10.1056/NEJMsa1901383
13. Frakt AB. Hospital consolidation isn't the key to lowering costs and raising quality. *JAMA*. 2015;313(4):345. doi: 10.1001/jama.2014.17412
14. Tsai TC, Jha AK. Hospital consolidation, competition, and quality: is bigger necessarily better? *JAMA*. 2014; 312(1):29–30. doi: 10.1001/jama.2014.4692
15. Wang E, Arnold S, Jones S, et al. Quality and safety outcomes of a hospital merger following a full integration at a safety net hospital. *JAMA Netw Open*. 2022;5(1):e2142382. doi: 10.1001/jamanetworkopen.2021.42382
16. Sheetz KH, Ryan AM, Ibrahim AM, Dimick JB. Association of hospital network participation with surgical outcomes and medicare expenditures. *Ann Surg*. 2019;270(2):288–294. doi: 10.1097/SLA.0000000000002791

17. Chhabra KR, Sheetz KH, Regenbogen SE, Dimick JB, Nathan H. Wide variation in surgical spending within hospital systems: a missed opportunity for bundled payment success. *Ann Surg*. 2021;274(6):e1078–e1084. doi: 10.1097/SLA.0000000000003741
18. Diaz A, Chhabra KR, Dimick JB, Nathan H. Variations in surgical spending within hospital systems for complex cancer surgery. *Cancer*. 2021;127(4):586–597. doi: 10.1002/cncr.33299
19. Sheetz KH, Ibrahim AM, Nathan H, Dimick JB. Variation in surgical outcomes across networks of the highest-rated US hospitals. *JAMA Surg*. 2019;154(6):510–515. doi: 10.1001/jamasurg.2019.0090
20. Sheetz KH, Dimick JB, Nathan H. Centralization of high-risk cancer surgery within existing hospital systems. *J Clin Oncol*. 2019;37(34):3234–3242. doi: 10.1200/JCO.18.02035
21. Gluckman TJ, Zelensky JK, Oseran DS. Cardiac surgery consolidation—improving value in care delivery. *NEJM Catalyst*. 2019;1(2). doi: 10.1056/CAT.20.0019
22. Elrod JK, Fortenberry JL, Jr. The hub-and-spoke organization design: an avenue for serving patients well. *BMC Health Serv Res*. 2017;17(Suppl 1):457. doi: 10.1186/s12913-017-2341-x

Disseminating Quality Standards Across a Hospital Network

17

CAROLINE E. REINKE AND MICHAEL BARRINGER

Clinical Delivery Challenge

Imagine two very similar patients who have decided to undergo elective laparoscopic sigmoid colectomy for recurrent, lifestyle-limiting diverticulitis. They compare notes after visiting their surgeon and are amazed at how similar the conversations were—the planned procedure, potential benefits, and risks/complications covered were the same. Yet they are shocked to discover that their preoperative instructions, guidance about postoperative recovery, and outlined expected length of stay were dramatically different. The explanation for this discordance is that one of the surgeons sees patients and operates in a hospital with a robust enhanced recovery program utilizing a colon bundle, while the other surgeon does not.

As healthcare systems develop, ongoing collaboration dissemination of quality standards across the network will support the implementation of best practices for all patients. In our health system, the implementation of a colon bundle across multiple settings was a clinical delivery challenge encountered early in our collaborative efforts. Best practices for enhanced recovery and use of surgical site infection (SSI) prevention bundles in colorectal surgery have been well established in the literature.[1,2] These interventions have been shown to reduce SSIs and promote early recovery.[1-3] However, utilization of enhanced recovery and SSI prevention standards is not routinely implemented, especially when comparing practices across a variety of facilities and practice types.

Our healthcare system spans multiple states, with the Greater Charlotte Region (GCR) including nine facilities that range in size (100–900 beds) and have a shared electronic medical record (EMR) and quality structure. Within the GCR, colon procedures are performed by both general surgeons and colorectal surgeons. The majority of the hospitals are not teaching hospitals, and surgeons have varied practice structures and group sizes. As efforts began across the general surgery service line (within our quality structure in the GCR), it became apparent that there was a disconnect between service line goals and facility-level goals. For example, colon SSIs were identified as a quality priority for the general surgery service line, yet at any specific hospital, there were often other quality initiatives that had higher visibility as established by facility-level leadership. The clinical delivery challenge, after gaining system leadership support, was to standardize the preoperative, intraoperative, and postoperative nontechnical aspects of care for patients undergoing colon surgery through the implementation of a standardized colon bundle to improve patient outcomes.

It is clear that hospitals are rapidly consolidating into networks. However, it is less clear how becoming part of the same network influences the quality standards at each site. Should they maintain their prior protocol and practice patterns? Should they converge to a common standard? If so, how could that be done? This chapter will explore disseminating quality standards across and newly formed hospital network.

● WORKUP

In order to think about how a quality standard may disseminate across our network, we need to first identify: current evidence, key stakeholders, and measurable outcomes and we might track the adoption of best practices (ie, process measures of care).

Current Evidence

To understand the baseline at the beginning of this initiative, a literature review of colon bundles and enhanced recovery practices for colon surgery was performed to identify what data needed to be collected. Process measures as recommended by multiple organizations were collated across the five phases of care and were presented to a surgeon leader from each hospital for evaluation and feedback on importance and feasibility (Table 17.1). The process elements reviewed included those recommended by the American College of Surgeons, the World Health Organization, the Centers for Disease Control and Prevention, and the International Enhanced Recovery After Surgery Society.[4–7]

The components chosen to implement and subsequently capture for tracking and trending are indicated with highlighting in Table 17.1.

Stakeholders

Representative surgeons from across the GCR who performed colon procedures participated in the development of a standardized approach to patients undergoing colon surgery. During regularly

Table 17.1   Process Measures Across the Five Phases of Care

Prehospital Phase	Immediate Preoperative	Intraoperative Phase	Postoperative Phase	Post-Discharge Phase
Enhanced nutritional support	Alvimopan	Chlorhexidine skin prep	Ambulate night of surgery and then TID	Short follow-up postoperative visit
Pre-admission education	Standardized anti-biotic prophylaxis	Normothermia	Gum chewing	Routine postop nurse phone call
Mechanical bowel prep	PONV prophylaxis	Wound protectors	Immediate postop-erative oral diet	Standardized discharge pain education
Oral antibiotics	Chlorhexidine wipes	Pre-closure glove/gown change	Routine bowel management medications	Standardized discharge pain medications
Carbohydrate load		Separate closing instruments	Limit PCA use	
Preoperative chlorhexidine showering		Redrape prior to closure	Continue Alvimopan	
Glucose control		Limiting OR traffic	Remove dressing at 48 hours	
Smoking cessation		Special wound dressing	Showering allowed at 48 hours	
2-hour NPO for clear liquids			Standardized dis-charge education	
Incentive spirome-ter training				

Abbreviations: TID, three times a day; NPO, nil per os (nothing by mouth).

Highlighted elements are those initially chosen for implementation and to track/trend going forward.

Table 17.2 — Outcome Measures Relevant to Selected Colon Bundle Components

NHSN	Premiere and Billing Data	NSQIP Colectomy
• Organ Space SSI	• Length of stay	• SSI
• Deep SSI	• Mortality	• Ventilator > 48 hours
• Superficial SSI	• Readmissions	• Morbidity
	• Variable cost	• Readmission

NHSN standards were used as the primary outcome target, and baseline metrics were used to compare SSI outcomes at all levels—system, facility, and provider. For system and facility data, they were also compared to national benchmarking. Quality metrics from Premier (https://products.premierinc.com/applied-sciences) were additionally used to evaluate the impact on length of stay, mortality, and readmissions. Though the National Surgical Quality Improvement Program (NSQIP) is not inclusive of all patients due to sampling and other exclusions (ie, trauma), all facilities were participating in NSQIP and this data was also utilized to triangulate outcomes.

scheduled meetings, specific components to be included in the pathway and tracked were chosen by consensus based on those which were felt to be both achievable and measurable. The meetings were held in person with a virtual option. Other stakeholders involved in the process included quality teammates, certified registered nurse anesthetists/anesthesia leadership, and nursing management representatives from across all phases of care.

Outcomes

We identified key outcomes that would be impacted by our quality standards. Specifically, we sought to identify outcomes that could readily be measured from sources of data we had access to for our institution. They are summarized in Table 17.2.

Tracking Process of Care

Notably, none of the available data sources provided information on process metrics. To overcome this challenge, our information and analytics services team developed forms to capture colon bundle-specific process measures as discreet variables within the EMR. These forms allowed specific colon bundle components to be recorded and our preoperative and intraoperative nurses were educated on how to complete these documents (Figures 17.1 and 17.2). Our data management team was then able to abstract the data and allow it to be presented in a comparative dashboard (PowerBI^{TM}).

● DIFFERENTIAL DIAGNOSIS

Factors contributing to challenges in implementing quality standards across a health system include differential education and surgeon-level interest, competing priorities, lack of system support, and the need to collaborate across departments. Development of standardized approaches to surgical care incorporating principles of early recovery is still relatively new and for many surgeons was not part of their surgical training. Depending on exposure to newer evidenced-based best practices (in training or through continuing medical education) and surgeon-specific adoption tendencies, new processes for care may be incorporated into a single surgeon's normal care pathway in a fragmented fashion. Collective planning of the day-to-day operational processes is not always part of the standard workflow for a surgeon, practice, hospital, or system. Varied facility environments (rural versus urban, teaching versus. non-teaching, etc) present significant challenges to initiation, and accomplishment of, a consistent pathway across different patient care departments. Additionally, each care department (outpatient clinic, inpatient operating room, and inpatient floor structures) often has somewhat siloed administrative leadership. Prioritizing the necessary time and effort to affect systemic change is rarely practical for an individual surgeon, even when knowledgeable and highly engaged. Therefore, a major barrier can

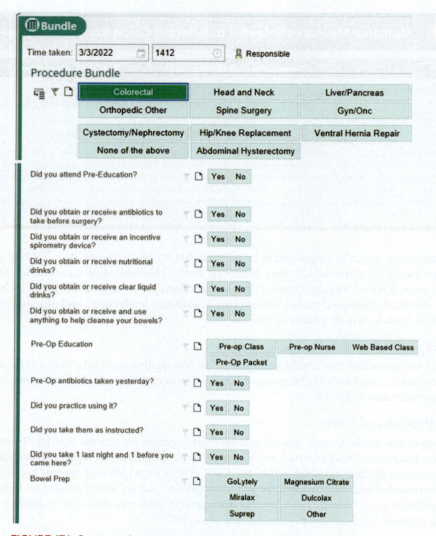

FIGURE 17.1 Capture of preoperative elements performed at home (captured by preoperative holding nurse).

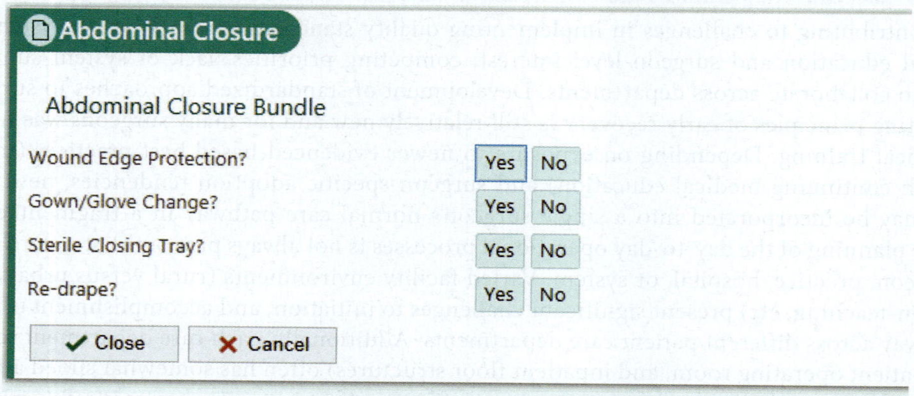

FIGURE 17.2 Capture of intraoperative elements (captured by circulating nurse).

be the absence of a formalized structure for developing new pathways at a facility or regional level. In addition, the solicitation of financial support from administrative leaders—with the ability to project the program's return on investment utilizing subjective estimates of reduced costs and improved quality metrics—may be associated with a negative perspective from surgeons trying to do the "best thing" for the patient. The development and maintenance of a fiscally responsible standardized quality improvement framework is a core challenge in itself and is not always recognized as an important goal during a unique pathway development effort.

● DIAGNOSIS AND TREATMENT

The highest leverage areas for improvement were those that were felt to have the greatest impact on patient care, as improving patient outcomes and reducing healthcare utilization are driving motivators for surgeons as well as all other involved caregivers and hospital administrations. Standardized and benchmarked data identifying an opportunity for improvement was utilized to inspire stakeholders to commit to the development of focused regional quality improvement processes.

Supporting a physician-led process with the necessary resources can facilitate surgeon engagement in the initiative. Utilizing consensus agreement for bundle components and maintaining the focus on improved patient care help minimize distractors. As the utilization of the individual components of the pathway is successfully increased, ongoing positive feedback and encouragement are critical to success. In addition, updating administrative leadership as to cost savings and improved nationally reported quality goals further ensures ongoing support for this and other similar projects.

The development of a solidly established and surgeon-supported pathway prior to the local facility rollouts was imperative. Accomplishing the spread of the pathway at individual sites provided another opportunity for the core team to encourage engagement by leading onsite collaborative meetings at each facility. Attended by a local surgeon champion; preoperative, intraoperative, and postoperative nursing caregivers; the anesthesia team members; and administrative leadership, the meeting allowed elements necessary for the implementation to be explained, questions concerning departmental roles and necessary interactivities to be answered, and potential obstacles to implementation addressed. Demonstrating the ability to track element completion and that participant engagement was necessary further encouraged those who would be part of the overall process to focus on the primary goal of improved patient outcomes.

● SCIENTIFIC PRINCIPLES AND EVIDENCE

Over the course of decades, reduction in SSIs has been a major quality metric focus across multiple initiatives with provider-level feedback and published facility comparisons available through National Healthcare Safety Network (NHSN).[8,9] Multiple individual studies have been performed looking at ways to reduce SSIs including bowel preparation, antibiotic choices, and more recently the technical aspects of colorectal procedures including proper cleansing of the skin, protection of the subcutaneous tissue, aspects of wound closure, and the care of the postoperative wound. Additional scientific information has led to the realization that the patient's biological condition including nutritional status, serum glucose, tissue oxygenation, and core temperature also play a role in reducing the risk of SSIs.

Enhanced recovery after surgery, including SSI-prevention bundles, has now become foundational to surgical care with the goal of reducing complications and improving outcomes. Quality metrics have expanded beyond SSI to include reduction in length of stay, readmission rates, and patient-reported outcomes. The involvement of the patient as an active participant in the surgical recovery process should now be the standard of care. Through educational preparation, the patient recognizes that nutritional support, glucose control, smoking cessation, skin cleansing, and perioperative physical activities including ambulation and incentive spirometry usage contribute to reducing their chances of complications and promoting a postoperative return to normalcy in a shorter length of time.

● IMPLEMENTING A SOLUTION

Change management is always a difficult endeavor and is especially so in environments where the proposed change requires coordination between multiple departments with different leadership structures. In addition, the implementation of a surgical care pathway is further complicated by competing priorities and opinions of highly focused and independent providers.

There are multiple change management models which vary in specific content, but most reflect similar principles despite their differences. Atrium Health has adopted the following as a template, but others are equally effective guides for the process (Figure 17.3).

Analyze and Approach

In this case, the analysis and approach have been outlined in detail earlier in this chapter. In our system, a surgeon-led review of the data and identification of an approach with high-level administrative and quality support was critical for broad engagement across our region. In contrast to top-down change which can be met with resistance, presenting key providers with the challenge of improving patient outcomes through a consensus-driven approach leads to a process with buy-in created during its development. In addition, when administrative support in the form of time and resources is provided for the proposed approach, a sense of recognized value given to the effort enhances the momentum of the process.

Aware, Aspire

Having the system surgeons and facilitators, who led the development, present the pathway at local meetings allows engagement with questions and fosters a community-driven effort focused on patient care. Additionally, the involvement of facility-level teammates in the process evolution provides an opportunity to clarify and identify any facility-specific barriers and allows upfront workflow modifications to enable integration of the new care pathway. Providing an open channel for follow-up questions, concerns and implementation assistance smooth the change process while revealing beneficial information that may assist other facilities.

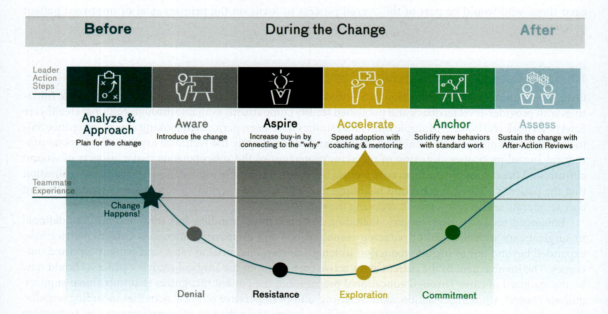

FIGURE 17.3 Change Acceleration Model (atriumhealthlearning.azurewebsites.net).

Accelerate

Once the new pathway had been created, introduced, and agreed upon by all stakeholders across sites, regular meetings to review data regarding the utilization of components and patient outcomes kept the work front-of-mind and allowed for increased uptake as barriers were identified and overcome. Additionally, being able to correlate process change with patient outcomes further encouraged utilization. Finally, surgeon-specific feedback on the utilization of compliance measures for cases with an identified SSI allowed for specific coaching.

Anchor and Assess

The modification of the EMR to capture the utilization of bundle elements hardwired the process and created standard work. Implementation of support processes such as having the preoperative elements available in the clinic as a package for patients and having stakeholders responsible for components of the pathway across different settings minimized the required action by any one group and allowed ongoing collaboration and teamwork.

Considerations in Equity

Having inequitable resource availability for facilities, practices, and patients should be recognized as a potential deficiency which can hinder the success of any improvement effort. Mechanisms to provide the essential supplies needed—in addition to providing supportive encouragement—were paramount to an effective implementation. The identified preoperative elements necessitated creating a pathway

Key Steps in Change Management and Potential Pitfalls

Key Steps in Change Management

	Colon Bundle Examples
1. Analyze and Approach	Analysis of available data Creating a coalition of providers, administration, nursing, and quality
2. Aware	Sharing outcomes and recommendations across settings
3. Aspire	Discussion of literature outlining the relationship between enhanced recovery and patient outcomes
4. Accelerate	Quickly scheduled facility visits
5. Anchor	Touchpoint revisits Dashboard review Surgeon-specific letters
6. Assess	Dashboard creation and feedback

Potential Pitfalls

1. Lack of structure to work collectively.
2. Resistance to consensus.
3. Lack of belief in literature findings based on personal experience or unique patient population.
4. Failure in attendance locally.
5. Workflow across departments.
6. Changes in personnel.
7. Information technology challenges.

for implementing patient education on enhanced recovery and providing nutritional support drinks, preoperative breathing exercises and tools, preoperative skin cleansing supplies, and preoperative bowel cleansing and oral antibiotic medications. To accomplish this for all patients, the system committed to providing the supplies necessary as a kit available to all patients free of charge.

After our initial focus on rollout in elective colon procedures, and based on an updated review of the literature, it was agreed that the pathway elements should also be offered to our nonelective cases as much as feasible given the patients' disease process. Knowing that there are many factors that may create barriers to achieving the necessary workup to prevent emergency colon cases, we believed that expansion of this pathway for all colon cases was important for improving equity in outcomes.

● MEASURING OUTCOMES

The key metrics to assess effectiveness were the utilization of pathway elements and patient outcomes. This was primarily achieved with the development of a PowerBI dashboard which allowed for a comparison of preoperative, intraoperative, and postoperative pathway element usage. These were merged with the aforementioned outcome metrics of SSIs, length of stay, readmissions, mortalities, and costs. The ability to compare compliance with outcomes at a system, facility, or provider level allowed consistent feedback and trending. Presentation of the outcomes and system- and local-level infection prevention and surgical quality meetings provided a mechanism to celebrate successes and well as troubleshoot any emerging barriers.

Potential unintended consequences of the pathway included canceled or delayed cases due to patients misunderstanding preoperative instructions or anesthesia providers uncomfortable with the 2-hour NPO rule for clear liquids. For postoperative care, early advancement of diet and early mobility had the potential for increasing postoperative nausea and vomiting (PONV), aspiration, and falls. These metrics are all regularly tracked within our healthcare system. Potential unintended consequences of implementing a bundle across all phases of care could be overwhelming participants or creating too many opportunities for "fallouts" that may discourage stakeholders. These were monitored for regular check-ins with the surgeons and stakeholders.

● FOLLOW-UP AND MAINTENANCE

Trending outcomes and utilization of pathway elements provided identification of opportunities for reeducation both at facility and provider levels. As this work progressed, we identified that we did not have a standardized way of onboarding new surgeons regarding the colon pathway, which turned out to be an important component of maintenance. Similar findings occurred with other stakeholders such as clinic staff, perioperative nursing, and surgical floor nurses. Ongoing evaluation of the data extraction and measurement tools identified additional opportunities to improve the accuracy of the data—including changes in coding, changes in the EMR, and ultimately a change from one EMR to another. Paramount to the success of the pathway was keeping the project visible to all involved stakeholders to ensure ongoing support.

REFERENCES

1. Keenan JE, Speicher PJ, Nussbaum DP, et al. Improving outcomes in colorectal surgery by sequential implementation of multiple standardized care programs. *J Am Coll Surg*. 2015;221:404–414 e401.
2. Keenan JE, Speicher PJ, Thacker JK, Walter M, Kuchibhatla M, Mantyh CR. The preventive surgical site infection bundle in colorectal surgery: an effective approach to surgical site infection reduction and health care cost savings. *JAMA Surg*. 2014;149:1045–1052.
3. Liu VX, Rosas E, Hwang J, et al. Enhanced recovery after surgery program implementation in 2 surgical populations in an integrated health care delivery system. *JAMA Surg*. 2017;152:e171032.
4. Berrios-Torres SI, Umscheid CA, Bratzler DW, et al. Centers for Disease Control and Prevention guideline for the prevention of surgical site infection. *JAMA Surg*. 2017;152:784–791.

5. Global guidelines for the prevention of surgical site infection, second edition. Geneva: World Health Organization 2018. Licence: CC BY-NC-SA 3.0 IGO.
6. DeHaas D, Aufderheide S, Gano J, Weigandt J, Ries J, Faust B. Colorectal surgical site infection reduction strategies. *Am J Surg*. 2016;212:175–177.
7. Gustafsson UO, Scott MJ, Hubner M, et al. Guidelines for perioperative care in elective colorectal surgery: Enhanced Recovery after Surgery (ERAS®) Society Recommendations: 2018. *World J Surg*. 2019;43:659–695.
8. Cataife G, Weinberg DA, Wong HH, Kahn KL. The effect of Surgical Care Improvement Project (SCIP) compliance on surgical site infections (SSI). *Med Care*. 2014;52:S66–73.
9. Surgical Site Infection (SSI) Events. Centers for Diseases Control and Prevention. January 2023. https://www.cdc.gov/nhsn/pdfs/pscmanual/9pscssicurrent.pdf. Accessed June 26, 2023.

Ensuring Quality while Exporting Brand to New Network Affiliates

RONALD B. HIRSCHL

Clinical Delivery Challenge

The past decade has seen considerable consolidation among healthcare systems in the United States. Consolidation and increasing scale among health systems have been accelerated by the thinner margins facing healthcare systems due to increasing costs, especially in an era of COVID-19 and associated workforce challenges, and involve opportunities to create economies of scale for clinical programs and back-office functions and to achieve success in alternative payment models that increasingly focus on value-based care and population health. Academic health centers (AHCs) have an additional rationale for consolidation and growth in that their educational and research programs often require access to large populations to continue to train providers and to care for and advance research around conditions with a low incidence. For example, estimates have suggested that access to a population of 3.5 million lives is required to support a liver transplantation program and the substrate necessary for accompanying training, a volume which an individual AHC frequently cannot command without mergers/affiliations. While some have argued that consolidation has the potential to drive improvements in quality, safety, and value delivery, studies on this aspect suggest that an affiliate acquisition by another hospital or hospital system is associated with modestly worse patient experience scores and no significant changes in readmission rates, although recent data suggest that mergers may be associated with improvement in mortality rates and other quality metrics.[1,2]

There are multiple challenges associated with affiliations related to differences in culture; levels of care expectations and standards; and available healthcare resources, in addition to wariness around intentions and trust. Affiliations may be associated with challenges related to new populations, unfamiliar infrastructure, and new settings with teams far from the AHC which leaves providers and patients alike potentially at risk.[3] There is also a challenge and risk associated with the reputation of AHCs and other large healthcare systems: that reputation is often of benefit to the affiliate in terms of joint marketing and co-branding, but unless the expectations around performance, safety, and quality are managed appropriately, there is a risk to the brand and reputation of the AHC. This is especially complicated when affiliations are isolated to segments of care (eg, limited only to children's care) such that the brand does not extend across the spectrum of care at the affiliate. Another challenge is in determining when the complexity of patient care exceeds that which is appropriate and safe given the resources available at the affiliate.[4] Some have suggested that the brand, along with names, logos, and slogans, is perhaps one of the most valuable assets of an AHC which, as with any asset, is at risk if not protected appropriately.[5] How the brand and associated logos are used and demonstrated is often a critical aspect of the marketing strategy of AHCs.[6]

Affiliations with other healthcare entities involve a spectrum from professional service agreements, perhaps for the provision of services by a single provider, to those that involve joint ventures around service lines and even full integration or acquisition with single hospitals or healthcare systems. We will use the example of a joint venture in children's care as a springboard for discussion of the challenges that are faced when extending the AHC brand.

Extension of a brand to a health system network affiliation creates expectations around performance, safety, and quality at the affiliate institution. Delivering these quality and performance expectations under a Marquis brand is not without challenges. We will use a joint venture in children's care as the illustrative scenario in this chapter to outline the issues that are faced when extending the brand to a partner affiliate.

CHAPTER 18 • Ensuring Quality while Exporting Brand to New Network Affiliates

● WORKUP

The initial challenge is in understanding existing resources and the quality of programs across the many sites of care within a newly formed system.

Evaluating Quality

Fortunately, there are regulatory bodies, medical societies, and interest groups which broadly evaluate the quality of healthcare entities and for which data are often publicly available. Examples include the Joint Commission evaluation, Leapfrog safety grades, Hospital Consumer Assessment of Healthcare Providers and Systems scores, and CMS Hospital Compare Overall Star Ratings.

Many areas of specialization have regional and national registries that allow assessment of quality of care, for example, the Society of Thoracic Surgeons National Database, although such databases may not always be in use at affiliate systems. Discussions with both clinical and administrative leaders is essential to identify areas of strengths and weaknesses, with a more detailed assessment obtained from clinicians in those areas of concern. Patient satisfaction data, such as from Press Ganey, frequently reveal areas of opportunity. Discussions with Graduate Medical Education (GME) directors around GME issues, when and where they are relevant, are also indicative of programs that may be struggling.

Evaluating Resources and Culture

Consultants may be retained during a "due-diligence" phase prior to closing on an affiliation, in part to provide a valuation of the enterprise at the affiliate, but that review may offer insight into quality gaps. Such assessments by independent entities offer a non-biased and unfettered view of both the opportunities and risks for both the AHC and the affiliate.

It is also critical to understand the fundamental culture and infrastructure associated with maintaining and enhancing safety and quality across the care spectrum of interest. The initial assessment should involve a physician with expertise in the clinical area of collaboration to identify key drivers of high-quality care and delineation of which of those drivers are in place or will need to be enhanced under the partnership. Discussions with quality and safety leadership and those managing such programs are vital. Analysis of the number and character of safety events as well as surveys on the culture of safety help to assess the safety and quality climate at the affiliate. With appropriate legal guardrails, assessment of relevant peer review and adverse event reports allows one to get a feel for provider-related concerns. It is important to document activities that demonstrate robust follow-up regarding safety reports and events and whether loop closure was implemented to realize necessary changes.

● DIFFERENTIAL DIAGNOSIS

The primary reasons for quality and safety concerns are often the same as those underlying the rationale for the relationship between the AHC and another health system, for example, gaps in care, financial challenges, resource constraints, and so on. The fundamental concern around brand use is the legal and reputation risk to the AHC. It is critical, therefore, that there be a robust analysis of those risks before marketing the brand at the affiliate. It is also key that the brand be selectively applied only to those areas of shared interest and participation in patient care as well as oversight and joint investment.

● DIAGNOSIS AND TREATMENT

It is important to have an ongoing assessment of gaps in care and development and enhancement of the quality and safety infrastructure. In establishing a children's care joint venture, large specialty-specific databases are not often available. However, other types of data may be helpful such as Vizient data for a broader service line quality assessment, Peds National Surgical Quality Improvement Program and the American College of Surgeons Children's Surgery Verification for surgical services, Improve Care Now for inflammatory bowel disease, and Vermont Oxford for neonatal ICU.

For our new joint venture, we reviewed many of these databases along with patient satisfaction data, and publicly available data reflecting hospital-wide care quality and performance. In Pediatrics, key drivers of high-quality care are often seen in the hospital-based specialties of Pediatric Anesthesia, Radiology, and Emergency Medicine, and the quality and safety profile of these services were specifically analyzed. Finally, we noted that children's care safety reporting was limited as was follow-up, mostly because such processes were part of and lost in the greater institutional, largely adult safety and quality efforts.

● SCIENTIFIC PRINCIPLES AND EVIDENCE

Often, the initial approach is to understand the general quality of care at the affiliate hospital, the programmatic gaps, and the safety and quality environment. Based on this analysis, the legal team will then help to develop a Licensing agreement and Conditions of Use (COU) for the brand that guides the application of the brand at the affiliate. Such COU provide a license to the affiliate to use the brand in connection with the proposed program, the specific circumstances under which the brand may be used, and the rights of the AHC as the owner of the brand to monitor use. In addition, the document details the quality standards and metrics which are required for ongoing brand use as well as the conditions under which the use of the brand may be revoked. Working closely with clinical leaders at the affiliate hospital, we developed a COU document at the initiation of our Pediatric joint venture which addressed areas of identified gaps and performance deficits that needed to be addressed for the brand to be used/ marketed.

We also developed a joint brand that featured and integrated the logos of the affiliate and our own. This joint brand has been outstanding at depicting the partnership, while also emphasizing that the brand is limited to children's care.

● IMPLEMENTATION OF A SOLUTION

Clinical leadership and service line management or co-management by faculty at the AHC are important features we think to drive high-quality care and further protect the brand. For our Pediatric joint venture, we implemented a joint clinical and administrative management team consisting of clinicians from both the AHC and the affiliate which, on a weekly basis, evaluated challenges and gaps in patient care, opportunities in patient satisfaction, and implemented changes to enhance care and communication. We are forming a separate Pediatric safety and quality program and are in the process of staffing the infrastructure to drive this work. Importantly, the committee which represents Pediatric quality and safety reports to the governing body overseeing the joint venture. We integrated the Pediatric quality and safety structure at Michigan Medicine with those at the affiliate to learn from and enhance the efforts at both sites and started to develop joint multicenter Pediatric clinical quality communities to share approaches and potential metrics toward enhancing quality. We are careful to apply our institution's brand only to those areas which are under our purview so that the extent of our influence and relationship is clear to both patients and providers.

What we also subsequently learned was that the initial COU document we developed was overly detailed, and included targets for quality measures, many of which we knew would be difficult to achieve. With subsequent affiliates, we have altered our approach to emphasize "hard" outcomes, that if not achieved would result in the removal of the brand: for example, failure to achieve Joint Commission accreditation and exclusion from a federal healthcare program. We further outline a "Quality Charter and Framework" which requires the implementation of robust quality processes to address safety and quality gaps and issues. Examples of this charter/framework include alignment between the AHC and the affiliate around credentialing requirements and various policies and practices, development of excellence in safety culture and employee engagement, and maintenance of high standards around quality improvement. The emphasis is placed, therefore, on the partnership working jointly on the quality and

> ## Key Steps in Change Management and Potential Pitfalls
>
> ### Key Steps in Change Management
>
> 1. Carry out a robust analysis of safety, quality, and risks before marketing the brand to the affiliate.
> 2. Evaluate challenges and gaps in patient care, opportunities in patient satisfaction, and implement changes to enhance care and communication.
> 3. Create clear Conditions of Brand Use that emphasizes "hard" outcomes.
> 4. Leverage the COU to require implementation of robust quality processes to address safety and quality gaps and issues, thus emphasizing the partnership working jointly on the quality and protection of the brand.
> 5. Develop a joint logo that communicates the partnership and the specific areas to which the brand may apply.
> 6. Implement a joint clinical and administrative management team to work on enhancing the partnership and patient care.
> 7. Create a separate Pediatric safety and quality program with staffing and infrastructure.
>
> ### Potential Pitfalls
>
> 1. Creating a COU that is detailed and aspirational, rather than realistic and directional, in terms of requirements or one that lacks "teeth."
> 2. Extending the brand beyond those areas of shared interest and oversight.
> 3. Failing to develop partnership and trust and joint enhancement in programmatic efforts.
> 4. Lack of development of a robust Pediatric safety and quality program and culture.

protection of the brand. Essentially, retraction of the brand would only be for substantial breaches or if the partnership around quality improvement processes were to be disrupted or not show meaningful progress over time.

MEASURING OUTCOMES

Important measures in networking/affiliation work include the following: (1) financial and political success of the affiliation, (2) closure of gaps in patient care, (3) performance on quality and safety metrics and change in the culture of safety over time, (4) maintenance of the brand without risk to the AHC, and (5) optimal marketing of the brand to the benefit of both entities.

Our Pediatric joint venture has been successful over the past 2–3 years with regional branding of our joint logo specifically around the Pediatric market; development of partnership and trust; joint enhancement in programmatic, subspecialty efforts around children's care; marked increases in Press Ganey patient satisfaction assessments; ongoing development of a robust Pediatric safety and quality program and culture; and maintenance of the brand. It is gratifying that we are now beginning to work as a system in terms of bed utilization; patient care resources; and transfer of patients between entities as the level of care requirements dictate, all to the advantage of both our institution and our affiliate. Finally, the ultimate winner is the patient and family for whom enhanced subspecialty care can be provided locally whenever possible.

FOLLOW-UP AND MAINTENANCE

Relationships between an AHC and an affiliate are constantly in flux. In many ways, one is continually threading the needle between differing agendas; developing compromises around the needs, vision, resources, and finances of differing entities; and relentlessly building high-quality programs and developing partnerships and trust. All of these ongoing efforts form the infrastructure that is the basis for the brand and its safe use.

REFERENCES

1. Beaulieu ND, Dafny LS, Landon BE, et al. Changes in quality of care after hospital mergers and Acquisitions. *NEJM*. 2020;382:51–59.
2. Wang E, Arnold S, and Jones S. Quality and safety outcomes of a hospital merger following a full integration at a safety net hospital. *JAMA Netw Open*. 2022;5(1):e2142382.
3. Haas S, Gawande A, Reynolds ME. The risks to patient safety from health system expansions. *JAMA*. 2018;319(17): 1765–1766. doi: 10.1001/jama.2018.2074
4. https://www.sfchronicle.com/bayarea/article/john-muir-medical-child-surgery-17057392.php
5. https://www.healthcaremarketinglaw.com
6. https://www.stanfordchildrens.org/content-public/pdf/brand-guidelines.pdf

Outreach and Referral Building at New Network Affiliates

19

BRENT D. MATTHEWS

Clinical Delivery Challenge

Atrium Health is an integrated, nonprofit health system headquartered in Charlotte, North Carolina, serving more than 7 million patients at 42 hospitals and more than 1,500 care locations across North Carolina, South Carolina, Georgia, Virginia, and Alabama. The Greater Charlotte Region (GCR) of Atrium Health includes nine hospitals, ranging from a 109-bed rural hospital to a 1100-bed, Level 1 trauma, academic medical center, Atrium Health Carolinas Medical Center. All locations in the GCR have open medical staffs merging Atrium Health Medical Group general surgeons with independent, affiliated surgery groups except the Level 1 trauma, academic medical center that has our Department of Surgery with Divisions of Abdominal Transplant Surgery, Acute Care Surgery, Surgical Oncology, General and Gastrointestinal Surgery, Pediatric Surgery, and Hepatopancreatic and Biliary Surgery performing the breadth of general surgery.

Providing surgery care locally through enhanced access to patient-focused quality care is a priority for the health system's regional hospital and predictably an accelerator for growth. Maintaining in-network referrals and increasing patient selection from primary and secondary markets are shared goals between the new network-affiliated general surgeons and regional hospitals. The challenges to do so with the new network-affiliated general surgeons are multifaceted, but primarily focused on surgeon engagement and alignment to data-driven, evidence-based care models and goal-oriented, metric-driven incentives. An internal challenge for the health system is the decision to diversify capabilities at the hospital through the redistribution of subspecialty surgery services from the academic medical center.

Operational efficiency, care coordination, cost containment, risk-based contracting, population health management, and service line or asset rationalization are drivers for affiliation in the healthcare marketplace.[1] Affiliations can be horizontal (hospital to hospital), vertical (hospital or health system to multispecialty or single-specialty group), or a combination of both. Examples of strategic affiliations include hospital or health system/physician group employment, clinical integration [Accountable Care Organization (ACO) or Clinically Integrated Network (CIN)], contractual arrangement (management or professional services agreements), and joint venture. As the convener, the network's outreach activities are critical to facilitate referrals for new network affiliates. Numerous data sources and engagement, alignment, marketing, and business development strategies guide the process. Envision a surgery group that is the exclusive provider of general surgery care at a new network, tertiary care hospital, yet remains independent with privileges at a competing health system's hospital in the primary service area (PSA). Maintaining in-network referrals and increasing patient selection from the primary and secondary markets are strategic imperatives.

Data Needed to Understand Surgical Care Across the Network

To understand current referral patterns, there are several primary data sources to review. Atrium Health Strategy Partners, a corporate services group for enterprise strategy, planning, and transformation, can provide estimated patient selection data for a PSA to a metropolitan statistical area (MSA) for outpatient and inpatient services. Trends for overall case volumes, PSA or MSA demand, network hospital growth or decline, and regional competitor hospital statistics are detailed according to the surgical services (HPB Surgery, Colorectal/Lower GI, Hernia Surgery, Bariatrics, Upper GI, etc.) provided. This is further subdivided into payor status (commercial, Medicare, Medicaid, and self-pay). Care alignment data in the PSA

121

or MSA is captured to delineate referrals from Atrium Health Primary Care and Atrium Health Specialty Care to Atrium Health Medical Group, affiliate, and nonaffiliate surgeons. Affiliate surgeons are defined by participation in the health systems CIN and ACO without employment through the Atrium Health Medical Group. Nonaffiliate surgeons are independent and do not participate in the CIN or ACO. These data sources are most accurate for in-network patients and directionally accurate for out-of-network patients and hospital competitor inpatient and outpatient surgery volumes.

Another critical data source is the American College of Surgeons (ACS) National Surgical Quality Improvement Program (NSQIP) semiannual reports. All nine of the GCR hospitals participate in ACS NSQIP bolstered by an Atrium Health ACS NSQIP Quality Collaborative of 13 hospitals across North Carolina, South Carolina, and Georgia (Figure 19.1). We can compare the risk-adjusted general

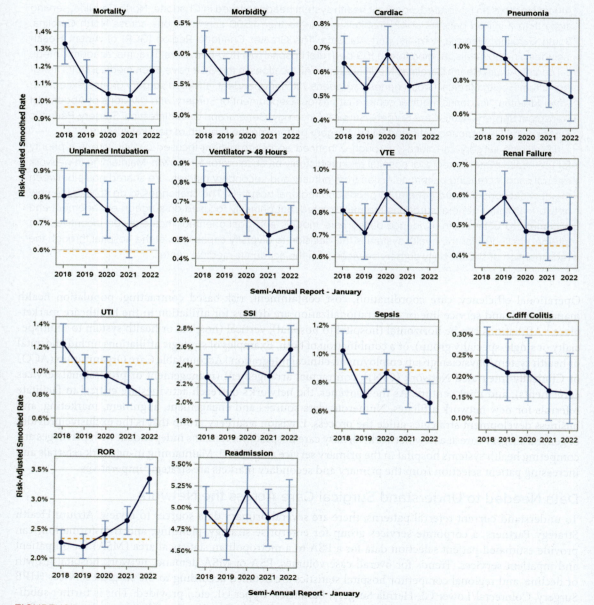

FIGURE 19.1 Atrium Health ACS NSQIP Collaborative 5-year outcome trends for 13 participating hospitals.

surgical occurrence at the new network hospital within the quality collaborative and identify areas needing performance improvement. Determining opportunities in subspecialty surgery care, Atrium Health Levine Cancer Institute provides Metrics Reports that detail case volumes, margin-free resections, preoperative tumor markers, nodal harvest, minimally invasive surgery rates, referral to medical oncology based on oncologic stage, reoperation/re-excision rates, consideration of reconstruction options, and tumor-specific care pathway compliance and patient outcomes for breast and colorectal cancer, respectively (Table 19.1).

Clinical Optimization is a physician-led program in Atrium Health to realize cost savings through the reduction in care variation.[2] Quarterly performance reports are provided for General Surgery leadership among many service lines. Atrium Health General Surgery Service Line primarily advances cost curve shifting through contractual negotiation to lower prices for disposable supplies (endomechanical, electrosurgical, trocars, etc.). Surgeon behaviors are revealed through cost-narrowing opportunities representing shifts in clinical practice toward single care standards (disposable supplies, care pathways, etc.) across General Surgery. Mean variable cost per case is calculated for every general surgeon in the GCR

Table 19.1	Levine Cancer Institute Colon Metric Report (January–July 2020) for Preoperative CEA Level, Margin-Free Resection Rate, and Mean Nodes Harvested for Colectomy		
Surgeon Name	Number of Planned Colectomies	Number of Planned Colectomies with Pre-Operative CEA Value	Planned Colectomies % with Pre-Operative CEA Value
D	1	0	0%
F	2	1	50%
R	2	1	50%
I	2	1	50%
X	12	8	67%
A	11	8	73%
BB	4	3	75%
AA	4	3	75%
B	13	12	92%
EE	3	3	100%
V	7	7	100%
G	1	1	100%
	21	21	100%
Y	1	1	100%
CC	2	2	100%
N	1	1	100%
L	2	2	100%
C	1	1	100%
FF	2	2	100%
E	1	1	100%
DD	2	2	100%
H	1	1	100%
Atrium Metro	96	82	85%

(continued)

Table 19.1 — Levine Cancer Institute Colon Metric Report (January–July 2020) for Preoperative CEA Level, Margin-Free Resection Rate, and Mean Nodes Harvested for Colectomy *(Continued)*

Surgeon Name	Number of Planned Colectomies	Number of Planned Colectomies (Margin-Free)	Planned Colectomies % Margin-Free
FF	2	1	50%
BB	4	2	50%
V	7	6	86%
A	11	10	91%
G	1	1	100%
Y	1	1	100%
N	1	1	100%
D	1	1	100%
C	1	1	100%
E	1	1	100%
H	1	1	100%
F	2	2	100%
R	2	2	100%
CC	2	2	100%
L	2	2	100%
DD	2	2	100%
I	2	2	100%
EE	3	3	100%
AA	4	4	100%
X	12	12	100%
B	13	13	100%
	21	21	100%
Atrium Metro	96	91	95%

Surgeon Name	Number of Planned Colectomies	Total Nodes (Median)	Total Nodes (Range)
L	2	5	4–6
A	11	14	10–69
BB	4	15	15–17
CC	2	15	14–16
B	13	15	13–24
DD	2	16	12–19
E	1	17	17
EE	3	20	16–21
C	1	20	20
R	2	23	21–24
FF	2	23	21–24
N	1	23	23

Table 19.1 — Levine Cancer Institute Colon Metric Report (January–July 2020) for Preoperative CEA Level, Margin-Free Resection Rate, and Mean Nodes Harvested for Colectomy *(Continued)*

Surgeon Name	Number of Planned Colectomies	Total Nodes (Median)	Total Nodes (Range)
H	1	24	24
I	2	25	22–27
F	2	29	15–43
AA	4	31	10–58
G	1	31	31
X	12	32	16–50
V	7	32	13–42
D	1	33	33
	21	34	8–83
Y	1	47	47
Atrium Metro	96	21	4–83

(Figure 19.2). The quality and cost data define baseline value metrics but also reveal opportunities for the affiliate general surgery group to participate in the CIN's Hospital Quality and Efficiency Program, a mechanism to create aligned incentives to support hospitals reduce costs associated with the delivery of care while financially rewarding surgeons for their role in reducing costs and maintaining predetermined quality outcomes metrics.

The Atrium Health Physician Connection Line (PCL) transfer center is a 24 hours a day, 7 days a week link between an inpatient or emergency department referring provider and a surgeon at Atrium Health. A transfer center specialist guides physicians through requests for consultation, transfer, and bed placement for a higher level of care and/or specialty services. Patient demographics, diagnosis, referring provider, accepting surgery service, and reason for transfer are recorded for patients transferred out of the facility. The PCL transfer data reveals not only volumes of patients transferred for surgical care from the network hospital but gives insight into resource constraints or technical skill gaps in general surgery at the new network hospital.

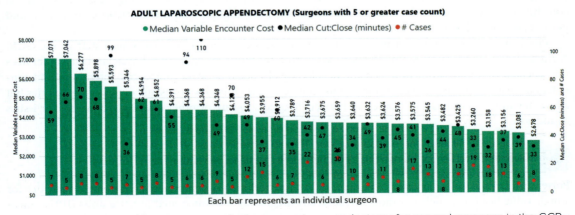

FIGURE 19.2 Mean variable cost per case for laparoscopic appendectomy for general surgeons in the GCR.

Stakeholders for Surgical Care Across the Network

A qualitative assessment through stakeholder interviews is critical to understanding perspectives, attitudes, and experiences to evaluate current state of general surgery care at the network hospital. The qualitative assessments are performed by Atrium Health Medical Group Surgery Care Division physician and administrative leadership. Stakeholders are identified and information needed and from whom is defined. The stakeholder group includes Atrium Health and affiliated primary care (Family Medicine, Internal Medicine, Gynecology), Gastroenterology, Emergency Medicine, Anesthesia, Critical Care, Radiology, facility executives, Chief Nursing and Medical Officers, and Perioperative leadership. The primary stakeholder group is the affiliated network of general surgeons.

● DIFFERENTIAL DIAGNOSIS

The affiliated general surgery group may have minimal tolerance for risk (change) considering the existing economic pressures of independent surgery practice. Relinquishing care for the emergency general surgery patient population detaches them from a predictable volume of patient consultations and surgery cases. Engagement and alignment to data-driven, evidence-based care models could be viewed as a diversion from standard workflow patterns. If the health system decides to diversify capabilities at the hospital through redistribution of subspecialty surgery services from the academic medical center, the affiliated general surgeons may disengage as a strategic partner because Atrium Health Medical Group general surgery could evolve into a competitor for patient referrals.

● DIAGNOSIS AND TREATMENT

The highest leverage area to approach the affiliated general surgeons will be aligned incentives and engagement through Atrium Health's culture commitments of creating a space where all belong, earning trust, working as one team, innovating to better the now and create the future, and driving for excellence always.

We can scale internal clinical strengths in general surgery through surgeon-led integration of standardized care pathways or alternative care models [prehabilitation, enhanced recovery after surgery (ERAS®), virtual care), participation in data-driven quality improvement processes (Atrium Health ACS NSQIP Collaborative), alignment and participation in multidisciplinary patient care structures (Levine Cancer Institute, Center for Digestive Health), and support them with electronic health information technology (IT). Although reducing disparities in outcomes, providing top quartile benchmarked quality, and providing highly reliable local care are alignment incentives to build patient referrals, we can employ financial incentives as well through participation in our CIN, Atrium Health Collaborative Physician Alliance (CPA), a physician-led care collaborative focusing on delivering efficient, affordable, coordinated care. Financial incentives (shared savings) are aligned with membership expectations and performance standards.

Physician liaisons are the primary contact for physicians, practice managers, and staff in the GCR. Atrium Health Corporate Communication, Marketing & Outreach (CCM&O) Physician Liaison Services is a crucial lever in providing outreach and developing physician network campaigns. Intentional and consistent outreach not only conveys information about relevant clinical services and evolving capabilities but allows for time-sensitive identification of barriers to access to care or other questions, concerns, or issues to address.

● SCIENTIFIC PRINCIPLES AND EVIDENCE

Porter and Lee's *The Strategy that Will Fix Health Care* outlines six components or strategic priorities for a high-value healthcare delivery model, specifically organizing into integrated practice units (IPUs), measuring outcomes and costs for every patient, moving to bundled payment for care cycles, integrated care delivery systems, expanded geographical reach, and building an enabling IT platform. Organizing into IPUs and measuring outcomes and cost being are the most critical to physicians.[3] The article states that "maintaining market share will be difficult for providers with nonemployed physicians if their inability to work together impedes progress in improving value ... hospitals with private-practice physicians will have to learn to function as a team to remain viable."

Research in healthcare organizational change has revealed critical steps to alignment that include seeking to understand why change does not align with existing culture and mission and to engage with data to explain and provide urgency.[4] Principles of Kotter's process for leading change include urgency, colalitions, creating and communicating a vision then empowering others to act on the vision, planning and creating short-term wins, consolidating improvements, and producing more change and institutionalizing (surgery groups behaviors to programmatic success) new approaches applies to this situation, but requires a phased approach, championed by surgery and hospital facility leadership in collaboration with an affiliated general surgery leader.[5]

U.S. general surgery consolidation is highlighted by a 21% reduction in unique general surgery practices and a 50% increase in general surgery practices affiliated with groups of 500 or more over the past decade.[6] Significant alteration in surgeon practice environments is occurring during an accelerated rate of hospital mergers and acquisitions. Hospital mergers and acquisitions have been associated with increased negotiated prices with commercial insurers, and modest deterioration in performance on patient experience with variable changes in readmission rates, mortality rates, or clinical-process measures.[7,8] Accepted evaluation frameworks do not exist to monitor or assess quality measures prior to and after hospital mergers and acquisitions, a fundamental gap to guide evolving care delivery models, structures, or collaborations.

An Athenahealth Physician Sentiment Index 2021 report revealed that providers going through a healthcare merger or acquisition are less likely to be willing to stay at their organization and more likely to experience physician burnout.[9] Other physicians reported feeling less positive about their collaboration with colleagues. Is this too much disruption for the affiliate general surgeons?

● IMPLEMENTING A SOLUTION

Organizational changes in healthcare delivery are bound by the responsibility to improve access, patient experience, quality, and affordability, but at the very least prevent regression in patient-centered outcomes. Successful change is characterized by giving the opportunity for physicians to influence the change, preparing them for the change, and demonstrating the value of change.[10] The Change Acceleration Model (CAM) is a resource available to physician leaders in Atrium Health that provides a structured, targeted approach to change that incorporates the elements of stakeholder participation, preparation, and value.

Analyze and Approach

This phase is dominated by conducting stakeholder interviews and reviewing primary data sources previously detailed. The analysis provides a framework for developing a project charter to organize and define fundamental project details including milestones, scope, success metrics, and a communication plan. In the current scenario, we determined that to increase referrals to the affiliated general surgeon to perform predominately elective, scheduled procedures, to participate in evidence-based care pathway redesign (ie, prehabilitation, ERAS) or quality collaborative initiatives, to partner fully with our Physician Liaison Service, and to build capabilities to participate in the CIN/ACO required minimizing their exposure to unscheduled, urgent, and emergent general surgery care at the hospital. This will also allow us to segment this more challenging population of patients to improve access and timeliness to care and patient outcomes or experience. Atrium Health Medical Group Regional General Surgery will provide emergency general surgery services within the GCR Acute Care Surgery Network. In addition, we concluded that subspecialty surgery services of breast surgical oncology and HPB surgery were essential to maintain in-network referrals and increase PSA referrals. The solutions for this will be disparate. We will support the recruitment of a breast surgical oncologist to be employed by the affiliated general surgery group but have a professional services agreement as a Levine Cancer Institute director and redistribute our HPB surgery program from the Level 1 trauma, academic center to the new network hospital supported by the recruitment of two fellowship-trained HPB surgeons employed through Atrium Health Department of Surgery.

Aware

This phase is highlighted by introducing change to the affiliate general surgery group and medical staff at the new network hospital and building awareness around the goals and anticipated outcomes. We also had to identify leadership who would champion the change. This includes leadership within the affiliated general surgery group, Atrium Health Primary and Specialty Care, and facility administration.

Aspire

Hesitation and resistance are natural responses to change, so it is important to share the "why" behind the change, increasing referrals to the affiliated general surgeons, reputation management (general surgeon and hospital), and economic health. It is important to involve the affiliated general surgeons in decisions and determine their attitudes toward the changes in emergency general surgery and HPB surgery coverage. This iterative process required regularly scheduled meetings with the affiliated general surgery group and other key stakeholders, primarily Atrium Health Primary Care and Specialty Care leadership, but also Atrium Health CCM&O and Physician Liaison Services.

Accelerate

To accelerate the initiatives outlined, we need to continuously identify and remove obstacles and barriers. Perhaps the most significant barrier was trust. Naturally, there was skepticism from the affiliated general surgery group. Can Atrium Health Medical Group build emergency general surgery and HPB surgery programs at the new network hospital while concurrently supporting the affiliated general surgery group to build a more robust referral network and a breast surgical oncology program? Would relinquishing the care of the emergency general surgery patient negatively impact their collaboration with the medical staff or group finances? Would all the workflow changes in patient care such as evidence-based care pathways or participation in performance improvement and quality collaboratives equate to increased patient referrals? The contrast of creating trust with the affiliate general surgeons while simultaneously having difficult conversations due to the change experienced was managed through appreciative inquiry, a method of asking questions to gather information for positive intent. Ultimately, we needed to foster relationships and increase the capacity for collaboration and change.

Anchor

At this stage during the adoption of change, the affiliated general surgery group has committed to the plan primarily based on positive initial results such as increased in-network referrals, increased surgery case volumes, improved operating room block utilization, and the cultivation of local physician referral relationships by the Physician Liaison Service. The affiliated general surgeons also witnessed their capacity to maintain the autonomy of group business decisions while realizing the efficiencies of a general surgery practice focused on elective, scheduled care.

Assess

Quantitative data guides the assessment of current state changes. The primary data sources were discussed previously. Key performance indicators such as the affiliated general surgeons' case volumes and operating room block utilization at the network hospital and associated ambulatory surgery center are monitored. On a yearly basis, estimated patient selection data for the PSA for outpatient and inpatient services will be refreshed to evaluate trends. Care alignment data in the PSA will be monitored to evaluate in-network referrals from Atrium Health Primary Care and Atrium Health Specialty Care.

The project management action plan has multiple strategic actions related to surgeon recruitment to support increasing referrals to the affiliated general surgeons. This includes (1) segmenting elective,

Key Steps in Change Management and Potential Pitfalls

Key Steps in Change Management	Increasing Referrals to Affiliated General Surgeon	Potential Pitfalls
Analyze & Approach	Stakeholder interviews, reviewing primary data sources, and formulating the project action plan	Not effectively assessing change readiness of the affiliated general surgeons
Aware	Reinforcing goals and anticipated outcomes of project action plan	Not identifying a change champion in the affiliated general surgery group; lack of consensus
Aspire	Communicate the "why" - increasing referrals to the affiliated general surgeons, reputation management (general surgeon and hospital), and economic health	Cynicism, skepticism of affiliated general surgery group inhibits engagement
Accelerate	Removing obstacles or barriers	Failure of primary care or specialty care to refer to affiliated general surgeons
Anchor	Commitment to change reinforced by an increase in network referrals, increased surgery case volumes, improved operating room block utilization, and the cultivation of local physician referral relationships by the Physician Liaison Service	Multiple stakeholder groups are required for success and internal financial metrics for affiliated general surgery group are proprietary
Assess	Data review and feedback	Sustainability dependent on long-term engagement of affiliated general surgery group and continuous process improvement of quality, evidence-base care

scheduled from unscheduled, urgent/emergent general surgery by developing an Atrium Health EGS program, (2) increasing retention of patients at and transfer into the new network hospital with pancreatic, biliary, and hepatic surgery condition by developing an Atrium Health HPB Surgery program, and (3) partnering with the affiliated general surgery group to recruit a breast surgical oncologist to minimize the previous high volume of patient referrals out of the PSA to the academic medical center or competing academic medical centers in North Carolina. It will be critical that all three of these strategic actions are managed with similar priority and focus to achieve project goals and objectives despite the financial investment being weighted to Atrium Health assets and resources.

● MEASURING OUTCOMES

The key performance metric is monthly and year-to-date general surgery case volumes at the new network hospital and ambulatory surgery center. This is not only for the affiliated general surgery group but for overall volumes to include developing programs for EGS and HPB surgeries. An unintended consequence could be "mission creep" with the EGS or HPB surgery groups competing for elective general surgery cases outside their core responsibilities. Initially, we anticipate increasing volumes at the ambulatory surgery center for the affiliate general surgery group. Transferring primary responsibility for emergency room calls and inpatient urgent or emergent consultations to an EGS group provides them the flexibility to utilize the off-campus ambulatory surgery center without unscheduled disruptions. Another unintended consequence as this model is implemented is the affiliated general surgeons feeling less fulfilled or professionally satisfied by relinquishing primary responsibility for the care of urgent or emergent surgical care. Nevertheless, as their referrals increase for higher acuity inpatient services and multidisciplinary breast surgical oncology patients, we project an increase in hospital-based surgical volumes. Estimated patient selection data for the PSA and care coordination data for Atrium Health Primary Care and Specialty Care will be utilized to evaluate referral trends and retention within the submarket. Additional performance metrics include semiannual patient outcomes reports and quarterly cost reports as measures of value-based care in preparation for participation in the CIN/ACO.

● FOLLOW-UP AND MAINTENANCE

We completed an after-action review to reflect on how the changes were implemented and to critically evaluate opportunities for sustainability. Ensuring that Atrium Health executive, Medical Group, surgery, finance, and facility leadership and corporate services (CCM&O, Liaison Services, etc.) continuously had situational awareness was challenging. The complexity of a matrixed leadership and resourced model would periodically lead to bureaucratic inertia or miscommunication with key stakeholder groups. Situational awareness, communication alignment, and coordinated action planning were fostered by implementing a bimonthly tactical market meeting. These serve as a forum to review key performance metrics, financial performance, care coordination data, PSA and MSA growth and demand for services, prioritize corrective actions, or coordinate tactics to advance growth and clinical integration strategies.

REFERENCES

1. Healthcare Financial Management Association. Acquisition and affiliation strategies: an HFMA Value Project Report Phase III. 2014.
2. Birnham EB, Riley J, Zweig M, et al. Achieving cost-savings goals through care variation reduction: Advisory Board Report. 2017.
3. Porter ME, Lee TH. The strategy that will fix health care. *Harv Bus Rev.* 2013;91:50–70.
4. Westra D, Angeli F, Kemp R, et al. If you say so: a mixed-method study of hospital mergers and quality of care. *Health Care Manage Rev.* 2022;47:37–48.
5. Kotter JP. Leading change: why transformation efforts fail. *Harv Bus Rev.* 1995;73:59–67.
6. Anderson ST, Hammond JB, Hogan JS, et al. Current trends in U.S. general surgery practice consolidation. *Am J Surg.* 2022;223:477–480.
7. Beaulieu ND, Dafny LS, Landon BE, et al. Changes in quality of care after hospital mergers and acquisitions. *N Engl J Med.* 2020;382:51–59.
8. Mariani M, Sisti LG, Isonne C, et al. Impact of hospital mergers: a systematic review focusing on healthcare quality measures. *Eur J Public Health.* 2022;2:191–199.
9. AthenaHealth. Physician Sentiment Index: insights into the physician experience. 2021.
10. Nilsen P, Seing I, Ericsson C, et al. Characteristics of successful changes in health care organizations: an interview study with physicians, registered nurses and assistant nurses. *BMC Health Serv Res.* 2020;20:147–155.

Coordinating Care and Referrals Across Affiliates

20

RYAN A. J. CAMPAGNA AND ANDREW C. CHANG

Clinical Delivery Challenge

The patient is a 33-year-old man who presents with a recently diagnosed distal esophageal adenocarcinoma. He has a history of spina bifida, myelomeningocele, and long-standing gastroesophageal reflux disease. A ventriculoperitoneal shunt was placed in childhood. He regularly consumes cigarettes, smokeless tobacco, and alcohol.

Despite advances in screening and risk-factor modification, esophageal cancer claims the lives of over 16,000 Americans annually.[1] Treatment of this deadly malignancy requires the integration of multiple healthcare specialists across a variable timeline. Surgical care is increasingly delivered at specific centers within a given health system, while medical and radiographic services are often accessed throughout the system. Additional stressors, such as the COVID-19 pandemic, have exacerbated care fragmentation across these complex networks.[2] Surgeons are often tasked with coordinating care within and between health systems during the perioperative period. To do so, we are challenged to align multiple provider networks with several data/information systems.

Over the course of the past three decades, the hospital landscape within the United States has significantly coalesced. The delivery of healthcare services has shifted from a multitude of siloed hospitals into local and regional healthcare systems.[3] This development has concomitantly improved access to advanced care modalities and introduced logistical challenges with coordinating intersystem care, especially for complex health conditions. Patients may suffer from suboptimal coordination between these systems, an effect known as care fragmentation.[4] This may contribute to worse clinical outcomes among patients with surgically treatable diseases, especially those with at-risk social determinants of health.[1,4] Herein, we use a case-based format to explore the challenges associated with coordinating care and referrals across affiliates of a health system.

● WORKUP

The requisite clinical data for a newly referred patient with esophageal cancer include a history and physical, diagnostic esophagogastroduodenoscopy, endoscopic ultrasound, and positron emission tomography (PET)/CT. Data obtained prior to the initial consultation is variably incorporated into the workup, as dictated by institutional practices of the referral center. For some organizations, studies obtained outside of the system are repeated internally as a rule. For others, incoming data is screened by a healthcare provider and/or their administrative staff for quality and recency. Based on the screening outcome, the studies are rejected and repeated, submitted for review by internal specialists (eg, pathology slides), or accepted in their current state. The integration of the electronic medical record between and within health systems has greatly facilitated data acquisition for referral patients. Nevertheless, the physical transfer of hard-copy records remains a common method for data transfer.

Stakeholders who navigate this process include patients, referring medical professionals, consultant medical professionals, office administrators, social workers, case managers, patient navigators, and other allied health professionals. Coordination between stakeholders takes place via post, telephone, and electronic means. Ensuring a shared understanding of the underlying institutional network can greatly facilitate communication among the stakeholders.

A useful taxonomy for the relationship of health system components was described by Shay and Mick.[5] The authors delineate *horizontal*, *vertical*, and *spatial differentiation* of local multihospital system (LMS) components, as depicted in Figure 20.1. *Horizontal differentiation* refers to the number of unique services offered by an LMS, whereas *vertical differentiation* refers to "qualitative variation in the complexity or level of care offered among organizational units."[5] *Spatial differentiation* is defined as the geographic relationship or layout of LMS components. Mapping out all three aspects of differentiation will in turn depict the *configuration* of a given LMS. The authors also define *integration* within a health system as the combination of differentiated components. *Horizontal integration* describes the incorporation of components with interchangeable outputs (eg, ambulatory care centers), whereas *vertical integration* involves the combination of non-substitutable components to produce a complete health service.[5] Navigating the patient experience across integrated and spatially differentiated LMS components requires *coordination* among healthcare professionals.

> The patient is wheelchair dependent and lives 120 miles from our institution's main quaternary care center. He is socially supported by his parents, who accompany him to medical visits and provide care at his home. All diagnostic studies were accessible via electronic medical records. Esophagogastroduodenoscopy/endoscopic ultrasound revealed a 2-cm friable mass in the distal esophagus consistent with a uT2N0 carcinoma. PET/CT demonstrated short segmental uptake in the distal esophagus without evidence of obvious metastatic disease.

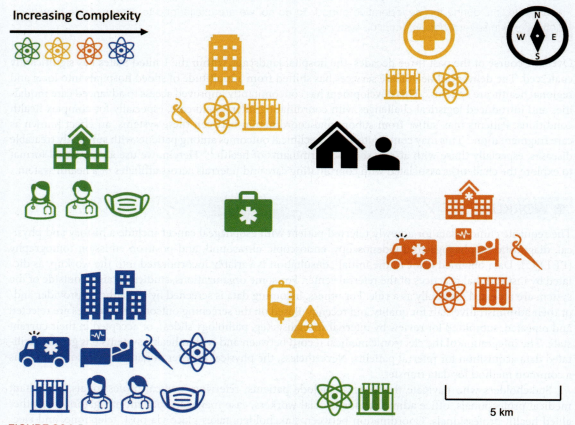

FIGURE 20.1 Patient-centered configuration of a theoretical LMS. Individual icons represent a health system component. Horizontal and vertical differentiation are denoted by icon illustrations and colors, respectively. Spatial differentiation is depicted by position on the map relative to the patient's home.

CHAPTER 20 • Coordinating Care and Referrals Across Affiliates

● DIFFERENTIAL DIAGNOSIS

Coordination within a health system is a function of its differentiation and integration. LMSs with limited differentiation may necessitate referral to outside healthcare systems, which often complicates communication and data exchange between providers. Highly differentiated systems offer care of varying complexity at several geographic locations, thereby improving patient access and limiting outside referrals. However, poor integration of system components may also lead to insufficient data exchange and provider communication. Therefore, systems at the highest risk of strained care coordination include those with limited differentiation and poor integration.

● DIAGNOSIS AND TREATMENT

The increasing prevalence and growing complexity of LMSs is a relatively recent phenomenon. However, the need to systematically assess a problem, develop a solution, and implement changes within a health system is not.

Performance intelligence is a framework used in health systems research to, "gather comparable data, develop indicators and identify optimal strategies for taking action."[2]

The first step in applying the performance intelligence framework to the coordination of care across health systems is obtaining the relevant data. Delineating the overall system structure, the identity and position of the key stakeholders within the system, and the available communication methods is crucial. Identifying current administrative practices for referral intake and information dissemination among providers is similarly important. Assessing clinical efficiency, as measured by care milestone intervals (eg, days from initial consultation to definitive treatment), number of patient and provider correspondences (eg, phone calls, print and electronic mails, EMR messaging), and other administrative metrics, is also warranted at this time. These data may serve as performance indicators throughout the implementation of a system intervention.

The second step in applying a performance intelligence framework to this clinical delivery challenge involves the analysis of the data gathered in the initial step. Key stakeholders review the data and apply their real-world experience to provide context and extract meaning. In doing so, they transform information into practical knowledge.[2] The latter informs decision-making and facilitates completion of the final step: action. Now that the stakeholders have gathered the appropriate data and applied their expertise to interpret the findings, they are able to construct meaningful interventions to the problem.

> The patient is slated for neoadjuvant chemoradiation followed by esophagectomy. His primary care, medical oncology, and radiation oncology providers are housed at separate clinics within our LMS. Electronic medical records from these encounters are accessible to all providers. The care clinics, infusion clinic, and radiography center are within 10 miles of his home. An oncology nurse navigator assists the patient remotely throughout his preoperative chemoradiation.

● SCIENTIFIC PRINCIPLES AND EVIDENCE

Two other frameworks deserve mention in addressing the coordination of care across health systems, both of which come from the Veterans Health Administration (VHA).[6,7] The VHA is a national integrated health system that serves millions of U.S. military veterans annually. These patients seek variably complex care in many practice settings, from routine outpatient health maintenance visits to advanced inpatient surgical admissions. As such, VHA providers have developed and studied numerous initiatives to integrate care across their network.

Atkins et al. describe the VHA's successful campaign for Patient Aligned Care Teams (PACTs) in the ambulatory setting.[6] PACTs are composed of various allied health professionals—primary care providers, nurse managers, pharmacists, and others—who aim to, "deliver coordinated, proactive team-based primary care to better address the needs of primary care patients, especially those with chronic diseases."[6] Services provided by PACTs promote provider coordination, patient education/self-management, and ancillary service utilization. The implementation of PACTs led to increased provider–patient communication and

SECTION 4 • Building Regional Networks

patient satisfaction. Moreover, sites utilizing PACTs experienced a decrease in emergency department utilization, increase in telehealth resources, and fewer inpatient admission for ambulatory-appropriate conditions.[6]

Another important VHA investigation was carried out by Rabin and colleagues.[7] They report on a multifaceted, ongoing quality initiative that spans various aspects of patient care. Two notable projects center on care transitions between health systems: one between out-of-network hospitals and network primary care providers, and the other between tertiary VHA hospitals and home PACTs.[7] Both projects utilize a data management framework to amass real-time feedback and implement iterative changes. The original framework, based on the constructs of Reach, Effectiveness, Adoption, Implementation, and Maintenance (RE-AIM), was simplified to reflect the *Who, What, When, Why,* and *How* of a given policy adaptation.[7,8] Periodic, semi-structured interviews are held with multiple stakeholders, during which the framework is used to gather data and make modifications in real time. This model is attractive due to its scalability and simplicity, and one can envisage its applicability to care transitions within the private sector. One important limitation of this method is the considerable cost of additional administrative support.

● IMPLEMENTING A SOLUTION

We advocate for a structured approach to identify and address care coordination challenges within an LMS. Given the complexity of the current healthcare landscape, a measured and reproducible approach is critical for affecting meaningful change. The essential steps of our proposed management plan are listed in Key Steps in Change Management and Potential Pitfalls. Developing a fundamental comprehension of the LMS's unique structure is the first step. Using standardized language, such as the taxonomy listed above, will help cement a shared understanding among stakeholders.[5] A diagram depicting the health system taxonomy is a useful adjunct. Next, one should apply a performance intelligence framework to gather the relevant health system data, construct indicators of performance, extract contextual information/knowledge, identify underlying deficiencies, and create an intervention.[2] Finally, employ a data acquisition and analysis plan, such as the modified RE-AIM framework, to monitor real-time progress and implement modifications via an iterative process.[7]

Key Steps in Change Management and Potential Pitfalls

Key Steps in Change Management

1. Outline your LMS structure using a standardized taxonomy.
2. Apply a performance intelligence framework:
   a. Gather relevant LMS data and metrics
   b. Construct indicators of performance
   c. Interpret the findings with stakeholders to extract information/knowledge
   d. Identify system deficiencies
   e. Create an intervention with measurable outcomes
3. Adopt a real-time data acquisition/analysis model to monitor progress and implement modifications.

Potential Pitfalls

1. Failure to identify LMS components.
2. Omission of system-wide, multilevel stakeholders.
3. Focusing primarily on indicators/deficiencies that affect a narrow stakeholder audience.
4. Failure to analyze and modify interventions iteratively.
5. Underestimating the cost of administrative support.
6. Neglecting modifications that address systemic inequities.

CHAPTER 20 • Coordinating Care and Referrals Across Affiliates

There are several potential pitfalls for this proposed management plan. A special note must be made for a pitfall especially germane to the United States. It is well documented that advances in cancer care over the past several decades have led to improved patient survival and quality of life. However, in the United States, these advances disproportionally benefit patients who identify as Non-Hispanic White and have a higher socioeconomic status.[1,9] Moreover, Non-White patients seeking oncologic surgery encounter significantly more care fragmentation as they navigate health systems, despite accounting for differences in cancer stage, medical comorbidities, and insurance status.[4,9] The American Cancer Society recently proposed interventions in the domains of surgical practice, research, and policy that address systemic inequities, and it behooves our profession to urgently assimilate these recommendations into our health systems.[9]

The patient successfully completed neoadjuvant chemoradiation near his home. He presented to our main quaternary care center for minimally invasive transhiatal esophagectomy and followed an uneventful postoperative course. He was discharged 8 days after surgery with home nursing services. Final pathology revealed a ypT2N0, Stage IIB adenocarcinoma of the gastroesophageal junction. He was evaluated 3 weeks after surgery at our affiliate clinic, at which time he was gaining weight and tolerating a soft diet.

● MEASURING OUTCOMES

Numerous metrics are available for process analysis, as dictated by the identified performance indicators and system deficiencies. Readily trackable data points include the number, frequency, and character of patient/provider correspondences, care milestone time intervals, patient satisfaction, and practice volume metrics. Using the iterative intervention methods outlined above, stakeholders can assess the progress of their interventions and adjust approaches as necessary.

● FOLLOW-UP AND MAINTENANCE

Patients with surgically treated distal esophageal adenocarcinoma should be evaluated clinically and radiographically at regular intervals, per published guidelines. Surgery clinics often remain the focal point of patient care for several months (if not years) after an oncologic operation. Ongoing care should be delivered close to the patient's home when possible, especially for those who are situated far from the system's main medical campus. An allied health navigator should contact the patient periodically between visits. Virtual video-based visits are used with increasing frequency in this patient population.

The patient receives adjuvant immunotherapy directed by his local oncologist. He attends virtual visits at our clinic at regular intervals and obtains appropriate radiographic follow-up, per national consensus guidelines.

REFERENCES

1. Corona E, Yang L, Esrailian E, et al. Trends in esophageal cancer mortality and stage at diagnosis by race and ethnicity in the United States. *Cancer Causes Control*. 2021;32(8):883–894.
2. Kringos D, Carinci F, Barbazza E, et al. Managing COVID-19 within and across health systems: why we need performance intelligence to coordinate a global response. *Health Res Policy Syst*. 2020;18(1):80.
3. Cutler DM, Scott Morton F. Hospitals, market share, and consolidation. *JAMA*. 2013;310(18):1964–1970.
4. Doose M, Sanchez JI, Cantor JC, et al. Fragmentation of care among black women with breast cancer and comorbidities: the role of health systems. *JCO Oncol Pract*. 2021;17(5):e637–e44.
5. Shay PD, Mick SF. Organizational and environmental factors associated with local multihospital systems: precipitants for coordination? *Health Care Manage Rev*. 2021;46(4):319–331.

6. Atkins D, Kilbourne AM, Shulkin D. Moving from discovery to system-wide change: the role of research in a learning health care system: experience from three decades of health systems research in the Veterans Health Administration. *Annu Rev Public Health*. 2017;38:467–487.
7. Rabin BA, McCreight M, Battaglia C, et al. Systematic, multimethod assessment of adaptations across four diverse health systems interventions. *Front Public Health*. 2018;6:102.
8. Hall TL, Holtrop JS, Dickinson LM, et al. Understanding adaptations to patient-centered medical home activities: the PCMH adaptations model. *Transl Behav Med*. 2017;7(4):861–872.
9. Alcaraz KI, Wiedt TL, Daniels EC, et al. Understanding and addressing social determinants to advance cancer health equity in the United States: a blueprint for practice, research, and policy. *CA Cancer J Clin*. 2020;70(1):31–46.

Investing in Health Outside the Hospital: Public and Community Infrastructure

21

POOJA CHANDRASHEKAR AND SACHIN H. JAIN

Clinical Delivery Challenge

The hospital staff knew Mr. N well. He was 65 years old, and in the past year, he had been hospitalized 6 times for a liver abscess that seemed to persist despite aggressive treatment. At first, his providers were perplexed, but a detailed social history soon shed light on the reasons for his vicious cycle of illness and hospitalization. Mr. N had immigrated to the United States almost 2 decades ago to escape war and poverty in Vietnam but had been unable to find stable employment and currently lived in a spare room in an acquaintance's basement. He had no access to reliable transportation and as a result, he was unable to pick up his medications after leaving the hospital. Finally, because Mr. N did not have a primary care physician (PCP) to discuss these concerns with, the local hospital's emergency department became his only option to access the care he needed.

Mr. N's case illustrates the importance of investing in health beyond the hospital's 4 walls. It is estimated that 20% of older adults are readmitted to the hospital within 30 days of discharge, in turn costing the Medicare program a staggering $24 billion each year. There are a number of reasons for this, including unmet medical, social, or behavioral health needs that make it challenging for patients to transition from the hospital to the community.

How can we address this delivery challenge, especially for patients recovering from surgery who have a greater need for rehabilitation, recuperation, symptom management, and continued medical management? In this chapter, we explore the 2 primary pieces to this puzzle: (1) streamlining the transition out of the hospital and to the next setting of care and (2) building the community-based infrastructure needed to help patients live healthy and independent lives in the long term.

● WORKUP

The first step to restructuring care for patients recovering from a surgical procedure is understanding the gaps that exist in the current system. Regarding the transition out of the hospital, it is important to understand how post-discharge needs are determined (eg, criteria used, which providers perform this assessment, to what extent patient and caregiver preferences are incorporated into this decision-making process) and discharge practices (eg, provision of patient-friendly discharge instructions, follow-up appointments, patient understanding of diagnosis, and satisfaction with discharge care).

Then, to understand the gaps in community-based infrastructure that lead to poor outcomes for surgical patients, it is important to understand the complex set of factors—both medical and nonmedical—that lead to these outcomes after discharge. Here we will use readmissions as our outcome of choice. It is fairly simple to use medical records, and insurance claims data to identify the most common diagnoses associated with readmissions, but it is more difficult (and arguably more important) to understand the social drivers. So far, few studies have asked patients to identify reasons for their own readmissions or examined patients' perspectives on reasons for readmission related to their clinical, social, and demographic characteristics. One way to address this gap in the existing literature is to survey patients readmitted within 30 days of discharge following a surgical procedure and query a wide range of potential factors contributing to readmission, including their ability to understand and follow discharge instructions, access to care, perceived challenges to staying healthy, caregiver support, and the social determinants of health (eg, transportation, stable housing, food security, and economic stability). These data will help us understand how best to design community-based health services to help patients stay healthy outside the hospital.

● DIFFERENTIAL DIAGNOSIS

In general, there are 3 "buckets" of root causes underlying the challenges associated with transitioning out of the hospital and to the community.

Discharge Planning

The first is poor discharge planning, including low rates of follow-up appointments and poor patient understanding of post-discharge care. In one study of older patients discharged home after hospitalization for acute coronary syndrome, heart failure, or pneumonia, over 40% of patients could not describe their diagnosis, warning symptoms, activity instructions, or diet guidelines in post-discharge interviews and over 26% of written discharge instructions were found to use language likely not intelligible or accessible to patients. In Mr. N's case, though the clinical staff consistently used an interpreter when speaking with him, he was discharged with written instructions in English, not Vietnamese—his first and preferred language.

Social or Behavioral Needs

The second "bucket" is unmet social or behavioral health needs. Patients may be connected to a social worker in the hospital (as Mr. N was, each time he was admitted), but this support often does not extend when they are discharged home or to another community-based care setting. One study of causes of readmissions found that substance use disorder, homelessness, or having 2 or more unmet social needs conferred more than twice the odds of having a preventable readmission.

Not Meeting the Patient Where They Are

The third "bucket" is care that does not meet patients where they are. This is often discussed in the context of care that is physically inaccessible to patients, but it is equally important to focus on *how* care is delivered and ensure it is culturally competent and aligned with patients' needs and preferences. That is, it is key for providers to understand how cultural elements such as ethnicity, race, language, cultural norms, and values intersect with patients' health needs and influence how patients prefer to communicate and participate in their care. There is growing evidence that receiving culturally competent care reduces hospital readmissions and improves outcomes, especially among patients with limited English proficiency or racial and ethnic minorities. This was true for Mr. N as well, where few providers took the time to understand his values (eg, he had struggled to find a Vietnamese community in Boston) and tailor interventions accordingly.

● DIAGNOSIS AND TREATMENT

Improving care for patients recovering from a surgical procedure requires transforming both the transition out of the hospital and the experience of receiving care in the community. In the transition out of the hospital, discharge planning and follow-up care remains a key obstacle.

One potential solution is enabling clinicians who care for patients in the hospital to also monitor patients in the outpatient setting. A good example of this is CareMore Health's Extensivist model, in which "extensivists" care for patients during and after a hospitalization in care centers and skilled nursing facilities until they are stable. If creating a new clinical role is not feasible, it is also possible to harness existing clinical staff to facilitate discharge planning. For example, at Rush University Medical Center's Enhanced Discharge Planning Program, social workers phone patients and caregivers after discharge to check in, identify any unanticipated needs, and connect them to healthcare providers and community-based services. Ultimately, both of these models prevent patients from falling through the cracks in our complex post-discharge system.

But it is not enough to stop there. Even after a successful transition out of the hospital, patients may fail to receive the care they need in the community. Of course, there are a number of reasons for this, but here

CHAPTER 21 • Investing in Health Outside the Hospital: Public and Community Infrastructure

we will focus on meeting patients where they are (referring to not just location, but also the importance of culturally sensitive care) and addressing patients' medical and nonmedical needs in tandem. One solution is to harness the underutilized potential of community health workers (CHWs) and better integrate them into outpatient models of care delivery. Because CHWs often hail from the same communities as their patients, they are able to serve as cultural brokers between communities and fragmented systems of care. They can leverage their cultural connectedness to provide tailored health coaching and support, identify social barriers that warrant a revised clinical assessment and plan that better addresses medical and nonmedical needs, and connect patients to community-based services. Integrating CHWs into community-based systems of care is supported by the literature—it is well established that CHWs can reduce the burden of illness among people with chronic disease and serious mental illness.

The crux of this puzzle is connecting these 2 pieces. Consider the following. Due to Mr. N's precarious social situation, he is deemed at high risk for readmission. At discharge, he receives written instructions in Vietnamese and speaks with a social worker who counsels him on post-discharge instructions and connects him to a PCP at a local community health center serving a predominantly East Asian population. The social worker speaks with the CHW at the community health center and tells her about Mr. N's medical and social needs, pointing out that he has trouble with transportation and may benefit from being connected to a cultural organization that serves the Vietnamese community in greater Boston. After Mr. N has settled in at home, the CHW reaches out, introducing herself, and asking if Mr. N needs assistance with transportation to make it to his PCP appointment. A week later, Mr. N receives a phone call from the same social worker, checking in and asking if he made it to his first PCP appointment. He says yes.

● SCIENTIFIC PRINCIPLES AND EVIDENCE

A useful framework to reference when tackling these problems is the Institute for Healthcare Improvement's (IHI) road map for improving transitions from the hospital to post-acute care settings to reduce avoidable rehospitalizations. Though this framework focuses specifically on the transition from hospital to post-acute care settings, it is a useful conceptual model to think about the process in 2 parts: the transition out of the hospital, and the activated and reliable reception into the next setting of care.

Furthermore, the IHI road map defines 4 pillars upon which to design solutions: patient and family engagement, cross-continuum team collaboration, evidence-based care in all clinical settings, and health information exchange and shared care plans. These 4 pillars informed the design of our solution, in which hospital social workers engage patients and caregivers both during and after a hospitalization, connect with CHWs to collaborate and share care plans, and CHWs work in tandem with clinicians to deliver evidence-based care that meets patients' complex medical and social needs.

● IMPLEMENTING A SOLUTION

In developing a solution that invests in patients' health outside the hospital, we referenced the IHI road map and divided the problem into 2 parts: how hospital-based health professionals can facilitate patients' transition to the community and how community-based health professionals can ensure patients stay healthy and connected to the appropriate resources in the long term. This allowed us to design a solution that took advantage of the resources that existed in both care settings—hospital and community. Finally, it is important that we connect these 2 pieces of the solution such that we are not creating more opportunities for information to fall through the cracks of an already fragmented system. We accomplished this by focusing on the "handoff" between the social worker and the CHW.

The key steps in change management are as follows: use EMR data to identify patients who have experienced readmission and then assess these patients' post-discharge needs, train clinicians in creating patient-friendly discharge materials as per the gaps identified through this assessment, develop a pilot a program for hospital social workers to phone call patients at high risk of readmission and connect them to clinical care (including "handoff" to CHW), collect feedback and iterate on the program design, and finally scale up the program to all patients at high risk of readmission while continuing to track outcomes (ie, readmissions).

SECTION 4 • Building Regional Networks

Key Steps in Change Management and Potential Pitfalls

Key Steps in Change Management

1. Use electronic medical record data to identify patients who have been readmitted to the hospital within 30 days following a surgical procedure.
2. Perform assessment (interview and chart review) of post-discharge needs for these patients to understand gaps in the discharge planning and follow-up process.
3. Train clinicians in creating patient-friendly discharge materials (eg, written instructions, oral counseling, etc.).
4. Develop a program for social workers to phone call patients at high risk of readmission and connect them to clinical care (including "handoff" to a CHW) after discharge.
5. Pilot the program with a small group of patients, refine based on feedback, and track readmissions for this group.
6. Scale up the program to all patients at high risk of readmission, continue tracking readmissions, and iterate on the process as necessary.

Potential Pitfalls

1. Ambiguous criteria for which patients should be followed by social workers.
2. Not speaking with social workers to understand if this program would be a meaningful use of their time or overextend their caseload.
3. Ineffective handoff between the hospital social worker and CHW in the next setting of care.
4. Not implementing a process to ensure that social workers' phone calls actually accomplish the aims of the program (ie, address unmet needs, connect to clinical care, "handoff" to CHW).
5. Scaling up the program too quickly without attention to staffing, resources, or need to adapt the program to different communities.

There are several pitfalls here that will be important to address. These include not defining clear criteria for identifying which patients are at high risk of readmission, not taking the time to understand what social workers need and want out of this program and how it will affect their caseloads, an ineffective handoff between social workers and CHWs (the crux of the program), not connecting the dots to ensure these phone calls actually reach patients and address identified goals, and scaling too quickly without attention to staffing and community needs.

● MEASURING OUTCOMES

For the purposes of this discussion, the primary outcome is 30-day hospital readmissions. This should be monitored as the program is rolled out to both ensure that the program is accomplishing its goals and inform adjustments as necessary. However, this metric does little to capture the nuances of patients' experience or monitor for unintended consequences. One potential solution is to send surveys to participating patients after the social workers' last phone call and assess patients' experience with the program, ability to access care, ability to reach a CHW, and perceived challenges to staying healthy.

● FOLLOW-UP AND MAINTENANCE

The success of this program depends on rigorous and regular assessment of the outcome at hand: readmissions among patients following a surgical procedure. This means that there must be oversight of patients' outcomes even after they leave the hospital and are receiving care in the community. Improving care for patients like Mr. N requires us to look beyond the hospital walls to where patients spend the vast majority of their lives. It requires us to build creative and evidence-based solutions that bridge the historical disconnect between hospitals and the communities they serve.

Working With Employers to Build Destination Programs for Complex Surgery

22

CAITLIN HALBERT

Clinical Delivery Challenge

Complex surgery is commonly reimbursed by insurers through 2 payment models: fee-for-service (FFS) system and bundled care payment models (BCPMs).

Traditional healthcare payment models are based on an FFS system where each individual service is paid in isolation. This model is dependent on the quantity of service and not necessarily the quality of the service. The service provided is independent of any other service and, in isolation, may contribute to overtreatment or even complications.

The rising costs of health care have encouraged insurers, healthcare systems, and policymakers alike to seek alternatives to the historic FFS model of reimbursement. The alternatives focus on value (the measure of health outcomes against the cost of delivering the outcomes) rather than quantity.[1] BCPMs are one such alternative designed to cover all costs surrounding an episode of care which inherently encourages value.[2]

Employers and healthcare organizations are both seeking innovative strategies to bring optimal health care to the patient. In doing so, employers and programs are coming together in partnership to create access to surgical programs. The employers are seeking the highest value partners and tend not to be geographically restricted in this search. Employers, and the conveners that manage these partnerships on their behalf, partner with healthcare programs from all over the country. Often, the partnership directs patients to programs not found in the patient's immediate location but potentially hundreds of miles away. These partnerships are considered destination programs for complex surgery or simply "destination programs." They are a departure from the traditional FFS model creating an innovative new way to deliver surgical care directly to patients. Destination programs should be differentiated from "medical tourism" where the patient, independent of their insurer, travels typically outside of their home country seeking health care.[3]

Destination programs are an evolving and expanding healthcare delivery model utilizing bundled payment reimbursement. The destination programs are created as a partnership with employers to provide high-quality care at low costs.

● WORKUP

Complex surgical programs, such as cancer care or bariatric surgery, involve a multidisciplinary approach before, during, and after the actual surgical intervention. Multispecialty consultations, lab work, imaging, preoperative procedures, patient and family education, postoperative care, and much more increase the complexity and cost of patient care. In an FFS model, each individual service is reimbursed which does not intrinsically encourage better outcomes. Alternatively, if the payments were bundled covering the entire episode of care, the programs would be incentivized to create an efficient system with little redundancy thus reducing costs. And if participation in these BCPMs were based on patient outcomes, programs would be motivated to improve overall value.

While in pursuit of an alternative payment model, the focus must not shift from patient care and access to healthcare resources. The concept of "access" has shifted in the modern era with the evolution of medical technology and telehealth. Health care is now more easily delivered from a distance, even across state lines. Patients participate in virtual education classes and small medical group sessions. Images can be uploaded and shared electronically. Asynchronous electronic communication has increased in use between providers and patients. Electronic medical record systems are integrating into larger statewide and regional systems to share health records among providers. In many instances, patients no longer must drive hours to see a specialist but rather log on from their home computer. Patients and providers alike are adjusting to a new norm for the delivery of health care. And the provider's "community" is ever expanding beyond their physical location.

One aspect of medical care that cannot be virtual, however, is the act of surgery. Destination surgical programs are the convergence of virtual health and the physical act of surgery. When developed in a thoughtful, patient-focused perspective, the results with regard to value, patient outcomes, and patient satisfaction can be equivalent to local surgical care.

A healthcare system interested in the development of a destination program needs to consider several key questions:

1. Is there an established program?
   Destination programs are often created as an expansion of a preexisting and successful "local" program. Best practices have been instituted and will carry into the development of the destination program. A strong quality improvement component ensures exceptional outcomes.
2. Is there support?
   The healthcare system must be supportive of the anticipated needs of the destination program. Creation of a destination program requires a dedicated leadership team working to, among other responsibilities, negotiate and maintain contracts and ensure proper staffing support for the expanded management of patients traveling for care. Staffing can include but is not limited to surgeons, advanced practice clinicians, concierge or nurse navigators, medical assistants, financial coordinators, and nurses.
3. Is there capacity?
   The destination program will bring an additional influx of patients, as expected, into the healthcare system. This anticipated increase in volume must be adequately accommodated with capacity in the schedule of the entire multidisciplinary team, surgical floor beds, operating room time, and so on. Additionally, the patient's interest must also be considered. Will patients be willing to travel to a distant location to meet their surgical needs? Both the insurer and the providers must consider how the patients will travel to foster high satisfaction and safety.

● DIFFERENTIAL DIAGNOSIS

To create a successful destination program, a strong alignment must be cultivated among the provider, the employer, and the patients. This can be particularly challenging in several ways. Providers and healthcare systems must be agreeable to shift from an FFS model to a BCPM. Insurers need to find and assess the available healthcare systems that would be interested in a partnership. And finally, the program must be designed to accommodate the patient, especially with respect to their travel expectations.[4] Without financial support of the traveling patient, access to partnered care may be significantly limited.

● DIAGNOSIS AND TREATMENT

The destination programs are partnerships between the employer and the provider in a BCMP. For many surgical programs and healthcare organizations, this is a shift from the traditional FFS model. It requires more than a new contract agreement, but a larger program-wide transformation focused on value-based healthcare delivery. This transition requires the establishment of strong relationships and collaborations among the multidisciplinary team. Efficient and effective protocols need to be developed based on strong evidence while being mindful of costs and redundancy. While this transition may be incremental in its implementation, the result will create a program poised to partner with employers.[5]

The employer will seek partnerships with interested surgical programs that meet predetermined selection criteria. The criteria can include a volume minimum (by surgeon and/or program) and a review of current outcomes data. The employer will work with the program to review all aspects of the episode of care

CHAPTER 22 • Working With Employers to Build Destination Programs for Complex Surgery

with an expectation for reproducible outcomes with predictable costs. The executed contracts can include, among other components, an agreement on price and volume, quality and cost targets, and the distribution of shared savings. It is important to specify eligibility for patients at the time of contract negotiations. This not only includes inclusion and exclusion criteria, but how those patients will be identified by the employer as a candidate.[5]

For many destination program patients, they will be given regional providers from which to choose. In some instances, their employer may have an exclusive partnership with a single provider. Regardless, patients may be required to travel a significant distance to receive care. The arranged partnership between the provider and the employer must take this distance into account. Providing traveling cost coverage for not only the patient but a caregiver, partnering with hotels, and providing local information for patients to find pharmacies, grocers, and so on is vital to patient access and experience. Additionally, providers need to determine the frequency and length of stay surrounding their episodes of care. Will the patient travel to meet the multidisciplinary team prior to scheduling the surgery date? Will the patient stay in a local hotel or apartment for a given amount of time after discharge from the hospital? These answers will depend on the type of destination program and the comfort and expectations of the providers.

● SCIENTIFIC PRINCIPLES AND EVIDENCE

BCPM seeks to provide a single reimbursement for an entire episode of care. Through this model, a healthcare system will receive a single payment for the entirety of care rendered for a particular condition. For example, in the management of joint care, this payment would cover all clinic visits, preoperative imaging, surgery, postoperative visits, and care up to a given number of days. While acute episodes may have a limited coverage to 90 days, chronic conditions may require longer coverage.

BCPM encourages the value of care within the healthcare system. If the costs related to the episode of care can be reduced while maintaining quality (thus increasing value), the healthcare system and the payer will be able to benefit from the single payment model. The Centers for Medicare and Medicaid Services (CMS) forayed into BCPM with the Bundled Payments for Care Improvement (BCPI) initiative which began in 2013. The first BCPI centered around lower extremity joint replacement, the most common Medicare inpatient surgical procedure. In 2014, joint replacements totaled over 450,000 cases at a cost of over $6 billion. Subsequent studies were undertaken comparing patients from hospitals that did and did not participate in the BCPI initiative. They found that for participating hospitals, a reduction in the acute surgical episode costs was noted while quality outcomes were maintained.[6]

Studies are lacking for BCPM through commercial insurances as compared to the CMS initiatives. One study compared a bundled-payment direct-to-employer destination program pre- and post-implementation. It estimated an over 10% reduction in procedure prices for 3 high-cost procedures—spinal fusion, major joint replacement, and bariatric surgery. This cost-saving can be passed to the patients, who may have their cost-sharing payments reduced or eliminated.[4]

● IMPLEMENTING A SOLUTION

The clinical delivery challenge for employers lies in how they can optimize the value of surgical care for their insured members. Some strategies have included price transparency platforms where patients seek lower-cost options and patient rewards systems. However, with a variable patient and provider participation and inconsistent improvement in costs and/or quality, these programs have not been widely adopted.[4,7] Through contracted destination programs, employers hold the provider responsible for an entire episode of care. The reimbursement covers care delivered during a given time frame before and after surgery. This puts the financial risk on the provider. Risks include postoperative complications and readmissions.[4]

For many employers seeking a destination surgery partnership, the time committed to searching for surgical program partners, vetting criteria and outcomes data, and negotiating a contract in partnership can be a significant barrier. Numerous "conveners" have emerged with experience to bring employers and surgical programs together in partnership.

Healthcare systems and providers may seek to develop destination programs for several reasons. First, they are interested in expanding access for patients within their community. If they are not participating in direct-to-employer partnerships, their local patients may be drawn out of their typical catchment area for care elsewhere. Second, providers may be looking for opportunities to increase patient referrals to their current programs. This is especially attractive in highly competitive areas. Through an increase in patient access and referrals, providers are poised to benefit financially from destination programs.[4]

Change Management to Create a Destination Program

The key change management steps in the development of a destination program include a great deal of preparation prior to the contracted partnership. Assessment of the current "local" surgical program is the first step. Current protocols and processes will need to be reviewed thoroughly through the lens of a BCPM. The development of a leadership team to negotiate partnership contracts on behalf of the institution's destination program is recommended. This team will be tasked with searching for, negotiating with, and establishment of partnerships with employers. The destination program will need to measure outcomes to ensure high-quality standards are consistently met. As the program matures, the expectations (including outcomes and costs) will need to be reassessed at a regular cadence with the partnered employer.

Potential Pitfalls when Creating a Destination Program

Several pitfalls must be considered when designing a destination program. First and foremost, the focus must be on the traveling patient. Destination programs will require patients and often a caregiver to travel to a distant location to receive their care. The provider and employer need to ensure safe and comfortable travel arrangements. The teams must be nimble and responsive to an array of novel challenges. Flight delays, hotel construction, pandemics, and much more must now be considered for the surgical patient. Routine meetings between the employer and provider are key to finding opportunities for improvement and addressing patient concerns. Open and frequent communication will encourage a healthy and agile partnership.

Many destination programs require that the patient has established a relationship with a primary care provider (PCP) in their hometown. This ensures an up-to-date assessment of the patient preoperatively but more importantly, allows for long-term follow-up postoperatively. Developing strategies to not only communicate to the PCP that a patient will be undergoing surgery but additionally how that surgery will impact their patient's long-term health and well-being can help improve the transition from the preoperative to the postoperative stage. PCP education regarding the planned operation delivered, for example, in the form of a provider letter or email or periodic live-streamed education sessions can be incredibly valuable.

Key Steps in Change Management and Potential Pitfalls

Key Steps in Change Management

1. Identify interest from the surgical program and leadership in pursuing a destination program partnership.
2. Review all components of the current "local" surgical program, including all protocols and processes. Analyze any opportunities to reduce inefficiency.
3. Create a value proposition that includes expected costs of care and surgical outcomes.
4. Seek out employers and conveners for partnership.
5. Create a process to identify appropriate patients for the destination program. This includes the creation of inclusion and exclusion criteria.
6. Track measurable outcomes.

Potential Pitfalls

1. Failure to anticipate the needs of a traveling patient.
2. Lack of communication among providers, employers, and patients.
3. Not anticipating capacity needs for the destination program.

When evaluating the "local" surgical program in preparation for a potential expansion to the destination, leadership must consider the capacity for additional patients and the anticipated support needed for a destination program. This encompasses not only the time needed for the clinical care of the patient from the multidisciplinary team but the dedicated staff who will be supporting the traveling patient.

MEASURING OUTCOMES

The destination program partnership will require an assessment of the value of the program by evaluating both outcomes and cost.

The patient clinical outcomes, both short and long term, should be maintained by the program and reviewed jointly with the employer. Patient satisfaction should also be routinely assessed by the provider and/or employer. Typical hospital-distributed patient surveys do not capture the nuances of a destination program, and it is recommended to find an additional source of patient feedback. Messaging applications tend to be successful in response rates while also returning quick results from which change can occur. Questions concerning travel or hotel accommodations, the provider and employer management teams, and so on should be asked in patient surveys.

As the program matures, reassessment of costs incurred throughout the patient's episode of care should occur on a regular cadence. There are often opportunities to reduce costs while maintaining high-quality outcomes. For example, transitioning patient education from an in-person individual to a group or virtual session may reduce costs while still delivering the same education to the patient.

FOLLOW-UP AND MAINTENANCE

After a healthcare system successfully implements a destination program, there are opportunities to expand to include additional surgical programs within the system. Bariatric surgery, gynecologic surgery, orthopedic surgery, cardiovascular surgery, and other complex surgical programs are proving to be successful in the BCPM. Through careful planning and preparation, patients can safely reach those high-quality programs, regardless of the distance.

REFERENCES

1. NEJM Catalyst. What is value-based healthcare? *NEJM Catalyst.* Published January 1, 2017. Accessed May 7, 2022. https://catalyst.nejm.org/doi/full/10.1056/CAT.17.0558?share=email&amp%3Bnb=1
2. NEJM Catalyst. What are bundled payments? *NEJM Catalyst.* February 28, 2018. Accessed May 4, 2023. https://catalyst.nejm.org/doi/full/10.1056/CAT.18.0247
3. Foley BM, Haglin JM, Tanzer JR, Eltorai AEM. Patient care without borders: a systematic review of medical and surgical tourism. *J Travel Med.* 2019;26(6):taz049. doi: 10.1093/jtm/taz049
4. Whaley CM, Dankert C, Richards M, Bravata D. An employer-provider direct payment program is associated with lower episode costs. *Health Affairs.* 2021;40(3):445–452. doi: 10.1377/hlthaff.2020.01488
5. Steenhuis S, Struijs J, Koolman X, Ket J, van der Hijden E. Unraveling the complexity in the design and implementation of bundle payments: a scoping review of key elements from a payer's perspective. *Milbank Q.* 2020;98(1):197–222.
6. Dummit LA, Kahvecioglu D, Marrufo G, et al. Association between hospital participation in a Medicare bundled payment initiative and payments and quality outcomes for lower extremity joint replacement episodes. *JAMA.* 2016;316(12):1267–1278. doi: 10.1001/jama.2016.12717
7. Whaley C, Schneider Chafen J, Pinkard S, et al. Association between availability of health service prices and payments for these services. *JAMA.* 2014;312(16):1670–1676. doi: 10.1001/jama.2014.13373

SECTION 5

Ensuring Quality and Safety

23 Ensuring Quality and Safety When Building a New Clinical Program
Anthony T. Petrick and Alvin Chang

24 Monitoring Quality and Safety Early in the Adoption of New Technology
Herbert J. Zeh and Melissa E. Hogg

25 Negotiating Turf Battles Between Specialties
Nicholas Osborne

26 Addressing Low Performance Outliers in Outcomes Monitoring Programs
Casey M. Silver, Karl Y. Bilimoria, and Anthony D. Yang

27 Managing a Surgeon With Demonstrated Poor Outcomes
Gerard Doherty

28 High-Volume Hospital With Low-Volume Surgeons
Patricia C. Conroy, Mohamed Abdelgadir Adam, and Julie Ann Sosa

29 High Variability in Surgical Teams
Sapan N. Ambani

30 Provider Burnout Impacting Clinical Care Delivery
Liane S. Feldman and Lawrence Lee

Ensuring Quality and Safety When Building a New Clinical Program

23

ANTHONY T. PETRICK AND ALVIN CHANG

Clinical Delivery Challenge

The American Society of Metabolic and Bariatric Surgery established national standards and a data collection system in 2003 through the Surgical Review Corporation (SRC) in response to national concerns about the variability in mortality and morbidity associated with bariatric procedures.[1] Despite these standards, 4 patient deaths were reported in 2013 after adjustable gastric band placement in southern California clinics associated with a high-profile marketing campaign.[2] In this chapter, we use Geisinger Health System's Proven Bariatric® as a case study to illustrate the methodology for incorporating national best practice standards to ensure quality and patient safety. Proven Bariatric was a 2-phased project designed and implemented over more than a decade. The first phase, ProvenCare Bariatric®, embeds best practices into the electronic health medical record system to minimize unwarranted variation in bariatric episodes of care. The design was started in 2006 and implemented in 2008. The second, Proven Recovery Bariatric®, is a perioperative enhanced recovery pathway designed and implemented in 2017. Both will be further described as case examples of how to ensure quality and safety when building new clinical programs.

Proven Bariatric® was developed around 5 core principles: (1) eliminate unjustified variation as a patient-safety issue; (2) ensure that justified variation is patient driven; (3) set a minimum level of reliability; (4) require clinicians to communicate and document exceptions; (5) measure outcomes and reasons for nonadherence.

Introducing new healthcare programs into complex medical systems presents significant quality and safety challenges. The National Academy of Medicine defines quality as the degree to which healthcare services for individuals and populations increase the likelihood of desired health outcomes and are consistent with current professional knowledge. In the landmark report, *Crossing the Quality Chasm*, the National Academy of Medicine identified 6 goals for healthcare delivery: (1) safe, (2) effective, (3) patient-centered, (4) timely, (5) efficient, and (6) equitable.[3] Reaching these goals requires stakeholders to design quality improvement projects utilizing either preexisting data collection tools or new ones. Key data fall into 3 categories: baseline performance, benchmarks, and performance post-implementation. The goal of this chapter is to establish the framework for a data-driven, high-quality care delivery system that meets the National Academy of Medicine's goals for healthcare delivery.

● WORKUP

There are many quality improvement process designs. The American College of Surgeons (ACS) division of quality offers guidance for surgical quality, including the Metabolic and Bariatric Surgery Quality Improvement Program (MBSAQIP), which uses DMAIC as the methodology for quality improvement. DMAIC is an acronym for define, measure, analyze, improve, and control. Proven Bariatric® was developed using DMAIC methodology to maintain alignment with our Geisinger ACS accreditation. Each of the DMAIC quality improvement methodologies will be highlighted in bold type as their use toward building the clinical program is described.

The first step toward the creation of a care delivery system is to identify key stakeholders. In health care, this includes providers, patients, administrators, and payers. For both Proven Bariatric® programs, key stakeholders were engaged to **define** the problem. The stakeholders included bariatric surgeons, medical bariatricians, dieticians, and behavioral specialists. Medical specialists included Cardiologists, Pulmonologists, Nephrologists, Pharmacists, and others to help guide pathways for perioperative management of the comorbid disease associated with obesity. Nurses and advanced practitioners provided not only clinical guidance but operational advice as they are responsible for many of the patient touchpoints. While clinical outcomes will be the focus of this chapter, the aims of Proven Bariatric® also included improving patient experience and reducing costs in the setting of a value-based payer program.[4] These objectives required engagement of additional stakeholders from administration, finance, and the Geisinger Health Plan.

Stakeholders reviewed national standards and best practices to determine key operational metrics as well as to understand the current state. These were defined as length of stay (LOS), extended length of stay (ELOS) >2 days, readmission within 30 days of discharge, reoperation within 30 days of surgery of discharge, intensive care unit (ICU) admission, major complications, and any complication. There was also consensus among stakeholders that measurement of provider adherence to care pathways was central to both understanding the effectiveness of implementation and the impact of care processes on outcomes.

Prior to process design, it is important to identify data sources to **measure** the current state. Data sources can be internal or external. Bariatric data were reported to be an external accreditation source, the SRC, when the program was conceived in 2006. These data were also collected internally and used to measure the current state of key process indicators (Table 23.1; Group α). No data sources were available to measure

Table 23.1	Clinical Outcomes of ProvenCare® Redesign Groups Versus Current State (Group α).[5]		
	Group α Current State	Group β Implementation Unreliable Care Delivery	Group Ω Implementation Reliable Care Delivery
Total (*n*)	429	448	1184
LOS (days)	3.2	2.6	2.2
Benchmark	2.0	p < 0.01	p < 0.01
ELOS (>2 days)	128 (29.8%)	109 (24.3%) p = 0.067	177 (14.9%) p < 0.0001
Readmission <30 days of discharge	50 (11.7%)	28 (6.3%)	67 (5.7%)
Benchmark	5%	p < 0.01	p < 0.0001
Reoperation <30 days of surgery	22 (5.1%)	14 (3.1%) p = 0.14	40 (3.4%) p = 0.107
ICU admission	17 (4.0%)	20 (4.5%) p = 0.71	25 (2.1%) p = 0.039
Major complication	32 (7.5%)	24 (5.4%) p = 0.20	56 (4.7%) p = 0.033
Any complication	95 (22.1%)	77 (17.2%) p = 0.065	155 (13.1%) p < 0.0001

Group α—current state
Group β—unreliable implementation of care redesign (<40%)
Group Ω—reliable implementation of care redesign (>90%)
Continuous data are presented as mean ± standard deviation and were compared using Student's t-test.
Categorical data were compared using chi-square test.
p-values represent a comparison against group α.

Adapted with permission from Petrick et al.[4]

CHAPTER 23 • Ensuring Quality and Safety When Building a New Clinical Program

adherence to care pathways, so these were developed internally. An informatic team was utilized to modify the electronic medical record creating standardized documentation as a source for electronic reports of adherence to all care pathway elements.

● DIFFERENTIAL DIAGNOSIS

The stakeholder group identified variability in care delivery as the key barrier to safe, effective, patient-centered, timely, and efficient bariatric care. Equity of care was primarily a function of payer status. National best practices and benchmarks were available for all 3 phases of care in which variability was identified. Consensus was developed that a program eliminating unwarranted variability would improve clinical outcomes, patient experience, and cost of care.

● DIAGNOSIS AND TREATMENT

Analysis of both internal and external data showed that current state LOS and readmission were both above national benchmarks with nearly 30% of patients having an ELOS (Table 23.1; Group α). These data identified the key operational metrics for improvement. Additional metrics were added based on their importance for compliance with national benchmarks for accreditation and payer center of excellence participation. These included reoperation, ICU utilization, and complications.

The primary care delivery challenge was to identify best care practices, and then design best practice care pathways to **improve** the quality of bariatric care. Care phases were divided into preoperative, perioperative, and postoperative inpatient and discharge phases. Stakeholder teams were formed to design care pathways for each.

The preoperative phase of care was primarily influenced by payers. Before authorizing bariatric surgery, most payers require 6 months of attempted medical weight loss and evaluations by a dietician and behavioral health specialists. The preoperative phase design was the most comprehensive in ProvenCare® Bariatric. The perioperative phase of care focused on medication management, antibiotic timing, venous thromboembolic prophylaxis, and glucose management. The postoperative inpatient design was similar, while the discharge phase design standardized follow-up care (Table 23.2).

Patients often get less than half the care intended by their providers.[5] There were no external benchmarks for provider adherence to processes. Stakeholders agreed to set an internal benchmark at 70% for adherence with an understanding that a more aggressive benchmark could be set after implementation.

● SCIENTIFIC PRINCIPLES AND EVIDENCE

Process tools vary widely in form, but all strive to empower providers with timely, necessary data to make changes in the process of healthcare delivery. Process improvement measurements are different from research measurements. Process improvement is a dynamic process with incremental changes and possesses its own unique challenges. It can be a costly endeavor and requires careful selection of measures, skilled team members for data collection and analysis, and long-term engagement and communication from all those involved. This is more crucial in the context of establishing a new clinical program where lack of experience in a setting with new team members may further hinder efforts of quality improvement.[6]

When gathering data, an essential tool is the electronic health record (EHR). The EHR allows an organization to collect systemic data in real time. Clinical data for ProvenCare® Bariatric was first collected from data inputted into the SRC data registry. As national bariatric accreditation moved to MBSAQIP, the data source moved to the MBSAQIP Registry which enabled ProvenCare® Bariatric to benefit from risk-adjusted benchmarks. Additional data sources available when designing new clinical programs include state Prescription Drug Monitoring Programs, in-house data registries, national

Table 23.2 ProvenCare® Bariatrics Best Practice Elements[5]

Preoperative Clinic/Preadmission

Patient attended bariatric nutrition class.
Patient attended behavior class.
Patient attended at least 2 bariatric group support meetings.
Patient given "green light" by Registered Dietitian.
Patient given "green light" by Behavioral Medicine.
Confirmation of an attempt at preoperative weight loss.
Confirmation of compliance with the medical program.
Patient had *Helicobacter pylori* testing.
Patient had *H. pylori* treatment, if applicable.
Patient had diabetes testing.
Surgical referral delayed if hemoglobin A1c is 12%.
Patient had cardiac evaluation as indicated.
Appropriate testing and/or cardiology consult completed.
Patients had completed an obstructive sleep apnea questionnaire.
Patients scoring 15 on sleep apnea questionnaire will have formal sleep evaluation by pulmonary medicine.
Cotinine/nicotine level was checked if the patient was smoking at the time of initial GI Nutrition evaluation.
Surgery postponed for positive nicotine/cotinine patients until the confirmation of smoking cessation and negative nicotine/cotinine testing.
Preoperative beta-blockers prescribed as indicated.
Confirmation of use of ACE/ARBs.
Patient underwent OS-MRS scoring.
Outpatient anticoagulation clinic referral.
Preoperative clinic/preadmission.
Patient attended bariatric nutrition class.

Perioperative

Confirmed that patient is off ACE/ARBs.
Correct type, dose, and timing of preoperative antibiotics.
Intraoperative glycemic monitoring and control per protocol.
Intraoperative DVT prophylaxis.

Postoperative Inpatient

Postoperative beta-blockers as indicated.
Postoperative glycemic monitoring and control per protocol for at least 24 hours.
Postoperative DVT prophylaxis as indicated.
Inpatient anticoagulation clinic referral.

Discharge/Post-Discharge

Post-discharge beta-blockers as indicated.
Patient had 7- to 14-day postoperative surgical visit.
Patient had 7- to 14-day postoperative GI Nutrition visit.
Patient had 30-day GI Nutrition visit.
Patient had 60-day GI Nutrition visit.
Inpatient anticoagulation clinic referral.

Abbreviations: ACE, angiotensin-converting enzyme inhibiting medications; ARB, angiotensin receptor blocking mediations; DVT, deep vein thrombosis; GI Nutrition, gastrointestinal nutritional support service; OS-RMS, Obesity Severity Mortality Risk Score.

Adapted with permission from Petrick et al.[4]

CHAPTER 23 • Ensuring Quality and Safety When Building a New Clinical Program

data registries, surveys, Patient-Reported Outcome Measures as well as interviews with patients and providers.

Each phase is critical to the quality and safety of surgical care and each is subject to quality improvement. We can apply Donabedian's 3 quality measures (structural, process, and outcome) to each phase. Structure is defined by the context of patient care (place, equipment, people, EHR). Process is the actions that are undertaken. Outcomes are the effects of the actions on the patient. As a patient transitions from the preoperative assessment to the post-discharge period, structure and processes change.[7]

● IMPLEMENTING A SOLUTION

After design, implementation represents the second key aspect of the **improvement** methodology in DMAIC. The EHR has become the cornerstone for implementing new clinical programs. The care pathways

Key Steps in Change Management and Potential Pitfalls

Key Steps in Change Management	ProvenCare Bariatric®
1. Identify a clear problem with a measurable outcome. 2. Understand the process and steps leading up to patients getting their procedure. 3. Spend time on the front line (eg, Gemba Walks) with key stakeholders involved. 4. Identify sources of quantitative data. 5. Introduce possible solutions to key stakeholders to test face validity and refine based on feedback. 6. Pilot the potential solution in a high-yield area and have regular opportunities to solicit feedback. 7. Track measurable outcomes.	• Bariatric surgical outcomes: LOS, ELOS, Readmission, Reoperation, ICU Admission, Complications. • Stakeholder meetings defining phases of care. • Stakeholder meetings with surgeons, bariatricians, dieticians, behavioral health specialists, trainees, administrators, and patients. • SRC and MBSAQIP Data Registries. • EMR as adherence data source, internal adherence dashboards. • Refinement of urine testing for smoking cessation based on timing and feasibility. • ProvenCare® and ProvenRecovery® Bariatric pathways with weekly adherence meetings. • Outcomes and adherence dashboards.

Potential Pitfalls	ProvenCare Bariatric®
1. Jumping straight to a solution. 2. Lack of a clear conceptual model for the process. 3. Not engaging enough of the correct stakeholders. 4. Forgetting to monitor for unintended consequences of your solution. 5. Broadly implementing your solution.	• Must collect and analyze data. • Core principles: eliminate unjustified variability in bariatric care. • Anesthesia developing parallel perioperative glucose management pathways. • Perioperative bradycardia in younger diabetic patients started on β-blockers. • Starting a bariatric program at a new hospital within the system. Personnel and resources are different affecting the alignment and timing of multidisciplinary care.

designed in Table 23.2 were embedded into the EHR by standardizing templates for clinic encounters, order sets, operative reports, progress notes, discharge summaries, and discharge instructions. Of these, order sets are the most critical element driving best practices. Care pathways should be aligned with data reporting registries and dashboards. If these performance metrics can be reported electronically, work effort and cost are reduced, while improving data accuracy.

A frequently stated mantra during the design and implementation of ProvenCare® Bariatrics was "make the right thing the easiest thing to do." The EHR facilitates this philosophy, but only if paired with frequent communication touchpoints to providers which ensures utilization of the tools.

Other standardized templates include telephone encounters and "episode of care" reports. The "episode" reports in the EHR list the care elements from Table 23.2. Providers responsible for each element are documented in a common report available to all bariatric providers. The field backgrounds turn to red, yellow, and green shading depending on the progress toward completion of the care element, thereby making it easier for providers to confirm care delivery.

An overview of the key steps to ensure safety and quality when building new programs is demonstrated in the table below with examples of each step from ProvenCare® Bariatric. Stakeholder expertise as well as continuous process control and communication is crucial to avoid unintended consequences that may undermine patient safety. One perioperative care element included in the initial ProvenCare Bariatric® elements was the initiation of perioperative beta-blockers for high-risk patients with long-term diabetes. Once implemented, we found that many younger diabetic patients came to the operating room bradycardic and required atropine, so the practice was quickly discontinued.

● MEASURING OUTCOMES

All processes are at risk of unintended consequences. Creating and utilizing tools to measure outcomes minimizes the risk of unintended consequences. Bariatric surgery data was entered into the MBSAQIP Registry and then exported to a Geisinger Bariatric Dashboard. Adherence data electronically reported from the EHR was continuously tracked on a separate dashboard created by Geisinger Analytics. Using this data, we were able to demonstrate that ELOS was significantly associated with unreliable adherence independent of operative approach (Figure 23.1). Any complication was significantly decreased with reliable adherence to care pathways (Figure 23.2). However, due to higher complications with open gastric bypass, this improvement was statistically significant only for open procedures. It is clear that simply developing best practices for clinical programs alone is not sufficient to improve quality of care.

● FOLLOW-UP AND MAINTENANCE

Active measurement of adherence to care pathways is necessary to effect changes in quality and safety, the **control** aspect of DMAIC. Sustainability can be the most difficult part of any quality improvement project. It is important that key stakeholders stay engaged and communicate regularly. These meetings should utilize a standing agenda. Accountable leads should review personnel and key process measures and assess threats to the progress of the program. Data dashboards are the cornerstone of evaluating measures. Opportunities for improvement must be frequently reassessed and maintained. Barriers need to be created against potential threats to success.

An example of a threat was experienced in our perioperative glucose control protocol. Several years into the program, the anesthesia department developed a parallel protocol for intraoperative glucose management. The clinical care delivery differed slightly, but the electronic tracking tools were not utilized resulting in dashboards reporting noncompliance. Because adherence was tracked in weekly meetings, the problem was quickly identified and the 2 care pathways easily aligned. Because structures and processes are

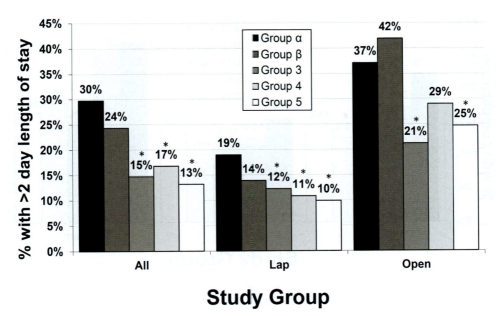

FIGURE 23.1 Association between ProvenCare® Redesign Groups and >2-day LOS for all patients and stratified by surgical access type.[5]
Group α—current state
Group β—unreliable adherence to care redesign (<40%)
Group Ω—reliable adherence to care redesign (>90%)
    Group 1—Group Ω year 1
    Group 2—Group Ω year 2
    Group 3—Group Ω year 3
*Indicates significant difference from Group α.
LOS was collected on 2061 ProvenCare® patients from May 2007 through April 2012. LOS was categorized into 2 groups (≤2 days and 3+ days) and chi-square tests were used to compare study groups to Group α.
Reprinted with permission from Petrick et al.[4]

constantly changing, stakeholders must continuously reassess to find potential opportunities and pitfalls to ensure fidelity of care pathways.

Nine years into the ProvenCare® Bariatric, it became clear to stakeholders that there were additional opportunities to improve surgical site infection rates and patient engagement as well as reduce opioid use by focusing on the perioperative and discharge periods. Stakeholders were reconvened and the DMAIC process was renewed. Care elements were **defined**, **measured**, and **analyzed**. Pathways were created, and then implemented, providing opportunities to **improve**. Dashboards were refined and the ProvenRecovery® Bariatric program was embedded across 2 hospitals. New outcome measures included tracking of opioid use as well as discharge opioid prescribing. Cost of care was also added to the updated dashboard.

In summary, building new clinical programs is a challenging endeavor. The increasing complexity of healthcare delivery creates more opportunities for missteps that can compromise patient safety. Program building cannot be done successfully by simply leveraging technology. Stakeholders must do the hard work of monitoring data and communicating regularly to ensure care processes continue to represent best practices and that providers remain aware and engaged in the process.

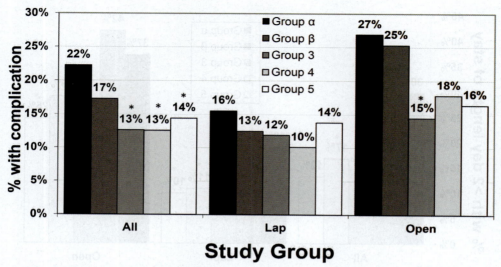

FIGURE 23.2 Association between ProvenCare® Redesign Groups and reduction in complications for all patients and stratified by surgical access type.[5]
Group α—current state
Group β—unreliable adherence to care redesign (<40%)
Group Ω—reliable adherence to care redesign (>90%)
  Group 1—Group Ω year 1
  Group 2—Group Ω year 2
  Group 3—Group Ω year 3
*Indicates significant difference from Group α.
Complications were collected on 2061 ProvenCare® patients from May 2008 through April 2012.
Complication data were defined as ≤30 day, and chi-square tests were used to compare study groups to Group α.
Reprinted with permission from Petrick et al.[4]

REFERENCES

1. American Society for Metabolic and Bariatric Surgery. ASMBS and SRC ink new contract for Bariatric Surgery Center of Excellence® program. *Newswise*. Accessed June 11, 2022. https://www.newswise.com/articles/asmbs-and-src-ink-new-contract-for-bariatric-surgery-center-of-excellence-program
2. Pfeifer S. Lap-Band clinic sued over death. *Los Angeles Times*. August 21, 2013. Accessed May 4, 2023. https://www.latimes.com/health/la-fi-lap-band-20110211-story.html
3. Institute of Medicine (US) Committee on Quality of Health Care in America. *Crossing the quality chasm: a new health system for the 21st century*. Washington, DC: National Academies Press; 2001.
4. Petrick AT, Still CD, Wood CG, et al. Feasibility and impact of an evidence-based program for gastric bypass surgery. *J Am Coll Surg*. 2015;220(5):855–862.
5. McGlynn EA, Asch SM, Adams J, et al. The quality of health care delivered in adults in the United States. *N Engl J Med*. 2003;342(26):2635–2645.
6. Dixon-Woods M, McNicol S, Martin G. Ten challenges in improving quality in healthcare: lessons from the Health Foundation's programme evaluations and relevant literature. *BMJ Qual Safety*. 2012;21(10):876–884. doi: 10.1136/bmjqs-2011-000760
7. Donabedian A. Evaluating the quality of medical care. 1966. *Milbank Q*. 2005;83(4):691–729. doi: 10.1111/j.1468-0009.2005.00397.x

Monitoring Quality and Safety Early in the Adoption of New Technology

24

HERBERT J. ZEH AND MELISSA E. HOGG

Clinical Delivery Challenge

One of the most common surgical operations performed in the United States is the repair of inguinal hernias (>500,000 each year).[1] The robotic approach to an inguinal hernia repair, first described by Dominguez et al. in 2015, is safe and feasible in the hands of highly proficient surgeons, as shown in a series from high-volume single institutions.[2,3] Indeed, this procedure appears to be increasing in popularity, driven largely by demand from surgeons, patients, and industry. The introduction of robotic technology into a hospital system requires an accurate modeling of the technology's risks and benefits and acceptable trade-offs in inefficiency and complications early in the learning curve for surgeons. The increased incorporation of the robotic platform across specialties in routine cases is an excellent case study for how healthcare leaders can address new surgical technology using available tools and emerging technology to minimize the impact on patient safety and potential litigation.

The overwhelming majority of healthcare systems will grant surgical privileges for specific procedures based on surrogate measures of surgeon competency, such as (1) the completion of an accredited residency, (2) certification by a surgical board, and (3) previous operative experience, which is assessed by the volume of procedures—not outcomes (Table 24.1). While these benchmarks are certainly requisite for surgeon privileging and credentialing, none of them speak to the specific competence of an individual surgeon to perform a given procedure. The analogy would be completing your pilot's training and getting your license and assuming that it qualifies you to fly any plane—clearly not the standard in the airline industry and not something the public would accept. The pathway to privileging new surgical technologies is even less robust. For robotic procedures like the inguinal hernia, the standard training in many places is attending a brief 48-hour industry-sponsored course. This is often enough to get you behind the robotic console while operating on a live person. While there is a proctor there to advise you, they are not allowed to "fly the plane." Thus, it is not surprising that the legal world is replete with examples of "planes going down" early in the roll-out of surgical robotics.[4,5] As the pace of surgical innovation and the demand from patients for new technology increases, the need to develop more objective and granular methods to assess surgical competency for credentialing cannot be overstated.

What can healthcare leaders use to assess the readiness of their "pilots" to perform specific procedures like robotic inguinal hernias? Case volume is certainly a reasonable starting point. The relationship between surgical outcomes and surgeon volume for a specific procedure has been well documented for several decades.[6,7] Providers who perform a higher volume of complex surgical procedures, such as esophagectomy and pancreaticoduodenectomy, have decreased mortality rates. The correlation between volume and outcomes for less complex procedures is clearly present but not so strong. However, the use of the volume of cases as a surrogate measure of proficiency is not possible when new technologies like robotics are being adopted by established surgeons—as all surgeons, by definition, will be low volume due to the technology's newness. A more granular and meaningful measure than case volume is needed to show a surgeon's proficiency.

Until recently, there was very little understanding of how to measure and quantify a surgeon's skill. There is now a body of literature that demonstrates that a surgeon's skill can be scored by video review and that this score directly correlates with risk-adjusted outcomes for patients.[8–12] The studies on this topic are provocative and have widespread implications for all levels of quality assessment and quality improvement for surgery. Unfortunately, the current paradigm of quality assessment, surgical education, and credentialing is not optimized to incorporate video-based review into privileging and credentialing pathways.

Table 24.1	Currently Accepted Metrics for Use in Credentialing and Privileging Surgeons for Specific Procedures
Metric	**Limitation**
Completion of surgical residency	• Currently technical proficiency-based metrics are underutilized and poorly standardized in U.S. surgical training programs
Board certification	• No assessment of technical skills is required for ABS certification at present
Surgical experience (previous volume)	• Reasonable surrogate but does not address outcomes of these procedures and threshold levels poorly defined • All surgeons will be low volume for new technology

How the surgical community ensures the safe introduction of new technologies has been the subject of great debate for the last several decades, which has been magnified by the introduction of laparoscopic and now robotic platforms. The adoption of these platforms seems to have been more driven by Brownian motion rather than a comprehensive policy to ensure the safety of the public. As a result, the number of bile duct injuries and complications from robotic platforms were arguably more than they should have been had the surgical community approached the roll-out of the new technology in a more organized fashion. In other industries, where high reliability is an expectation, such a disorganized introduction would not be tolerated by the public. For example, the Federal Aviation Administration (FAA) strictly regulates the airline industry to ensure that new airplanes are safe and that pilots have the necessary training to safely navigate new technology. Despite some notable exceptions[13] most people would argue that the bureaucratic burden for aviation has been a worth trade-off for public safety. Currently, the U.S. Food & Drug Administration only oversees the approval process of new surgical devices and has little to no oversight over the roll-out of these devices once approved. The onus to confirm a surgeon's competency with new surgical technologies lies with institutions and the individual surgeon.[14] In healthcare settings in the United States, there appears to be little appetite to develop an FAA-like approach, and much weight is given to the autonomy of medical practitioners to do what they perceive to be in the best interest of their patients. Given this, how can healthcare leaders assess the readiness of an individual surgeon to safely utilize emerging technologies?

● WORKUP

To better assess a surgeon's competency to "fly certain aircraft," we will have to reimagine our current credentialing and privileging pathways for innovative surgical procedures (and for well-established operations). Borrowing again from other high-reliability industries, such as aviation and the military, we can improve our processes by better incorporation of (1) simulation, (2) coaching, and (3) more comprehensive data collection from the operating room (OR).

Our scenario of the adoption of robotic surgery for inguinal hernia is an ideal example of how systems can shift toward privileging that is proficiency based.[15] To master a surgical procedure, a surgeon must move through several domains: (1) mastery of the instrument, (2) mastery of handling tissues and understanding dissection planes, (3) mastery of the specific steps of the procedure, (4) optimal psychomotor performance, and (5) judgment regarding when a procedure should be applied (Figure 24.1). In robotic surgery, mastery of the instrument can easily be assessed and quantified with the widespread availability of simulators. A large body of data exist on the performance of surgeons using these simulators.[16,17] We propose setting a threshold score for proficiency on the simulator or completing a mastery-based simulation curriculum as the starting point for hospital privileging committees before allowing surgeons to begin robotic procedures.[15] Currently, very few, if any, systems employ such an approach.

CHAPTER 24 • Monitoring Quality and Safety Early in the Adoption of New Technology

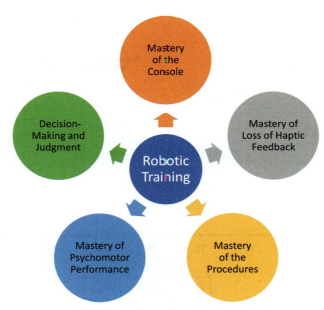

FIGURE 24.1 Crucial steps in the mastery of a surgical procedure.

Simulation can also be used to create high-fidelity inanimate bioartificial drills for surgeons that are videotaped and scored for surgical performance. Proficiency in these drills in an inanimate environment can serve as a surrogate measure of tissue or procedure mastery and technical proficiency. We have developed several bioartificial drills for robotic general surgery and surgical oncology procedures. These "flight simulators" can be used to grade performance, differentiate skills, and set benchmarks that can be used to determine when surgeons have reached adequate proficiency to begin performing robotic procedures on patients.[18]

● SCIENTIFIC PRINCIPLES AND EVIDENCE

We have previously reported the success of this pathway in a large tertiary care healthcare system, demonstrating that the adoption of a proficiency-based curriculum resulted in a statistically significant decrease in the learning curve and financial savings for the system.[15] In our study, a nonrandomized control group of surgeons followed the standard pathway of taking an industry-sponsored introductory course on the use of a robot—a course that was not proficiency based and in which everybody passes (nobody has ever failed an industry-sponsored robotics course). Following the 2-day course, the surgeons were allowed to "fly the plane" in 3 proctored cases. The proctor for these cases was only there as a consultant with no ability to intervene if the "flight" ran into difficulty. In contrast, the intervention group in our study underwent proficiency-based training, starting with virtual simulators and doing graded drills in bioartificial inanimate simulation. After achieving threshold scores on the biotissue drills, the trainees were allowed to proceed to live proctored cases. We demonstrated that the proficiency-based group was 20–30 cases ahead of the industry-sponsored group on the learning curve in terms of OR times. Moreover, even after 40 cases, the control group had still not approached the performance of the proficiency-trained group (Figure 24.2). Equally as important, the proficiency-trained and credentialed group had, on average, a $1500 case savings in OR time and equipment costs.

The final piece of this new approach is a better assessment of ongoing surgical performance. A surgeon's technical performance is strongly linked to patient outcomes, and recognizing this fact is driving the development of new technology that will fully assess the myriad factors that contribute to performance, including technical skills, the OR environment (distractions), and team dynamics. One such technology, developed by Surgical Safety Technologies (Toronto, Canada), is called the OR Black Box™, and it combines the comprehensive collection of data from the OR with advanced machine-learning algorithms to identify safety threats and optimize "flight safety".[19] The OR Black Box™ uses artificial

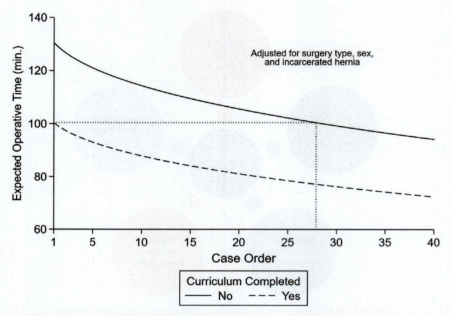

FIGURE 24.2 Expected operative time by case order and curriculum completion status. Expected operative times are adjusted for surgery type (bilateral vs. unilateral), patient sex, and hernia incarceration. Curriculum non-trainees (solid line) required an estimated 28 additional cases to match the starting proficiency of trainees (dashed line). Reprinted from Tam et al. Copyright © 2019 Elsevier. With permission.[15]

intelligence to identify patients in real time who are at risk for bad outcomes—either from physiologic outliers or from performance outliers.

Next-generation analytics from the OR (flight data) will include integrated measurements of patient physiology (vital signs), patient "omics" (which predict how a patient is responding to the controlled trauma of surgery), OR time (the duration of the trauma), team engagement (compliance with checklists), weather (environmental distractions), operational deviations (in-room flagging by teams), equipment utilization and failures, and lastly, surgeon technical performance (an automated, artificial intelligence–driven score). The integration of these data will allow the unprecedented identification of safety threats. With the deployment of this technology, we can imagine being able to identify patients who are at high risk for adverse events and take steps to mitigate the risk in real time. Indeed the final destination of this technology would be to provide the surgeon and surgical teams with real-time over-the-shoulder monitoring for safety threats similar to the modern-day cock pit. Patients, the OR team, surgeons, administration, and leadership are all key stakeholders in the development and utilization of these metrics.

● DIFFERENTIAL DIAGNOSIS

The ability to implement proficiency-based credentialing and ongoing monitoring of operative performance is rapidly evolving, and many obstacles to their more widespread adoption are being addressed. First of these challenges, the scoring metrics to determine threshold proficiency will need to be validated with real patient outcomes. For some procedures with low risk—such as our example of robotic inguinal hernia—consensus will need to be developed around surrogate end points for safety and proficiency. Second, the proficiency thresholds will need to be examined and validated across different settings, including in different locations (ie, geographic) and types of medical centers. Third, the infrastructure necessary to capture videos from training sessions and live operative procedures needs to be developed, as does the means for making the videos accessible and ready for scoring and for storing them digitally. The American College of Surgeons is currently conducting a pilot program of video-based review in collaboration with several potential vendors. Undoubtedly, there will need to be more innovation in this area to fully recognize its potential.

● DIAGNOSIS AND TREATMENT

To address the challenge of safely introducing new surgical technology, we must accept that the current system is insufficient, unsustainable, and be willing to support a substantial change in the culture of safety in surgery. To transition ourselves to a culture of high reliability, the following characteristics will be critical: (1) following safety rules will be considered normal behavior, (2) ongoing monitoring for safety threats, (3) frequent candid communication, (4) error reporting will be encouraged, and (5) a preoccupation with safety. Furthermore, the transition to proficiency-based assessment using video review for credentialing and privileging will require substantial administrative and financial support.

● SCIENTIFIC PRINCIPLES AND EVIDENCE

If training can improve technical skills and technical skills translate to patient outcomes, then training improves technical skills. It is very hard to study and isolate 1 factor and how this can translate singularly to patient outcomes. Many clinical papers have been written to assess the risk of a pancreatic fistula after a Whipple procedure. Using video review and technical grading, we asked the question of whether technical scores could also predict fistulas and be additive to clinical factors alone. This study found that surgeon factors "aka technical skills" as assessed by Objective Structured Assessment of Technical Skills grading were additive to patient clinical factors, including the fistula risk score in determining fistula risk after a Whipple.[9] It stands to reason then that if not all patient factors can be changed, there is the possibility to change for the better surgeon factors.

Many studies have looked at learning curves for different procedures, especially robotic procedures. These tend to have the theme that with more time and volume outcomes become better. This is a key step toward monitoring quality and safety early in the adoption of new technology. However, with early adopters comes mentees and dissemination. Another key strategy needs to be how early adopters are teaching the next generation, how effective this teaching is in terms of patient safety, and how ongoing value is being assessed. Monitoring second- and third-generation learning curves is a relatively new concept that has not been published in a widespread fashion because it is hard to quantify. However, with the institution of a proficiency-based robotic training system, there is evidence of improving outcomes when (1) training the next generation of surgeons in a hospital system,[20] (2) training next generation as they start a new program,[18] and (3) transplanting that system to another country and disseminating it.[21] The true goal of proficiency-based training would be to eliminate a "learning curve" because this would happen prior to the OR like pilots have in simulation prior to their first flight. Studies to translate this robotic hernia training program to the next generation are ongoing.[22]

● IMPLEMENTATION OF A SOLUTION

The implications of incorporating this proficiency-based credentialing and privileging pathway is transformative and disruptive. Most importantly, patients will benefit from improved clinical outcomes because we will be ensuring the technical competence of our surgical teams. Patients will be confident that they are under the care of proficient surgeons with capable teams. Hospitals will have a new and valuable tool to ensure that surgeons have reached an accepted level of competence. Insurance and government funding agencies can decrease expenditures through safer, more cost-effective procedures. Additionally, reimbursement for surgeons and procedures can be tied to training and compliance of institutions. Lastly, we as surgeons, partners, and colleagues will assure the public that we can self-assess, train, and enhance our skills to deliver the best possible outcomes for our patients.

We have previously proposed a proficiency-based curriculum that deploys 3 levels of surgical proficiency review (Figure 24.3).[15] The first level is experience as measured by case volume in the preceding

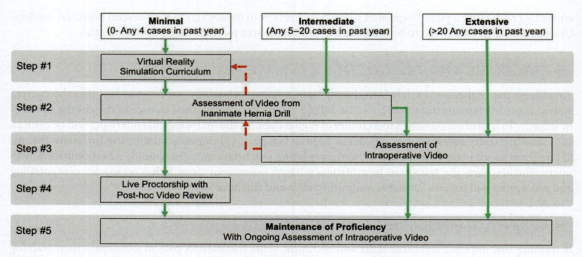

FIGURE 24.3 Proposed proficiency-based privileging schema. Three levels of surgical proficiency review are incorporated. The starting point is volume-based proficiency, and video review is the final step. Surgeons with minimal experience will be required to complete the entire pathway. Surgeons with extensive experience may begin with a video review and, if proficient, become credentialed. Surgeons with intermediate experience will be assessed to determine whether they need the entire pathway or can test into the video-review cohort. The solid arrows represent advancement. Remediation (dashed arrows) will be offered to surgeons not deemed proficient on video review. Reproduced with permission from Tam et al. Copyright © 2017 American Medical Association. All rights reserved.[23]

12 months. The second is performance in simulation and the third is a video-based review of current skills to credential a practitioner for a surgical procedure.

In our framework, surgeons or newly graduating trainees would be required to complete a multipart training pathway to become proficient in a procedure and must reach established performance thresholds to advance themselves. The pathway involves virtual simulation, videotaped and scored inanimate biotissue drills, and lastly, a video-based review of actual surgical performance. Surgeons with extensive experience may begin with a video review, and if proficient, become credentialed. Remediation will be offered to surgeons not deemed proficient after video review.

In our published work, we have provided proof of principle that such a framework can be deployed for robotic inguinal hernia and result in a substantial decrease in the learning curve as measured by OR time and the cost to a healthcare system. The general framework is expected to be applicable to complex low-volume procedures and a variety of technologies (eg, laparoscopy, robotics, and endoscopy).

Key Steps in Change Management and Potential Pitfalls

Key Steps in Change Management
1. Identify the technology's risks and benefits and acceptable trade-offs.
2. Identify inefficiencies and complications attributed to the learning curve for surgeons.
3. Create pathways for surgeons to shorten the learning curve outside of the OR.
4. Assess surgeon competency through video review.

Potential Pitfalls
1. Lack of validation between in situ technical skills and real-world outcomes.
2. Infrastructure for video-based review, including storage and scalability of scoring.

CHAPTER 24 • Monitoring Quality and Safety Early in the Adoption of New Technology

● MEASURING OUTCOMES

You cannot improve what you do not measure. Collaboration and centralization would be beneficial to widespread adoption as every center would not have the know-how, infrastructure, or desire. These simulations would need to be videotaped and analyzed with movement toward an automated system with artificial intelligence being the best way to make this scalable over person-powered video review. Finally, the use of sophisticated electronic medical record systems to automate or use synoptic operative, discharge, and follow-up reporting will help glean relevant data.

● FOLLOW-UP AND MAINTENANCE

The IDEAL framework discusses a progression from (1) Idea to (2) Development to (3) Exploration and (4) Assessment with eventual (5) Long-term surveillance. Monitoring quality and safety early in the adoption of new technology fits perfectly within this framework.[24,25] Currently, this would be through the idea and development phase and now within exploration and assessment. Proof of principle is available and dissemination of the playbook to other programs for the robotic inguinal hernia or comparable procedures with new dedicated technology is now essential. Randomization for such an endeavor would be difficult but setting up comparative studies for outcomes with those who have and have not undergone the proficiency-based training on a broader, multi-institutional level with evaluation for possible ways to improve would be the next key follow-up step.

REFERENCES

1. Aiolfi A, Cavalli M, Del Ferraro S, et al., Treatment of inguinal hernia: systematic review and updated network meta-analysis of randomized controlled trials. *Ann Surg*. 2021;274(6): 954–961.
2. Escobar Dominguez JE, Gonzalez A, Donkor C. Robotic inguinal hernia repair. *J Surg Oncol*. 2015;112(3): 310–314.
3. Miller BT, Prabhu AS, Petro CC, et al. Laparoscopic versus robotic inguinal hernia repair: 1- and 2-year outcomes from the RIVAL trial. *Surg Endosc*. 2022;37(1):723–728.
4. De Ravin E, Sell EA, Newman JG, Rajasekaran K. Medical malpractice in robotic surgery: a Westlaw database analysis. *J Robot Surg*. 2022;17(1):191–196.
5. Pradarelli JC, Campbell, DA, Jr, Dimick JB. Hospital credentialing and privileging of surgeons: a potential safety blind spot. *JAMA*. 2015;313(13):1313–1314.
6. Finks JF, Osborne NH, Birkmeyer JD. Trends in hospital volume and operative mortality for high-risk surgery. *N Engl J Med*. 2011;364(22): 2128–2137.
7. Reames BN, Ghaferi AA, Birkmeyer JD, Dimick JB. Hospital volume and operative mortality in the modern era. *Ann Surg*. 2014;260(2):244–251.
8. Birkmeyer JD, Finks JF, O'Reilly A, et al. Surgical skill and complication rates after bariatric surgery. *N Engl J Med*. 2013;369(15):1434–1442.
9. Hogg ME, Zenati M, Novak S, et al. Grading of surgeon technical performance predicts postoperative pancreatic fistula for pancreaticoduodenectomy independent of patient-related variables. *Ann Surg*. 2016;264(3):482–491.
10. Goldenberg MG, Goldenberg L, Grantcharov TP. Surgeon performance predicts early continence after robot-assisted radical prostatectomy. *J Endourol*. 2017;31(9):858–863.
11. Goldenberg MG, Grantcharov TP. A novel method of setting performance standards in surgery using patient outcomes. *Ann Surg*. 2019;269(1):79–82.
12. Stulberg JJ, Huang R, Kreutzer L, et al. Association between surgeon technical skills and patient outcomes. *JAMA Surg*. 2020;155(10): 960–968.
13. Shepardson D. U.S. lawmakers seek review of FAA Boeing 737 MAX oversight. *Reuters*. February 16, 2022. Accessed May 5, 2023. https://www.reuters.com/business/aerospace-defense/us-lawmakers-seek-review-faa-boeing-737-max-oversight-2022-02-15/
14. Pradarelli JC, Thornton JP, Dimick JB. Who is responsible for the safe introduction of new surgical technology?: an important legal precedent from the da Vinci surgical system trials. *JAMA Surg*. 2017;152(8):717–718.
15. Tam V, Borrebach J, Dunn SA, et al. Proficiency-based training and credentialing can improve patient outcomes and decrease cost to a hospital system. *Am J Surg*. 2019;217(4):591–596.

16. Hogg ME, Tam V, Zenati M, et al. Mastery-based virtual reality robotic simulation curriculum: the first step toward operative robotic proficiency. *J Surg Educ*. 2017;74(3):477–485.
17. Ahmad SB, Rice MJ, Chang C, Zureikat AH, Zeh HJ, 3rd, Hogg ME. dV-Trainer vs. da Vinci simulator: comparison of virtual reality platforms for robotic surgery. *J Surg Res*. 2021;267:695–704. doi: 10.1016/j.jss.2021.06.036
18. Schmidt CR, Harris BR, Musgrove KA, et al. Formal robotic training diminishes the learning curve for robotic pancreatoduodenectomy: implications for new programs in complex robotic surgery. *J Surg Oncol*. 2021;123(2):375–380.
19. Nensi A, Palter V, Reed C, et al. Utilizing the operating room Black Box to characterize intraoperative delays, distractions, and threats in the gynecology operating room: a pilot study. *Cureus*. 2021;13(7):e16218.
20. Rice MK, Hodges JC, Bellon J, et al. Association of mentorship and a formal robotic proficiency skills curriculum with subsequent generations' learning curve and safety for robotic pancreaticoduodenectomy. *JAMA Surg*. 2020;155(7):607–615.
21. Zwart MJW, Nota CLM, de Rooij T, et al. Outcomes of a multicenter training program in robotic pancreatoduodenectomy (LAELAPS-3). *Ann Surg*. 2022;276(6):e886–e895.
22. Al Abbas AI, Wang C, Hamad AB, et al. Mentorship and formal robotic proficiency skills curriculum improve subsequent generations' learning curve for the robotic distal pancreatectomy. *HPB (Oxford)*. 2021;23(12):1849–1855.
23. Tam V, Zeh HJ III, Hogg ME. Incorporating metrics of surgical proficiency into credentialing and privileging pathways. *JAMA Surg*. 2017;152(5):494–495.
24. Khachane A, Philippou Y, Hirst A, McCulloch P. Appraising the uptake and use of the IDEAL framework and recommendations: a review of the literature. *Int J Surg*. 2018;57:84–90. doi: 10.1016/j.ijsu.2018.07.008
25. McCulloch P, Altman DG, Campbell WB, et al. No surgical innovation without evaluation: the IDEAL recommendations. *Lancet*. 2009;374(9695):1105–1112.

Negotiating Turf Battles Between Specialties

25

NICHOLAS OSBORNE

Clinical Delivery Challenge

Within an academic-affiliated medical center, the sudden departure of 2 very experienced interventional radiologists has created an acute void in the clinical care of patients with vascular disease. Historically, this hospital has provided advanced vascular care including open surgery (offered by the vascular surgeons) and endovascular therapies (offered by the invasive cardiologists and interventional radiologists). To meet the clinical need, the hospital has temporarily asked the vascular surgeons to provide endovascular care to these patients.

Interdepartmental conflicts, "Turf wars," are commonplace in medicine. As specialties have evolved with overlapping diagnostic and therapeutic skills, turf wars often arise because of financial pressures, ego, and power. These turf wars can result in fragmented and nonstandardized care, inappropriate care, and stifled creativity and innovation. We will consider a scenario common to many medical centers navigating turf between specialties.

● WORKUP

To understand the clinical challenge, we will first explore the current paradigm. In the previous 2 years, the 2 interventional radiologists have provided care across the spectrum of interventional radiology, including visceral and vascular interventional radiology (including over 400 vascular procedures per year).

The hospital serves as an important training site for all 3 training programs (invasive cardiology, interventional radiology, and vascular surgery). The vascular procedures performed at this hospital are an important source of endovascular procedures performed for these training programs. Interventional radiology has looked to this site as the primary training site for peripheral interventions as vascular surgery has taken over most arterial procedures at the academic hospital.

In the immediate term, interventional radiology currently is being staffed with 1 vascular surgeon and temporary IR physicians. Recruitment of experienced permanent radiologists has been challenging. Invasive cardiology is under-resourced and has decided to focus on structural heart programs. The vascular surgeons are in the process of recruiting additional surgeons with expertise in the endovascular space; however, they are limited by OR availability.

● DIFFERENTIAL DIAGNOSIS

When considering why the hospital is suffering from such an unanticipated staffing dilemma, we must examine the underlying culture and relationships between departments. Although not particular to this situation, this scenario is an example of how specialties across medicine develop competing structures for care instead of developing a collaborative approach to care. Traditionally, access to the interventional radiology suite has been limited to radiologists. The invasive cardiologists who perform these studies have become overextended with the expansion of other clinical programs and withdrawn from this clinical space.

Vascular surgery, although well trained in endovascular procedures, has been limited by inaccessibility to the cath lab or interventional suite. This siloed approach to care has led to the current paradigm with no existing mechanisms to mitigate this loss in staffing.

● DIAGNOSIS AND TREATMENT

Considering the acute need: Patients requiring vascular procedures must be treated promptly and appropriately. How this hospital can develop a plan to leverage the loss of 2 established providers to create a healthier and more resilient treatment paradigm is ideal. However, this will require careful negotiations between competing specialties to develop an equitable plan. The competing interests can be broken down into specific domains:

1. Educational threats/opportunities (how to maintain access for both interventional radiology and vascular surgery trainees to these cases).
2. Territorialism/turf wars (eg, "these procedures are mine").
3. Infrastructure and structural challenges (space limitations).
4. Financial pressures (revenue loss from moving cases out of IR).

● EDUCATIONAL THREATS/OPPORTUNITIES

First, educational threats and opportunities must be directly addressed. The viability of robust training programs is vital to academic medical centers. Stakeholders extend beyond the affiliated hospital to the program directors and educational leaders at the main academic center. These negotiations will need to identify not only the threats to education but also opportunities to expand the educational opportunities for training programs. As these negotiations progress, involving the educational leadership of both vascular surgery and interventional radiology will be vital. In an ideal situation, both training programs can benefit from a shared model of staffing of endovascular cases. The diversity of approaches that trainees can be exposed to in a multidisciplinary model will help both programs produce the best trained product.

● TERRITORIALISM/TURF WARS

Turf wars and conflict between departments within a healthcare system frequently involve a variety of emotions and "cultural differences." Providers and departments often view their approach as the best approach. Threats to their practice will be met with apprehension and aggression. A recent study of collaboration and conflict between vascular surgeons and interventional radiologists identified that cultural differences between specialties seemed more important than ego and financial drivers.[1]

● INFRASTRUCTURE AND STRUCTURAL CHALLENGES

Infrastructure and structural challenges may seem to be the easiest problem to tackle; however, changes to infrastructure or sharing of resources can create significant discord. Hospitals frequently are balancing the distribution of scarce resources. Recognizing the current limitations of infrastructure and the consequences of distributing these resources will be critical for negotiation effectively.

● FINANCIAL PRESSURES

Financial pressures are a strong barrier to collaboration between specialties. Reimbursement models in hospitals that create provider or specialty incentives tied to volume may exacerbate existing tensions between groups. The pressures of billing can be alleviated by leadership restructuring incentives to reward collaboration through multidisciplinary care, or quality.

CHAPTER 25 • Negotiating Turf Battles Between Specialties

● SCIENTIFIC PRINCIPLES AND EVIDENCE

Approaching the negotiations, we will review the literature surrounding negotiation and collaboration. There has been a significant effort to discuss navigating these difficult relationships in the business world. We will consider several useful components below.

Emotion

Emotion is a crucial component of negotiation. Traditionally, we have focused on developing a "game plan" for negotiation involving offers and counteroffers, but we have dedicated insufficient effort to understanding how emotion can influence negotiation, especially in charged situations. Alison Wood Brooks writes about how emotion affects negotiations and how to anticipate the impact of emotion on negotiations in her Harvard Business Review article, "Emotion and the Art of Negotiation."[2] Dr. Brooks details the impact of anxiety, anger, excitement, disappointment, sadness, and regret on negotiations. Anxiety, as Dr. Brooks details, may lead to a desire to end negotiations and worse outcomes of negotiations. Avoiding anxiety requires planning, practicing, and rehearsing. In situations where anxiety seems unavoidable, a third-party negotiator can help mitigate these emotions. Anger is probably a more common emotion in negotiating "turf wars." Anger often is seen as useful emotion, but unfortunately, it is counterproductive to building a collaborative team or environment. In competitive environments, where participants view negotiations as "all or none," Dr. Brooks writes that anger often leads to escalation of conflict, biasing of perceptions, and impasses.[2] The repercussions of negotiations often lead to conflicting emotions of excitement, disappointment, sadness, and regret. Understanding not only your own emotions but the emotions of the persons on the other side of the table can lead to more effective negotiations. Through your negotiations, you must strive to involve all parties and give them ample time to have their voice heard. The best negotiators, as Dr. Brooks writes, not only improve outcomes for themselves, but also help their counterparts feel as though they too have "won" even when they have not benefited as greatly.[2]

Hardwiring Collaboration or Coaching Conflict

Organizations may try to increase collaboration through team-building exercises and trying to "hardwire collaboration," but often overlook the role of conflict in breakdowns within organizations. This is no different in health care. As Jeff Weiss and Jonathan Hughes write in their Harvard Business Review article, "Want Collaboration—Accept and Actively Manage Conflict,"[3] many executives underappreciate the inevitability and value of conflict. As they detail, effective organizations not only understand that conflict can result in improved outcomes but try to equip their teams with tools to manage conflict. Although the hospital leadership may want to own this conflict, escalation of conflict beyond the immediate players, in this case, the vascular surgery and interventional radiology leaders, may strip them of an opportunity to gain important experience in negotiation. Allowing the 2 groups to manage this conflict will hopefully result in more satisfaction with the outcomes, than if the decisions are simply handed down by management.[4]

● IMPLEMENTING A SOLUTION

Negotiation is critical to the success of the patients. Having a data-driven and methodical approach to your negotiations will lead to a more prepared negotiation and hopefully improved outcomes for all parties.

Key Steps

The first steps of negotiation must describe the current state. The team must identify the clinical needs and goals of all stakeholders. This must include not only a focus on the clinical needs but also any educational needs, research needs, and opportunities and financial incentives. After developing an understanding of the current scenario, it is important to explore the implications of any solutions on the stakeholders (both short and long term). During negotiations, the more prepared you are, the more likely you will have a successful outcome. Anticipation of the implications of change to all stakeholders will lead to a more prepared and effective negotiation. The negotiations will undoubtedly be much more successful if the stakeholders feel their voice is heard and appreciated. As you prepare, it will also be important to identify the barriers to change. In this example, barriers may be cultural (a lack of collaboration) or structural (lack of available time for procedures in the interventional suite). When negotiating, it will be important to be an active observer. Paying attention to your counterpart's body language and behavior will help you lead the discussion in the desired direction. Do not allow emotion to spoil the negotiations. Successfully negotiating your outcomes, try to start small and expand after reflection and evaluation. After successfully trialing the solution, have a plan for implementation more broadly.

Potential Pitfalls

When negotiating, make sure that everyone has a seat at the table. Excluding key groups will only lead to resentment and potentially jeopardize your success in implementation. After bringing everyone to the table, another potential pitfall is rushing to a solution. It is important to acknowledge all stakeholders' interests and give them equal weight. Rushing negotiations may lead to escalating tension or eventual disappointment with the outcome. Anger, as outlined above, is a common emotion in negotiations. It frequently is a defense when feeling threatened. You must avoid anger in your own negotiation, but you must also be prepared to defuse an angry counterpart. If anger is introduced, try to acknowledge their frustrations, and validate them, but try to lead them away. If, despite these strategies, tensions continue to rise, take a break to cool off. When you return to your negotiations, hopefully, some of the emotion will have dissipated. Similarly, entering a negotiation with anxiety or a desire to avoid conflict may lead to unsuccessful negotiations and concessions. Preparing ahead may help to alleviate your anxiety. Conflict must also be recognized, and understood, but not avoided. Reading the room, you need to also observe your counterparts' behavior and recognize when anxiety is driving their negotiation. Your thorough preparation will help to lead away from these anxieties and hopefully toward a positive outcome.

Key Steps in Change Management and Potential Pitfalls

Key Steps in Change Management

1. Describe the current clinical paradigm.
2. Engage the leaders within each department to understand the clinical, education, research, and financial needs and goals.
3. Understand and identify the implications of change to the clinical paradigm to all involved parties (patients, trainees, providers, departments, hospitals).
4. Identify barriers to collaboration and discuss openly solutions to these barriers.
5. Prepare for negotiations—plan and rehearse your negotiation.
6. Be observant of your counterpart's behavior and emotion—harness emotional intelligence.
7. Trail the solution within a specific time frame with planned evaluation following this trial period, engaging all parties in the evaluation.

Potential Pitfalls

1. Excluding key stakeholders from the negotiation.
2. Rushing the negotiation and developing a plan without critical input from all involved.
3. Allowing anger to interfere with successful negotiation.
4. Avoiding conflict and allowing anxiety to prevent successful negotiations.
5. Failing to follow up following the implementation of the solution.

MEASURING OUTCOMES

The success of these negotiations may not be obvious immediately. It will be important not only to determine metrics for success a priori but also to set a timetable for assessment. The success of reorganizing the care of patients undergoing endovascular procedures should be first determined by metrics of access, room utilization, and quality outcomes. The success of collaboration between IR and vascular surgery requires regular assessment of collaboration and regular meetings between IR and vascular providers. Since these changes impact educational programs for both programs, evaluations of the rotation should be openly examined by both vascular surgery and IR educational leadership and site representatives. Goals specific to this example are the following:

1. Wait times for procedures of less than 4 weeks for elective procedures and 1 week for urgent procedures.
2. Successful collaboration assessed by multidisciplinary meetings between groups and increased participation in cross-departmental programs.
3. Stable or improved trainee evaluations of the site rotation for both IR and vascular trainees.

FOLLOW-UP AND MAINTENANCE

To address this clinical shortfall, multiple strategies for treating patients with vascular disease were entertained. The options included the following: (1) Hiring interventional radiologists to maintain the current structure. (2) Closing the interventional radiology suite to vascular patients and shifting these patients to other services (cardiology and vascular surgery). (3) Opening the interventional suite to other services (vascular surgery and cardiology). (4) Creating a multidisciplinary team for the treatment of vascular disease that utilizes the OR and IR space.

After negotiations between hospital administration, vascular surgery, and IR, a multidisciplinary approach to patient care was developed. This included expanded collaboration between IR and vascular surgery to treat patients needing endovascular procedures. Vascular surgery was granted regular access to the IR suite to perform endovascular procedures. IR will continue to share in the care of patients requiring endovascular procedures. Junior faculty recruited to fill the IR vacancies will be mentored by both IR and vascular surgery faculty. The training programs for both IR and vascular surgery will benefit from collaboration. The trainees of both programs will staff cases regardless of specialty in the IR suite. This newly encouraged training across specialties will spur increased collaboration and improved training diversity. Although financial concerns may have been the most obvious concern, the focus on building a multidisciplinary offered a different incentive. Vascular surgery's presence in the IR suite has pulled revenue away from the radiology department; however, the access of IR to a multidisciplinary clinic and the promise of future avenues for patients offered a greater incentive to the IR team. The hospital administration has tied incentives to the development of this multidisciplinary program and has committed additional faculty positions and support to developing a multidisciplinary program that includes both IR and vascular surgery.

REFERENCES

1. Keller EJ, Collins JD, Crowley-Makota M, Chrisman HB, Milad MP, Vogelzang RL. Why vascular surgeons and interventional radiologists collaborate or compete: a look at endovascular stent placements. *Cardiovasc Inter Radiol.* 2017;40(6):814–821.
2. Brooks AW. Emotion and the art of negotiation: how to use your feelings to your advantage. *Harvard Business Review.* 2015;56–64.
3. Weiss J, Hughes J. Want collaboration—accept and actively manage conflict. *Harvard Business Review.* 2005; 93–101.
4. Saltman DC, O'Dea NA, Kidd MR. Conflict management: a primer for doctors in training. *Postgrad Med J.* 2006;82(963):9–12.

Addressing Low Performance Outliers in Outcomes Monitoring Programs

26

CASEY M. SILVER, KARL Y. BILIMORIA, AND ANTHONY D. YANG

Clinical Delivery Challenge

Upon reviewing a quality report, such as the American College of Surgeons National Surgical Quality Improvement Program (ACS NSQIP) Semiannual Report (SAR), a hospital learns that while they have performed well in most areas, their rates of postoperative venous thromboembolism (VTE) are higher than those at other hospitals, ranking in the bottom quartile of performance and as a statistically significant low performance outlier. VTE, including pulmonary embolism (PE) and deep vein thrombosis (DVT), represents a leading cause of preventable death in surgical patients, and it is therefore a common target of quality improvement (QI) efforts.[1] Surgeons reviewing the report consider possible explanations for their poor VTE outcomes. A convenient, often-used explanation for poor-quality performance is: "Our patients are sicker or more complicated than everyone else's." However, ACS NSQIP's data are risk adjusted, and thus differences in characteristics of patients treated in their hospital compared with others are likely already accounted for. The data are also case-mix adjusted, accounting for differences in the complexity of operations performed at the hospital. As a result, the explanation "Our patients are sicker than everyone else's" is unlikely to apply. Therefore, rather than searching for excuses or seeking to blame others for their poor VTE outcomes, the effective surgical QI team must take time for thoughtful reflection and ask themselves, "Why are our rates of VTE higher than those at other hospitals?" and "How can our VTE rates be reduced?"[2]

Outcomes monitoring initiatives have been instrumental in driving QI. Programs such as the ACS NSQIP collect risk-adjusted, patient-level data on surgical complications ranging from readmission to surgical site infection to mortality. Advantages of surgical registries over administrative data (eg, Medicare and insurance claims) include accurate data collection directly from patient records by trained clinical reviewers, outcomes measured to 30 days after surgery, and rigorous risk adjustment.[3] These data empower hospitals to measure and evaluate their performance relative to other similar facilities, and can help hospitals easily identify outcomes for which they are statistically significant poor-quality outliers. Once such an outlier has been identified, focused QI initiatives may be undertaken to correct the outlier and improve surgical care and patient outcomes. However, hospitals often find it difficult to understand how to improve performance based on outcome measure data alone.

● WORKUP

Upon the identification of a poor-quality outlier outcome, a thorough "workup" must be undertaken to understand the issues driving the low performance. First, it is important to recognize that while outcome measures are excellent in identifying distinct performance problems, it is usually difficult to understand the root causes underlying suboptimal care delivery based on outcome measures alone. *Process of care measures* (process measures) are often more useful metrics in identifying modifiable root causes of a poor outcome that can then be addressed in focused QI initiatives. Process measures are practices that, when performed or omitted, contribute either positively or negatively to a particular outcome.[4] In this case, VTE rates are the outcome measure, and associated process measures include administration of mechanical or chemical prophylaxis, which have been shown to reduce VTE rates by up to 80%. The successful or unsuccessful provision of postoperative prophylaxis will therefore likely be a major driver of VTE rates at any institution.[5] Many process measures are described in the literature, but are very specific to each outcome, the evidence-based care practices associated with that outcome, and the processes of care at each institution.

When trying to understand the underlying drivers of a particular poor outcome, process improvement methodologies (see the "Scientific Principles and Evidence" section) provide important, data-driven frameworks to identify process metrics and root causes that may be central to improving a poor outcome. A particularly useful tool from process improvement methodologies is *process mapping* that can aid in visualizing and detailing the steps and personnel involved in a specific care process such as the administration of VTE prophylaxis. Commonly used in business and manufacturing, as well as in health care, process mapping diagrams the inputs and outputs of a process in a table form, which can help identify potential care failure points (eg, VTE chemoprophylaxis never ordered or never administered) that might underlie a particular poor outcome.[6] A sample process map for the administration of VTE chemoprophylaxis is shown in Figure 26.1. Each step in the process map, in which a modifiable failure in care (eg, chemoprophylaxis not ordered) can lead to the adverse outcome (VTE), can be chosen as a process measure that can be addressed through a QI initiative.

A thorough data analysis is also needed to gain a better understanding of the current state of both outcome and process measures. Identifying patients who have suffered the adverse outcome (in this example, DVT and PE) and evaluating these patients for common failures in care based on the process map may offer a valuable starting point. Did these patients undergo the same or similar operations? Did they recover on the same unit postoperatively? Data sources that may be leveraged to answer these questions include not only ACS NSQIP SAR but also those that offer more granular data such as patient charts.

Forming a multidisciplinary QI team is vital to conducting a thorough, thoughtful assessment. Such a team should consist of relevant stakeholders at all levels and may include nursing leaders, physicians,

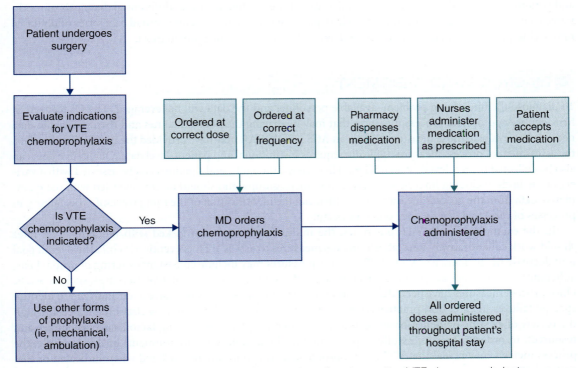

FIGURE 26.1 Example of a process map for administration of postoperative VTE chemoprophylaxis.

pharmacists, QI staff, and administrators, each of whom will contribute a range of experience and expertise. Health-care providers, including nurses, physicians, and trainees, will be able to assist with process mapping and help generate hypotheses about where failures in care may be occurring. Data abstractors may offer useful insights into not only the coding of the complication and whether or not changes to clinical documentation may have contributed to apparent increased rates of the complication but also, more importantly, help identify patterns of failure that they may have noticed while abstracting data. Hospital administrators and hospital quality leadership should also be engaged early to secure resources and ongoing support throughout the project lifecycle. Aligning the poor outlier outcome with a specific hospital strategic priority may help garner support and resources for a specific project. For instance, improving VTE outcomes will reduce the institution's Medicare Hospital-Acquired Condition penalties and improve its Leapfrog Hospital Safety Grade. Finally, direct observations of the care process and interviews with patients themselves can provide surgical QI teams with valuable insights into care processes and failures.

● DIFFERENTIAL DIAGNOSIS

Potential root causes underlying a poor performance outlier are varied and can usually be traced to one or more particular failure points in the process map. For instance, it is possible that most of the events occurred within a particular patient population. In the case of VTE rates, though the American College of Chest Physicians recommends VTE chemoprophylaxis throughout the entire inpatient hospitalization, studies have shown that up to 33% of surgical patients do not receive appropriate VTE chemoprophylaxis.[7] When digging deeper, the team may find that most of the events occurred within patients of a particular surgical department or hospital floor. When complications appear to be clustered, they may be due to intrahospital cultural or educational differences. For example, nurses may believe that sequential compression devices (SCDs) increase a patient's risk of falling. Other common reasons for failure to provide comprehensive VTE prophylaxis include patient refusal, medication not ordered or ordered at an incorrect dose or frequency, and patient off unit at the designated administration time.[7] While the exact differential diagnosis of modifiable root causes driving a poor outcome will depend on the specific outcome, broad categories of potential underlying problems—data, patients, providers, and processes—will apply to most.

● DIAGNOSIS AND TREATMENT

To diagnose the underlying problem, available personnel and the data will be leveraged. The QI team must first identify appropriate process measures that may be driving the poor outcomes and then gather the data necessary to evaluate those measures. While an ACS NSQIP SAR may have provided the initial outcome data, the assessment of process measures typically requires institutional and patient-level data. Qualitative data can also be collected from relevant stakeholders. Their views, thoughts, and opinions can be assessed with a variety of methods, including interviews, surveys, and focus groups, and should be corroborated with the quantitative data from the process measures. Only then can the identification of the root problem(s) (ie, failures in processes of care) that drive a poor outcome occur.

In the example of poor VTE outcomes, the multidisciplinary team tasked with reducing VTE rates should work collaboratively to establish process measures to assess VTE prevention. While the overall goal is to decrease the incidence of VTE, VTE process measures may include consistent ordering of prophylaxis, adherence to guidelines across all surgical floors, and use of adjunct preventative measures, such as SCDs. Once process measures have been defined and the data from these measures have been analyzed to identify specific failures in care, best practice solutions to address these failures may be first established through the review of existing evidence-based solutions and then adapted, considering factors such as culture and resources, in order to be successfully implemented in the unique care environment. In this example, the process metrics may reveal that VTE chemoprophylaxis is commonly not ordered when indicated or that patients often refuse chemoprophylaxis.

SCIENTIFIC PRINCIPLES AND EVIDENCE

Process improvement methodologies are varied and well described throughout both industry and health care. Plan-Do-Study-Act, Six Sigma, and Define-Measure-Analyze-Improve-Control (DMAIC) represent some of the most common frameworks, and though they differ in their exact terminology and methodology, they share a similar approach to improving processes of care and subsequent health outcomes. Each uses a stepwise approach to use data to guide change.[8]

QI initiatives in health care are often instigated by the identification of a problem of poor performance on a given outcome metric (if using DMAIC terminology, the Define phase), which prompts a more detailed investigation to uncover the root cause driving the performance problem (the Measure and Analyze phases). Activities performed within these initial three DMAIC steps are described in the "Workup" and "Diagnosis" sections of this chapter. In most cases, there can be a number of root causes, each accounting for a different portion of the overall problem. The Pareto principle (80/20 rule) postulates that 80% of problematic outcomes come from 20% of the underlying causes.[9] Assessment of the relative contributions of each root cause to the overall problem can thus be valuable in identifying which causes may be the highest yield to target for improvement. Once the underlying root causes have been identified, a plan for solving the problem is developed and then implemented (the Improve phase in DMAIC, described in the "Diagnosis and Treatment" and "Implementing a Solution" sections). Crucial to each framework is the subsequent evaluation of the effectiveness of the changes in improving both outcome and process measures. Results of these evaluations are then used to guide adaptation and create a plan for maintenance improvements in performance over time (the DMAIC Control phase, described in the "Follow-Up and Maintenance" section).

IMPLEMENTING A SOLUTION

Factors to consider when deciding which solutions to implement include the potential for benefit, the available evidence, and the simplicity and/or cost. While all causes for error should be considered as possible points of intervention and improvement, the Pareto principle dictates that some causes will contribute more to the outcome than others. Those root causes that account for the largest proportion of errors are often the best targets for improvement because they carry the largest potential benefit. The evidence supporting different interventions should also be considered. For many outcome measures, possible strategies for improvement are described in peer-reviewed publications and provide rigorous supportive for the efficacy of the intervention; however, the adaptation of the intervention may be required for it to be effective locally at each institution. Existing resources, such as best practice guidelines and toolkits, are available from organizations, such as the ACS, the Agency for Healthcare Research and Quality (AHRQ), and the Joint Commission. These resources can also be tailored to help meet the needs of individual hospitals, and some provide guidance for the adaptation of interventions. Solutions should also be evaluated for simplicity to determine if the effort of implementation is worth the possible benefit. For example, in the case of reducing VTE rates, a surgical QI team could consider enacting a new protocol to require and enforce the use of SCDs 24 hours a day postoperatively. However, this solution may ultimately be deemed lower priority due to an unfavorable effort to benefit ratio. Associated costs of proposed solutions should similarly be considered. Finally, failure to anticipate unintended consequences of introducing an intervention can lead to other, unexpected negative outcomes. In the aforementioned example, constant SCD use may lead to a higher fall rate. Simplicity, cost, effort and resources required to implement, and possible consequences should all be weighed carefully when deciding which solutions to implement.

Once the intervention(s) to be implemented have been agreed upon, there are a number of key *change management* steps that should be undertaken for implementation. First, buy-in from the relevant stakeholders is necessary. Specific stakeholders will vary depending on the intervention but will likely include nurses, physicians, billing specialists, and/or hospital administrators. When engaging with stakeholders, it is important to provide both evidence of the need for improvement as well as information on the possible benefits, and risks, of the proposed interventions.

SECTION 5 • Ensuring Quality and Safety

> ### Key Steps in Change Management and Potential Pitfalls
>
> #### Key Steps in Change Management
>
> 1. Form a multidisciplinary quality improvement team.
> 2. Speak with relevant stakeholders, including surgeons, trainees, nurses, administrators, data abstractors, and patients.
> 3. Understand potential root causes of the poor outcome and identify process measures that contribute to the outcome measure.
> 4. Gather and evaluate quantitative and qualitative data on the process measures that you have identified.
> 5. Formulate potential solutions based on available practice guidelines and feedback from stakeholders and devise a protocol for implementation.
> 6. Pilot the solution(s) in one smaller area to evaluate the feasibility, effectiveness, and potential unintended consequences. Gather data on both the relevant process measures and the overall outcome measure.
> 7. Scale the solution.
>
> #### Potential Pitfalls
>
> 1. Lack of a clear process map of possible root causes that may have contributed to the poor outcome measure.
> 2. Not getting buy-in from the stakeholders.
> 3. Failing to consider how changes will be maintained in the long term.

An implementation plan is also required. In many cases, it is useful to pilot the change in one smaller area, such as a single department or unit, to evaluate the feasibility, effectiveness, and potential unintended consequences before scaling the intervention to include a larger number of patients and providers. If multiple interventions are required, then the QI team will need to decide if they can be implemented simultaneously or sequentially. Finally, it is also important to prospectively plan for sustaining the improvements that are made, which might necessitate considerations of long-term changes to budgets, protocols, and outcomes monitoring processes.

● MEASURING OUTCOMES

Measuring the effectiveness of a QI initiative will require assessing performance over time (pre- to post-implementation) on not only the overall outcome measure but also the individual process measures addressed by the chosen interventions. In this case, the ACS NSQIP postoperative VTE rate will be the ultimate arbiter of success of the QI initiative, but changes in adherence to the relevant process measures pre- and postimplementation will also be key to understanding whether the initiative has been successful. It is also important to monitor for unintended consequences, which may require using data from other sources. Ongoing qualitative data collection (eg, follow-up interviews) may also be useful to assess how the solutions are being perceived by both patients and front-line providers affected by the interventions and whether or not there have been any challenges in their implementation.

● FOLLOW-UP AND MAINTENANCE

Follow-up is critical for sustaining and building on improvements that have been made. This "Control Phase" of a QI initiative (using DMAIC terminology) is undertaken when ongoing data collection occurs to monitor performance on both the key outcome and process measures over time to ensure that improvements are sustained. In many cases, an initial improvement may be followed by a decline in performance or adherence to a process. Thresholds for when performance declines enough to prompt a review should be set. Follow-up may require repeated iterative cycles of implementation, including either reinforcement

CHAPTER 26 • Addressing Low Performance Outliers in Outcomes Monitoring Programs

of one of the first initiatives or modification to an initiative in order to address an unintended consequence or a challenge in its implementation. QI is an iterative process that requires relevant and high-quality data, a multidisciplinary team with an effective leader, and the application of rigorous improvement methodology to improve processes of care and outcomes. With these elements, QI efforts may successfully create lasting improvement in surgical care when poor-quality performance outliers are identified.

REFERENCES

1. Gould MK, Garcia DA, Wren SM, et al. Prevention of VTE in nonorthopedic surgical patients: antithrombotic therapy and prevention of thrombosis: American College of Chest Physicians Evidence-Based Clinical Practice Guidelines. *Chest.* 2012;141(Suppl 2):e227S–e277S.
2. Yang AD, Bilimoria KY. Accurately measuring hospital venous thromboembolism prevention efforts. *JAMA.* 2016;315(19):2113–2114. doi: 10.1001/jama.2016.5422
3. About ACS NSQIP. Accessed May 6, 2022. https://www.facs.org/quality-programs/data-and-registries/acs-nsqip/about-acs-nsqip/
4. Birkmeyer JD, Dimick JB, Birkmeyer NJ. Measuring the quality of surgical care: structure, process, or outcomes? *J Am Coll Surg.* 2004;198(4):626–632. doi: 10.1016/j.jamcollsurg.2003.11.017
5. Khorfan R, Kreutzer L, Love R, et al. Association between missed doses of chemoprophylaxis and VTE incidence in a statewide colectomy cohort. *Ann Surg.* 2021;273(4):e151–e152. doi: 10.1097/SLA.0000000000004349
6. Antonacci G, Lennox L, Barlow J, Evans L, Reed J. Process mapping in healthcare: a systematic review. *BMC Health Serv Res.* 2021;21(1):342. doi: 10.1186/s12913-021-06254-1
7. Yang AD, Hewitt DB, Blay E, Jr., et al. Multi-institution evaluation of adherence to comprehensive postoperative VTE chemoprophylaxis. *Ann Surg.* 2020;271(6):1072–1079. doi: 10.1097/sla.0000000000003124
8. Minami CA, Sheils CR, Bilimoria KY, et al. Process improvement in surgery. *Curr Probl Surg.* 2016;53(2):62–96. doi: 10.1067/j.cpsurg.2015.11.001
9. Bates DW. Distribution of problems, medications and lab results in electronic health records: the Pareto principle at work. *Appl Clin Inform.* 2010;1(1):32–37.

Managing a Surgeon With Demonstrated Poor Outcomes

27

GERARD DOHERTY

> ### Clinical Delivery Challenge
>
> At 8:30 AM on a Tuesday, Dr. Tomaso, the section chief for Breast Surgery in the Division of Plastic Surgery laid out the data for the chair of the department. "Dr. Harper is now in her third year of practice," she noted, "but she is just not up to the task. Her results for wound infections, reoperations and patient satisfaction all deviate from the rest of us, and her reputation with the breast surgical oncologists is suffering." Dr. Tomaso presented 6 months of quality improvement data to support that. She concluded, "I am bringing this directly to you because she was a prize recruit for our division chief, and I am afraid that my impression that she is failing won't be well-received or appropriately addressed if I go to my chief."

The chair puzzled over the dimensions of this. The area of practice was outside of his direct expertise, but a variety of issues were swirling for him. Breast reconstruction was complex and multidisciplinary, involving opportunities for errors in judgment, technique, and patient relations. Junior faculty members often take some time to mature as independent surgeons; it was not uncommon for there to be a learning curve to their development. It was true that occasionally someone would fail, but that was unusual. He also knew that there was some rivalry within this division, and he was concerned about Dr. Tomaso's choice to bypass the division chief.

● WORKUP

The key first step in triaging a report of poor clinical outcomes—whether the report is connected to a surgeon, or to a service—is to assess the situation for risk of patient harm to determine whether the current activity can continue. If the risk is substantial, then the interests of patients, the surgeon, and the institution are generally aligned in suspending the activity.[1] For example, the death of a healthy donor during an organ harvest for transplantation should trigger a suspension of activity until the event can be thoroughly investigated and any program revisions implemented. In contrast, a cluster of wound infections following pancreas surgery may be expeditiously investigated while the planned activity continues under close observation. Though this embraces some risk that the cluster will be extended, the risk of harm from a wound infection is balanced by the harms of delaying care. This judgment must be made as the workup is planned: to continue activity or to suspend it.

Regarding a quality concern for a single surgeon, it may be possible to limit the risk to patients during evaluation. Depending on the circumstances and practice area, the surgeon may be restricted from doing some portfolio of high-risk cases. Alternatively, she or he may be asked to have a colleague do preoperative review of the plan or to act as a co-surgeon in the operating room while the evaluation is ongoing. This plan to prevent patient harm is dictated by the initial impression of the safety risk.

The second task is to determine whether, and to what extent, a problem exists. The evaluation of clinical quality data should be done professionally and as impartially as possible. It is usually preferable to involve institutional quality structures to aid this. Some areas of surgery may have pre-existing quality collaborative datasets that can be useful (eg, cardiac surgery, bariatric surgery, or transplant surgery), whereas others may require some collection of primary data or cross-referencing of existing datasets, such as hospital infection data, blood usage, or OR times, to develop a clear picture of surgeon performance and patient outcomes. Involvement of hospital patient safety/quality improvement experts can avoid the selective use of data (eg, too short a time period, inappropriate comparison group) that can be skewed to either level or refute a claim of poor outcomes. Finally, the weaponization of safety reporting has been used to damage surgeons for a variety of motivations (examples include personal or research disputes, clinical practice competition, or political rivalry). The assurance of fair evaluation of outcomes is critical to making the correct judgments and selecting the best interventions.

> By the end of the meeting, the chair determined that this report required further evaluation, but that there was no immediate danger to patients. He had some concerns about the possible inappropriate targeting of Dr. Harper by this quality report, but was equally concerned with the perception that the division chief might prefer to suppress the evaluation. He asked Dr. Tomaso to do 3 things: (1) review Dr. Harper's scheduled cases for the next few weeks to ensure appropriate preoperative decision-making; (2) meet with the Plastic Surgery division chief to review the same data that she had brought today; and (3) return the following week for a meeting with the Plastic Surgery division chief and the department representative from the Quality & Patient Safety department so that the 4 of them could plan an assessment.

● DIFFERENTIAL DIAGNOSIS

Patient outcomes that are worse than expected can occur over short periods due to bad luck, but even that requires demonstration that there are no underlying issues. The 4 basic areas that contribute to the patient outcomes attributable to a single surgeon can be divided into the following: **Judgment**, **technical skills**, **nontechnical skills**, and **service function** (Figure 27.1). Any of these can contribute; typically more than 1 is involved and requires attention. All of them should be evaluated in order to develop a complete diagnosis of the issue and a comprehensive intervention. Finally, the possibility that there is no defect in care and that in fact there is an ulterior motive for the safety reporting must always be considered.

> The meeting with Dr. Tomaso, Karen Najjar (a nurse from the Quality & Patient Safety department) and the Plastic Surgery division chief went reasonably well. Though the division chief was initially defensive and clearly a bit miffed by the report from Dr. Tomaso, Karen's discussion of how they might do an objective and confidential assessment calmed things down. Though that work would require a few weeks to complete, her review of the preliminary data and some back-channel information from the OR was both reassuring and informative. She did see evidence that Dr. Harper's operations were slower than others'. The OR nursing staff volunteered that she was "not very fast, but loses a lot of blood," but was also thought to be careful and typical of a junior surgeon. This led Karen to suggest 3 things that should be proposed publicly and led by Dr. Tomaso without targeting Dr. Harper: (1) implement and lead a weekly preoperative conference; (2) plan 360-degree evaluations by the hospital HR department as a service QI project, with the first 3 subjects including Drs. Harper and Tomaso, and the service-lead nurse in the OR; and (3) prepare a service manual for breast reconstruction, to detail their standard reconstructive ladder for breast cancer patients. The chair considered the highlight of the meeting to be Dr. Tomaso's observation that each of the other members of the Breast Surgery section trained in the department, and so it could be that Dr. Harper was finding some of their practices unclear.

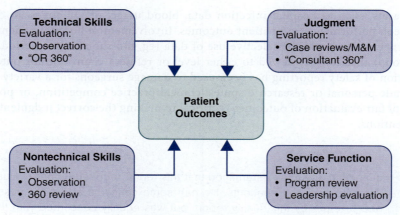

FIGURE 27.1 Surgeon-focused impacts to patient outcomes.

● DIAGNOSIS AND TREATMENT

The evaluation of a practitioner with suspect outcomes includes an assessment of each of the 4 domains in question, using approaches appropriate to the area. **Judgment** includes both preoperative and intraoperative decision-making, and the impact of each varies by specialty. The choices of whether a patient can benefit from an operation, and then which operative approach will work best, are complex. Wrong choices often cannot be overcome through technical skills. Determination of whether a surgeon judgment is responsible for poor patient outcomes usually requires an expert review of cases and is often a qualitative assessment. Additional information may be gleaned from consultant views of provider judgment, often collected by including them in a 360-degree evaluation process. Although technical errors are often determined to be the most common errors in patient care, many consider judgment errors to be the more important in creating the opportunity for subsequent technical mistakes.

Technical skills are often the primary problem identified by review, but less likely the predominant issue unless there has been the development of a physical impediment, as may more often happen with an aging surgeon.[2,3] Assessment of this usually requires direct OR observation or video review, or a review of observations by those frequently close to the technical performance, such as OR nurses, technicians, and trainees.[4] **Nontechnical OR skills** include communication, teamwork, leadership, and decision-making; deficits may be important to diagnose and improve, but are rarely the primary issue leading to poor patient outcomes. More frequently, nontechnical skill deficits amplify shortcomings in judgment or technical ability. Junior surgeons often take time to learn how to lead an OR team through an efficient day.[5]

Finally, **service function** can be a protective or injurious feature; surgeons are typically not isolated practitioners in our multidisciplinary practices. The impact of the practice environment must be included as a possible factor affecting patient outcomes. Are there structures in place to support best practices in preoperative planning (eg, tumor boards, service conferences)? Are there effective onboarding and mentoring structures for new faculty members to support their development? The role of service leadership should be included in any assessment of individual surgeon performance.

The review from Karen in Quality & Patient Safety was not great. With a full year of data, and including all of her cases, Dr. Harper did have worse outcomes; her patients, though recovered in the end, went through much longer operations and had more major (though mostly recoverable) complications. A records review of her cases by a senior plastic surgeon had shown no egregious planning errors, but a few cases that, in retrospect, might have been managed differently by others. In the 8 weeks since Dr. Tomaso's initial report, the preoperative conference had gotten started and met twice, the 360-degree evaluation questionnaires had been sent out by HR, but not yet analyzed, and one of the Plastic Surgery chief residents had produced a draft of a service standard document that others were currently reviewing. However, none of these plans seemed expedient enough to match what the chair now knew for certain about the patient results.

Dr. Harper was very worried to get a meeting invitation to see the chair and her division chief. She was even more concerned when she saw Karen in the conference room, as she only knew her previously from a sentinel event review. The chair had chosen the participants carefully; this would be an intimidating meeting for anyone. He wanted to keep the section chief out of this initial meeting because he wanted her to be a trusted part of the solution, and he included Karen because she could be a calming and objective influence. He and the division chief had to be there—it was their job, and they were ultimately the ones who needed to take responsibility for this.

After pleasantries, Karen reviewed the service results, and Dr. Harper's results in comparison. This was not news to Dr. Harper as she knew she was struggling to get patients recovered smoothly; in the moment she was horrified and assumed that she would be asked to find a new job. Upon later reflection, she was relieved by the plan for a 6-month Focused Professional Practice Evaluation (FPPE). The FPPE would require her to review each of her breast reconstruction cases at least a week ahead of time with Dr. Tomaso to finalize the OR plan and to have a co-attending surgeon with no trainees for all free-flap reconstructions. It would be a bit awkward with the residents, but those relationships were strained already; she had heard the whispers about how long she took in the OR, and how much of the case she did herself. At the end of the 6 months, Drs. Tomaso and Harper would return to review progress as measured by Karen's updated data, and they would decide whether the FPPE could end.

● SCIENTIFIC PRINCIPLES AND EVIDENCE

The most common deficit that causes a surgeon to have poorer than typical patient outcomes is errors in judgment; though case reviews often show technical errors as the most proximate mistake, many surgeons would point to judgment errors creating the context for that failing. This can manifest in a variety of ways, with surgeons, especially earlier in their experience, planning operations that their more seasoned colleagues might recognize as unlikely to succeed. As more experience accumulates, surgeons may experience a different effect, as their overall good outcomes may cause them to stretch the envelope to plan a big intervention when a more prudent plan might be a limited or foregone operation. Finally, in contrast, a senior surgeon who has taken on the role as a last resort for some patients may appropriately have measurably worse outcomes if risk adjustments do not reflect this status.

The intervention for all of these situations is the robust implementation of preoperative, multidisciplinary decision-making structures. These may include tumor boards for cancer practices, preoperative conferences for vascular or bariatric surgical services, and so on. The goal of these conferences is to provide an opportunity for group input in the operative plan. This is educational for the junior surgeon to protect against misjudgments, provides guardrails for the surgeon whose experience puts her or him at risk of becoming cavalier, and is protective for the surgeon who is knowingly assuming high-risk cases.

To intervene for the surgeon who either does not have access to this type of structure or whose results reveal deficits in spite of this, a mandatory, structured preoperative review of cases with a senior colleague can be helpful. This allows the adjustment of operative plans to the patient's benefit and provides education for the surgeon. In cases where this is necessary based on patient outcomes, it is often best for the surgeon, the mentor, and the institution for this to be done as a part of an FPPE process.[6] The FPPE must be a written plan with a time frame and metrics for resolution of the need for the FPPE. This deliberate structure is helpful in maintaining the initial momentum of the plan.

Technical skills are less often the primary issue in surgical patient outcomes, though they can be in some circumstances. For example, a junior surgeon may be tasked with taking on complex operations that they

180   SECTION 5 • Ensuring Quality and Safety

are not capable of completing in a reasonable time, thus leading to complications; or a surgeon may attempt to perform procedures using techniques that they are not skilled in (eg, a surgeon skilled at open hernia repair may be technically inadequate with the laparoscopic approach); or if they develop some physical deficit. Technical deficits can be overcome with training or coaching, and may require using a co-surgeon for a time, or require obtaining some remedial or proctored training. An FPPE, especially for utilizing new technology, may be useful. For surgeons with new physical impediments to operating, the resolution can usually only be achieved by removing them from that situation.

Nontechnical skills deficits are often related to the other deficits. Surgeons who are performing inadequately are often defensive and ineffective as communicators and team leaders in that moment. Nontechnical skills can be taught and learned, for example, through team-training exercises, but this training is most effective if combined with correction of the underlying deficiency.

Any assessment of the deficiencies of an individual surgeon should be combined with the evaluation of the function of the service. To what extent does the service support the safe practice of surgery and the introduction of new practitioners into the system? How can this be improved?

> After 3 months, Dr. Tomaso brought an interim report to the chair. "Dr. Harper is doing well; she was a bit reluctant at first to take on complex cases, but we got through that. I've been doing most of the co-surgeon duty, and frankly we've both been enjoying the chance to operate with another attending. It's been fun to show her some ways to manage the OR that move things along more quickly." At the 6 month mark, Karen pulled the data for the cases and compared them to previous. Dr. Harper's median OR times had come down to about 120% of the group median and her complications were on par with the group. In a meeting with the chair and division chief, the FPPE was determined to be resolved and was formally lifted. Monitoring would continue, and Dr. Tomaso resolved to maintain the service preoperative conference and the formal reconstructive ladder document for their group. She also noted that, in the future, she would establish a more involved process for bringing on and orienting a new surgeon to the group.

● IMPLEMENTING A SOLUTION

The key to making the proper plan is to make the proper assessment, followed by the proper intervention. The involvement of the Quality & Patient Safety department provides some arms-length protection, and with the right personnel can ensure a thorough assessment. In this case, the key to a positive resolution was gaining the personal involvement of Dr. Tomaso, the section chief, who was responsible for the function of the service. She may have initially thought that her responsibility was solely to report the issue, however, in what may have been a learning opportunity for her, the chair made it clear that her role also included the responsibility to intervene given her content expertise and leadership role. This was a measure of her ability to manage the function of the service.

The pitfalls and risks in a situation like this are several. First, there is a risk to the faculty member (Dr. Harper, in this case) that this episode could be damaging in a career-changing way. There are certainly cases in which the evaluated faculty member chooses to leave the institution for a fresh start, rather than engaging in a constructive process. There is also a risk of leadership responding in too limited a way. In scenarios such as this one, many people are aware of the shortcomings of the surgeon, and if those are left unaddressed, it reflects very negatively on the leadership. Finally, there is a risk that, in spite of sincere effort through FPPE, coaching, and other forms of remediation, the surgeon cannot perform at the required level. This FPPE may be followed by a reassessment of the surgeon's career plans, which can lead to any change along a spectrum extending from changing clinical focus to a more amenable area, to leaving surgery altogether. Though these events are troubling for all involved, if that is the right answer, it is better to reach that conclusion sooner than later.

Key Steps in Change Management and Potential Pitfalls

Key Steps in Change Management

Step	Details
Evaluate the immediate risk to patients	Suspend activity (surgeon or service) or continue during evaluation?
Obtain objective, valid measurement of quality data to assess/document perceived issue	Involve Quality & Patient Safety professionals in the assessment
Review reasons for surgeon quality deficit	
1. Assess surgeon judgment	Case reviews; M&M Conference; 360-degree evaluation including clinical staff and trainees
2. Assess surgeon technical skills	OR observation; 360-degree evaluation including OR staff and trainees
3. Assess surgeon nontechnical skills	Observation in and out of OR; 360-degree evaluation
4. Assess service function	Service review; leadership evaluation
Intervene on items 1–4 as needed	Liberal use of FPPE—constructive, not punitive
Monitor ongoing outcomes	Special attention to outcomes in service quality evaluations
Maintenance	Maintain any service function improvements that have been built into the change process

Potential Pitfalls

Pitfall	Risk
Surgeon perceives targeting rather than a constructive process	Surgeon may leave the institution when they should have been retained and improved
Leadership underreacts to information leading to persistence of quality issues	Patients suffer from persistent quality deficits; leadership viewed as ineffective by others in the institution
Surgeon incapable of performing at necessary level; role or responsibilities modified	Loss of investment in surgeons balanced by reduction of patient harm through resolving the misjudgment

● MEASURING OUTCOMES, FOLLOW-UP, AND MAINTENANCE

Quality measurement should be a routine part of managing a surgical practice. In a case such as this, with a known history of quality issues, there should certainly be careful attention to the outcomes of this surgeon in the future. However, in the best-case scenario, that attention diminishes over time as the results consistently blend with the rest of the group.

Most importantly, however, the service function aspects that were changed in order to support this improvement should be maintained. In addition, any lessons learned about bringing on new surgeons should be applied for future recruits.

REFERENCES

1. Enumah SJ, Resnick AS, David C, Chang DC. Association of measured quality with financial health among U.S. hospitals. *PLoS One*. 2022;17(4):e0266696.
2. Marsh KM, Turrentine FE, Schenk WG, et al. Errors in surgery: a case control study. *Ann Surg*. 2022;276(5):e347–e352.
3. Rosengart TK, Doherty G, Higgins R, Kibbe MR, Mosenthal AC. Transition planning for the senior surgeon: guidance and recommendations from the Society of Surgical Chairs. *JAMA Surg*. 2019;154(7):647–653.
4. Chhabra KR, Thumma JR, Varban OA, Dimick JB. Associations between video evaluations of surgical technique and outcomes of laparoscopic sleeve gastrectomy. *JAMA Surg*. 2021;156(2):e205532.
5. Sinyard RD, Rentas CM, Gunn EG, et al. Managing a team in the operating room: the science of teamwork and non-technical skills for surgeons. *Curr Probl Surg*. 2022;59(7):101172.
6. Focused Professional Practice Evaluation (FPPE)—Understanding the Requirements. What are the key elements organizations need to understand regarding the Focused Professional Practice Evaluation requirements? Accessed August 21, 2022. https://www.jointcommission.org/standards/standard-faqs/hospital-and-hospital-clinics/medical-staff-ms/000001485/

High-Volume Hospital With Low-Volume Surgeons

28

PATRICIA C. CONROY, MOHAMED ABDELGADIR ADAM, AND JULIE ANN SOSA

Clinical Delivery Challenge

At a high-volume quaternary academic medical center, various surgeons take acute care surgery call. On any given day, the attending surgeon on call may be a general surgeon, an acute care surgeon, or a subspecialized minimally invasive, hepato-pancreato-biliary, colorectal, breast, or endocrine surgeon. One evening, a patient presents to the emergency department with a 6 cm pelvic abscess secondary to complicated diverticulitis (Hinchey II) without peritonitis. The on-call attending has an elective practice focused primarily on minimally invasive foregut surgery. The patient is admitted to the general surgery service, and interventional radiology is consulted to place a percutaneous drain. Three days later, the patient has not improved despite adequate drainage, and the decision is made to proceed to the operating room (OR). However, the admitting surgeon rarely performs non-emergent colorectal procedures

When considering **low-volume surgeons** at **high-volume centers**, how can we ensure (1) optimal patient outcomes, (2) patient access to complex operations, and (3) surgeons are able to develop and maintain skills for complex operations?

Surgical treatment at **high-volume hospitals** and by **high-volume surgeons** has been shown to be associated with improved outcomes for many surgical procedures.[1,2] Surgeons with low volumes for a specific procedure but high volumes for related procedures appear to have similar or at least improved outcomes compared to overall low-volume surgeons.[3] However, the relative importance of hospital volume versus surgeon volume seems to differ based on the surgical procedure.

● WORKUP

Several key components of this clinical delivery challenge revolve around **surgeon-level operational data**. A detailed review of the surgeon call schedule should be performed, including a review of which surgeons are taking call and how often. Comparing the operations surgeons are performing while on-call to their practice's field will be important to understand. Analysis of variability of the cost associated with on-call procedures and subsequent hospitalizations by surgeon and surgeon specialty is critical, as is reviewing the work relative value units (wRVUs) of surgeons' on-call versus elective operations. Depending on the payer mix, profitability has been shown to reflect outcomes.[4] Major postoperative complications are associated with increased hospital costs[5] and a lower hospital contribution margin depending on patients' insurance coverage.[4] Consequently, patient-level outcomes data by surgeon, including metrics such as operative duration, estimated blood loss, hospital length of stay, reoperation, readmission, and overall complication indices are important to understand. Institution-level data from established programs such as the American College of Surgeons National Surgical Quality Improvement Program (ACS-NSQIP) also may be helpful in understanding patient-level outcomes by surgeons. Information regarding the impact of operation-specialty mismatch on clinical outcomes and profitability at each institution will be helpful to understand the hospital-specific extent of the problem.

Data regarding **staffing** and **resource availability** are critical. If subspecialized surgeons have no redundancy in their schedules in order to take on urgent cases, the system will be limited in its ability to triage

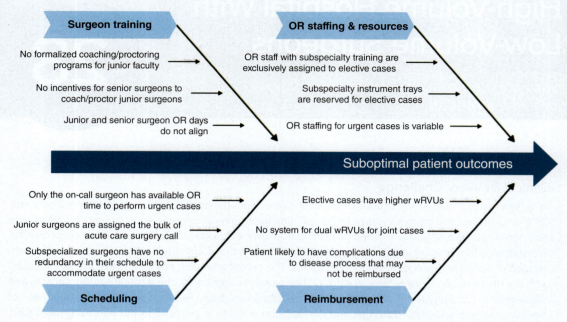

FIGURE 28.1 Example fishbone diagram to identify areas for improvement when low-volume surgeons are performing complex operations at high-volume centers leading to suboptimal patient outcomes.

nonelective cases to its high-volume surgeons. Leadership from different departments and divisions within the same institution are key stakeholders and may have different philosophies regarding how their surgeons spend their time. Individual surgeons may have different motivators; it is important to understand surgeon-level concerns from both low-volume and high-volume surgeons' perspectives. Availability of OR staffing is also an important consideration. Inexperienced OR staff working with a low-volume surgeon may lead to inefficiencies and adverse outcomes.

Several process tools may be helpful to identify target areas for improvement. A fishbone diagram (also known as an Ishikawa diagram) may be particularly helpful given the wide range of stakeholders when considering low-volume surgeons at high-volume centers. An example fishbone diagram is shown in Figure 28.1.

Return to Scenario

The admitting surgeon is interested in obtaining more experience with colorectal operations. However, because the patient will likely need a Hartmann's procedure and subsequent complex takedown, the admitting surgeon would like to involve a colorectal surgeon in this patient's care. This process can be facilitated and supported by hospital leadership and administration, motivated by the demonstration of improved outcomes and profitability.

● DIFFERENTIAL DIAGNOSIS

There are several potential challenges in involving a colorectal surgeon in this patient's care while also keeping the admitting, low-volume (non-colorectal) surgeon involved. The subspecialized surgeon may not have OR time to accommodate an urgent case. There may be **limited incentives** for both surgeons to remain involved in the patient's care. For example, performing a joint case may not be lucrative for the subspecialized surgeon, who may be reimbursed at a higher rate for performing an elective case on their own. Similarly, if the low-volume surgeon is not the primary surgeon for this patient's operation, the low-volume surgeon may not be compensated for the preoperative care they have already provided.

DIAGNOSIS AND TREATMENT

Optimizing scheduling strategies is critical to solving this challenge. Including strategic redundancy in surgeons' schedules to accommodate adding on urgent operations will allow for intra-institutional centralization of complex cases and high-volume surgeons to be involved when the need arises. This could include call schedule redundancy, where there are both a primary surgeon on call and subspecialty surgeons available for intradepartmental referral. If such redundancy already exists within the hospital, the process for intradepartmental referral should be formalized in order to leverage existing systems. This also ensures broader patient access to care because it does not require that patients are transferred to another institution to receive high-volume care. Centralized scheduling for OR time and staffing should also be considered. Establishing dedicated rooms and/or time for urgent cases can be helpful to ensure availability. Such strategies will require multidisciplinary participation by nursing, OR staff, and anesthesiologists to ensure appropriate levels of specialized support are in place to facilitate complex operations.

Incentives will need to be in place to encourage joint participation by both low-volume and high-volume surgeons. Allowing for dual wRVUs is a potential strategy to ensure both surgeons are adequately compensated for their time. Introducing some flexibility in surgeons' OR time may allow for increased willingness to accommodate urgent add-ons which may be disruptive to a surgeon's schedule. Aligning operative days so that junior surgeons have access to senior partners for intraoperative consultation on challenging cases is an important strategy that minimizes the burden on both surgeons. Formalizing coaching/proctoring programs for junior surgeons by senior surgeons leverages existing expertise at the institutional level. Formal mentoring programs at the professional societal level may also mitigate some of these challenges. For example, early career mentorship programs for fellowship-trained hepato-pancreato-biliary surgeons have been developed to aid in optimizing patient outcomes in laparoscopic hepato-pancreato-biliary surgery.

Surgeon-specific factors are also important to consider. If a surgeon's low volume is a consequence of their poor or no longer contemporary skill set, this is a problematic challenge to overcome. In this situation, the difficult but appropriate solution may require that the surgeon no longer practice. In contrast, if a surgeon's low volume is a consequence of their early career stage without an established referral network, strategies such as institution-sponsored marketing may be helpful. Similarly, expansion and regionalization of the healthcare system to grow overall volume may be considered. For example, in the setting of a crowded marketplace for a low-volume surgeon who is new to an academic medical center, the addition of an affiliated platform may allow the surgeon to build their practice while also bringing complex cases to the institution. If this approach is taken, it is important that the affiliate have a system in place to support complex cases. Sometimes, complex cases necessarily are done at the academic medical center due to the systems expertise needed.

SCIENTIFIC PRINCIPLES AND EVIDENCE

Hospital and surgeon volume have been shown to be key predictors of surgical outcomes.[1,2] The relative importance of center volume varies according to procedure type, and differences in outcomes based on hospital volume are generally greater for more complex operations.[1] For example, outcomes after esophagectomy, pancreatectomy, and abdominal aortic aneurysm repair have been shown to be better when the operations are performed at high-volume hospitals. This effect is likely due to more consistent processes for postoperative care, better-staffed intensive care units, and greater access to resources for managing complications. In contrast, for less complex operations where patients are relatively healthy and the risk of complications is lower, superior patient outcomes do not require a large perioperative team of surgeons, intensivists, consultants, and complex care teams. In these cases, high surgeon volume may be more protective than high hospital volume.[6] Consequently, a low-volume surgeon practicing at a high-volume center poses a clinical delivery challenge. **Potential solutions will leverage the infrastructure present at the high-volume center and the expertise of its high-volume surgeons to bolster patient safety and improve outcomes for low-volume surgeons.**

When approaching this problem, there are various key stakeholders who may have differing priorities. Consequently, it is important to produce objective, easily understandable data that illustrate the underlying problem and potential solutions. In the case of low-volume surgeons practicing at high-volume hospitals, the underlying problems are suboptimal resource use and patient outcomes. To directly compare surgeon performance, statistical process controls (SPC), where statistical methods are applied in order to control a process to evaluate quality, can be used to evaluate performance data by a surgeon.[7] A key step in SPC is creating a control chart, and risk-adjusted cumulative sum (CUSUM) charts have been successfully employed to study quality in surgical care.[8] When thoughtfully constructed, CUSUM charts are intuitive and easily interpretable. In parallel, surgical auditing has been shown to facilitate both quality improvement and cost reduction and can be employed to increase stakeholder buy-in.[9]

Return to Scenario

The colorectal surgeon is willing to be involved in the patient's index operation and assume their long-term care and eventual ostomy takedown. However, the colorectal surgeon had to reschedule elective patients and is frustrated because this is a recurring issue. The Department of Surgery initiates a review of the acute care surgery call system and surgeon-specific performance evaluations using SPC. These data are used to initiate discussions with the surgical division chiefs to create a backup subspecialty call system and a policy for dual wRVUs for combined acute care surgery cases.

● IMPLEMENTING A SOLUTION

Solutions to this clinical delivery challenge should be crafted to achieve 3 major objectives. First, optimizing patient outcomes should be at the forefront of decision-making. Second, ensuring broad patient access to complex care is a priority. Limiting procedures to only high-volume surgeons at high-volume hospitals disproportionately affects patients with limited access to care.[10] It is important to establish pathways to broaden access to surgical care without compromising the quality of care. Third, surgeons should be given opportunities to safely develop and maintain their skills. In this scenario of a low-volume surgeon at a high-volume center, the necessary expertise is available at the medical center in question to achieve these 3 objectives. Creating a subspecialist intradepartmental referral system and ensuring strategic redundancy in subspecialists' schedules to accommodate urgent and potentially emergent cases reduces the burden on the subspecialist to assist with care. Depending on surgeon preference, it is possible to create pathways to transfer patients to the care of subspecialized surgeons within the same institution. Alternatively, establishing a dual wRVU system may incentivize collaboration between surgeons and encourage joint cases. The ultimate goal is to establish processes that encourage and ensure smooth cross-specialty intradepartmental collaboration. These approaches allow for intrainstitutional centralization of complex cases without needing to transfer patients to other centers to receive their care.

Effectively implementing this change will require a systematic approach. First, the faculty in the Department should be made aware that discussions are ongoing to create an intradepartmental referral system. Faculty should be given opportunities to voice their concerns and provide input on how such a system might be created. Residents, schedulers, administrators, and nursing staff should also be given an opportunity to participate in these discussions. Once all key stakeholders have had a chance to provide input, leadership should craft both a long-term vision and a clear plan for implementing and troubleshooting an intradepartmental referral system. Part of this process should include a literature review and consultation with experts in the field. After the plans have been sufficiently distributed, the changes should be implemented at a smaller scale. Instead of initiating a referral system for all subspecialties, the Department should choose the subspecialty which is most often burdened by the current system and pilot the changes for that group. After a trial period, the results of the pilot should be analyzed to determine what changes should be made before widely implementing the new system across divisions. Finally, key metrics of success should be shared widely with the Department and key stakeholders.

Key Steps in Change Management and Potential Pitfalls

Key Steps in Change Management

1. Communicate with key stakeholders that a problem has been identified and discussions are ongoing regarding how best to address it.
2. Broadly elicit feedback and input from faculty, residents, schedulers, administrators, nursing staff, and others who may be affected.
3. Craft a plan for implementing and troubleshooting the proposed change with a clear vision of what the goals are.
4. Distribute the plans and overarching vision to key stakeholders.
5. Pilot the potential changes at a smaller scale in an area most likely to be affected (eg, implement an intradepartmental referral schedule for colorectal surgery only).
6. Analyze the results of the pilot using predetermined metrics and make changes as appropriate.
7. Broadly implement the revised changes.
8. Share key metrics of success with key stakeholders.

Potential Pitfalls

1. Not involving key stakeholders in decision-making; crafting a solution that does not meet stakeholder needs and instead increases their work burden.
2. Widespread implementation of a change without first piloting changes at a smaller scale.
3. Not planning for periodic reviews after implementation to adapt solutions as needs arise.

There are several pitfalls to be aware of when crafting and implementing a solution to this problem. It is critical to engage team members who will be most affected by these changes. A solution that does not meet their needs and potentially increases burdens on their work will not be successful. There will likely be unanticipated issues that need to be worked out; it is critical to pilot changes before widespread implementation. Creating and implementing solutions to these clinical challenges are iterative. It is important to plan for periodic reviews to adapt solutions as needs arise.

● MEASURING OUTCOMES

The key metrics to assess the effectiveness of the solution should include a careful review of patient-level outcomes data and surgeon-level productivity data. Comparing aggregate outcomes data, including metrics such as hospital length of stay, reoperation, readmission, and overall complications indices before and after implementation, will be important to identify both positive and negative effects of any changes. Hospital-level data on costs associated with procedures and hospitalizations associated with the acute care surgery service should be reviewed. Similarly, surgeon operative volume and cumulative wRVUs are important metrics to ensure surgeon productivity has not been negatively affected. Outcomes data should be broadly reviewed at regularly defined intervals to identify unintended consequences, particularly with regard to interests outside of the Division or Department, including the overarching health system and other perioperative departments.

● FOLLOW-UP AND MAINTENANCE

New challenges are likely to arise, and the department should remain adaptable. Particular attention should be paid when hiring new faculty who may have different levels of expertise and case volumes, which could affect the current structure. The same metrics that are used to evaluate outcomes should be periodically reviewed at regular intervals with a focused lens on optimizing patient access to high-volume care.

REFERENCES

1. Birkmeyer JD, Siewers AE, Finlayson EV, et al. Hospital volume and surgical mortality in the United States. *N Engl J Med*. 2002;346(15):1128–1137. doi: 10.1056/NEJMsa012337
2. Birkmeyer JD, Stukel TA, Siewers AE, Goodney PP, Wennberg DE, Lucas FL. Surgeon volume and operative mortality in the United States. *N Engl J Med*. 2003;349(22):2117–2127. doi: 10.1056/NEJMsa035205
3. Modrall JG, Minter RM, Minhajuddin A, et al. The surgeon volume-outcome relationship: not yet ready for policy. *Ann Surg*. 2018;267(5):863–867. doi: 10.1097/SLA.0000000000002334
4. Eappen S, Lane BH, Rosenberg B, et al. Relationship between occurrence of surgical complications and hospital finances. *JAMA*. 2013;309(15):1599–1606. doi: 10.1001/jama.2013.2773
5. Dimick JB, Chen SL, Taheri PA, Henderson WG, Khuri SF, Campbell DA. Hospital costs associated with surgical complications: a report from the private-sector National Surgical Quality Improvement Program. *J Am Coll Surg*. 2004;199(4):531–537. doi: 10.1016/j.jamcollsurg.2004.05.276
6. Sosa JA, Bowman HM, Tielsch JM, Powe NR, Gordon TA, Udelsman R. The importance of surgeon experience for clinical and economic outcomes from thyroidectomy. *Ann Surg*. 1998;228(3):320–330. doi: 10.1097/00000658-199809000-00005
7. Chen TT, Chang YJ, Ku SL, Chung KP. Statistical process control as a tool for controlling operating room performance: retrospective analysis and benchmarking. *J Eval Clin Pract*. 2010;16(5):905–910. doi: 10.1111/j.1365-2753.2009.01213.x
8. Rogers CA, Reeves BC, Caputo M, Ganesh JS, Bonser RS, Angelini GD. Control chart methods for monitoring cardiac surgical performance and their interpretation. *J Thorac Cardiovasc Surg*. 2004;128(6):811–819. doi: 10.1016/j.jtcvs.2004.03.011
9. Govaert JA, van Bommel AC, van Dijk WA, van Leersum NJ, Tollenaar RA, Wouters MW. Reducing healthcare costs facilitated by surgical auditing: a systematic review. *World J Surg*. 2015;39(7):1672–1680. doi: 10.1007/s00268-015-3005-9
10. Reames BN, Ghaferi AA, Birkmeyer JD, Dimick JB. Hospital volume and operative mortality in the modern era. *Ann Surg*. 2014;260(2):244–251. doi: 10.1097/SLA.0000000000000375

High Variability in Surgical Teams

29

SAPAN N. AMBANI

"If your actions inspire others to dream more, learn more, do more, and become more, you are a leader."
—John Quincy Adams

Clinical Delivery Challenge

An established surgeon is assigned to a new surgical site within a healthcare system, consisting of team members new to a practice. The surgeon previously benefited from a dedicated, established team of operating room (OR) staff who have routinely performed the same surgical procedures for years. Each unique individual of the team knew the other team member's strengths, weaknesses, and sequences of events. In these surgical cases, team members were able to anticipate and fill in the gaps of others. The surgeon's outcomes were on par with established benchmarks and national averages.

In addition to a new site, the COVID-19 pandemic led to significant changes that affected the stability of the health system workforce. Furloughs, employee displacement to different systems or geographic locations, or an exit of workforce members permanently, led to a lack of consistency in the local workforce.[1]

High-quality surgical care hinges on solid teamwork. The goal of a surgical team is to shepherd a patient through an invasive surgical procedure and ensure that the harm of treatment is minimized while the benefit is maximized. Surgery must work as an efficient fine-tuned machine, consisting of many parts (team members). They must work in synchrony to achieve a high-quality outcome. Just as a complex machine, frequent part exchange may lead to misalignment threatening overall performance and may lead to unsatisfactory patient outcomes. In this chapter, we will explore pitfalls that may accompany a highly variable surgical team and provide strategies to safeguard patient care.

● WORKUP

With a new location and a variable team, it is important to define the team members. What number of staff are considered temporary (eg, agency or traveling staff) versus those in permanent positions? How many of those in permanent positions belong to a team as opposed to floating to cover different service lines?

Simultaneously, quantitative and qualitative data collection should commence to ensure patient outcomes remain similar to previous standards. Quantitative data metrics should include well-accepted patient outcomes with root cause analysis. In addition to patient outcomes data, OR efficiency metrics should be gathered. These metrics can be analyzed across surgery sites and include different surgical staff, surgeons, and anesthesia providers to determine whether any consistent points of variance are identified.

Metrics that are commonly used to assess OR efficiency include the following Figure 29.1:

- Intraoperative time: wheels in and out (the total time a patient spends in the OR). This is influenced by the surgical team, anesthesia team, and OR nurse/technicians, but can also be affected by equipment (eg, central supply processing, equipment stocking) and ancillary services (eg, fluoroscopy, laser, pharmacy).

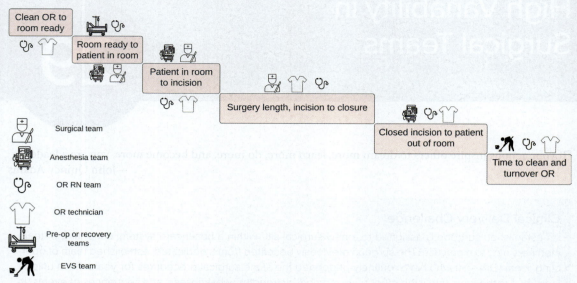

FIGURE 29.1 Peri- and intraoperative time per patient.

- Turnover time (the time from "wheels out" of a patient to "wheels in"). This is primarily influenced by the Preoperative/Postanesthesia team, OR nurse/technicians, anesthesia team, surgical team, environmental services, and patient complexity, but can also be affected by equipment (eg, central supply processing, equipment availability) and ancillary services (eg, pharmacy, specimen processing).
- OR ready for patient in the room, preoperative. This is primarily influenced by the anesthesia team, OR RN/technicians, and preoperative team. Patient factors can also affect this metric such as unforeseen patient complexity requiring additional preoperative testing (EKG, electrolyte blood testing, etc.) or patient anatomy (difficult IV or difficulty with preoperative pain blocks).
- Patient in the room to incision, preoperative. This is primarily influenced by the anesthesia team for induction, surgical team for patient positioning, OR RN/technicians, and patient complexity. This is the point where all personnel in the OR are responsible for a safe, effective pre-incision verification and time-out procedure(s).
- Closure of the incision to the patient out of the room, postoperative. This is influenced by the surgical team, anesthesia team, OR RN/technician, and patient complexity
- Total operative time. This is influenced by the surgical team and OR team. Sometimes additional equipment requirements can lead to delays when they require delivery by central supply and procurement by the OR RN or OR technicians.

In each of these time points, OR staff all have fluid roles, and the primary leader of the team will shift. Listing every point of observed variability is beyond the scope of this chapter and institution dependent; however, we will describe a couple of common points of variability among each position.

OR surgical technician staff—responsible for removal, obtainment, and preparation of instruments for each case. They ensure instruments are properly accounted for before and after each case.

- Inexperience with surgical teams leading to inefficient movements during surgery.
- Unfamiliarity with OR RN staff, which may lead to suboptimal communication when accounting for instruments.

OR RN staff—They are responsible for patient safety during different phases of patient care from pre-op, intra-op, and Postanesthesia Care Unit.

- Ineffective communication between OR RN, anesthesia, and surgical teams can lead to a preoperative delay if the patient is not marked, or documentation is not properly performed.

- Patient and/or procedural complexity outside their usual scope of practice. OR RNs assigned to unfamiliar service lines may not be aware of special equipment outside of a pick sheet, variations in documentation, or relevant patient details.

Anesthesia staff—responsible for workup, administration of safe anesthesia, and real-time monitoring.

- Additional requests for more invasive treatment or monitoring not previously discussed until the time of surgery which may include arterial line placement, paralysis during surgery, or rapid transfusion equipment.
- Ineffective communication between surgical teams and anesthesia staff. Unawareness of surgery completion can lead to prolonged procedure end to extubation time.

Surgical staff—responsible for proper patient selection and preparation, documentation of the necessity of the procedure, and the surgical procedure itself.

- Unfamiliar surgical teams between the surgeon and resident surgeon/first assistant where the flow of the surgery requires additional communication for simple and complex steps.
- Patient complexity. Difficult patient anatomy or complexity can prolong surgical time and may not be accounted for preoperatively.

Environmental services (EVS) staff—responsible for room sanitization between surgical procedures and removal of hazardous waste from the previous surgery.

- Notification delay. If the environmental services staff are delayed in notification that the patient has departed the OR, room turnover will be delayed.
- Staffing shortage. A shortage of EVS personnel can lead to longer individual cleanings of each OR due to increased personal responsibilities and/or delays in arrival.

All the key stakeholders above and the hospital or OR leadership can review the time points when significant variability occurs. It is then the responsibility of the team members and administration to qualitatively investigate the outlier cases to obtain the points of view of the personnel involved. Trends and themes may emerge in cases that finish in shorter and longer amounts of time. A root cause analysis can lead to actionable items from a high-functioning team that could be adopted across other surgical cases. In addition, when negative outcomes are observed, protective actions or factors could be put into place to prevent additional or recurrent negative events.

● DIFFERENTIAL DIAGNOSIS

Variability in surgical teams is an inevitable event in modern medicine, especially when moving to a new location. As the new environment comes online, new relationships will have to be formed between all OR stakeholders. New and unpredictable combinations of coworkers will frequently occur. A team in the OR needs to ensure clear, consistent, and concise communication occurs as well as be knowledgeable about the surgical case and their role in the delivery of surgical care.

Another point of variability could be different policies from the original location. It is important that leaders, surgeons, and staff review the new policies and procedures that can accompany a new location even if within the same healthcare system. Emergency and routine procedures for operations management can vary greatly.

● DIAGNOSIS AND TREATMENT

At a new site, data should be heavily reviewed to ensure patient outcomes are consistent and to correct non-desirable outcomes before they become habits that engrain themselves into the workplace culture. As before, a quantitative review of OR time stamps can clue the team members and administration into positive and negative outcomes. However, direct observation by a third-party member and qualitative interviews with the OR staff will more clearly identify the specific problems or issues that may occur. Direct observation and interviews are time intensive; however, their utility cannot be understated. To treat an ever-changing team, the broad culture of an institution or new location must be addressed. The social interaction, norms, and knowledge of the team members must be supported and enriched to build a cohesive network of personnel that make up variable teams. Team members must be educated and empowered, including at the time of hire, to speak freely and challenge a situation that they feel may harm patient care. A recent narrative, or qualitative systematic review, found that education, empowerment, and a culture of hierarchy flattening are essential to have a sustained environment of safety reporting.[2]

● SCIENTIFIC PRINCIPLES AND EVIDENCE

A systematic review of teamwork between healthcare teams found that teams who engaged in teamwork processes in simulated and real environments are 2.8 times more likely to achieve high performance than teams who do not.[3] Teamwork processes were defined as communication, coordination, and/or decision-making. The authors found that team training in routine situations, such as elective surgery, had a benefit in addition to emergency training. Increased teamwork had a significant improvement in the reduction of morbidity and mortality and improvement of patient outcomes. Team training and clinical event debriefings can lead to system improvement and improved teamwork.

A prospective observation study sought to evaluate factors that influence the expected length of surgery. In their observations and analysis, they concluded that communication failures between OR staff members are common and occurred in 57% of their observed surgical procedures across all surgical and surgical subspecialties which led to longer surgical times outside of the expected time allotment. Closed-loop communication, defined as feedback or a statement from the sender confirmed by the recipient, was also found to reduce communication failures. They also noted that when there was a lack of information or a lack of knowledge, communication was more likely to break down between team members.[4]

A qualitative investigation of effective teamwork in the ORs has been analyzed through semi-structured anonymous interviews with all team members of the OR. The found that ineffective team dynamics can increase errors and decrease patient safety, which increases morbidity and mortality. The authors described for major themes for effective OR performance and teams with expert-level performances.

1. Smooth flow. This describes a team where individuals have clear job duties, yet also understand the duties of the other team members in the OR. Individual team members monitor the performance of others, unburden overworked coworkers through shared work, adapt to changes, and have a shared mental model of the primary objective of the surgery.
2. United effort. This describes a team where there is a shared mutual trust between team members as they work together. A flattened hierarchy allows team members to speak up without reparation when a problem is occurring or about to occur.
3. Communication. This describes a team that has been introduced to each other by name to decrease communication barriers. This also focuses on direct and clear verbal information exchange between team members.
4. Positive attitude. This describes the shared respect that must be present between team members to minimize tension. A positive attitude helps foster communication during high-stress situations. This also includes a positive culture in the work environment that is meant to transcend the usual "hierarchy" role system.

The findings above were confirmed to apply to highly reliable, high-performing surgical teams that were also highly variable (citation). They found that fostering a positive OR environment, initiated by the surgeon, led to surgeries that performed well in terms of efficiency and outcomes. A work environment focusing on team behavior allowed for greater adaptability. In situations where the unexpected occurred (which is often the case in the OR), a supportive environment accommodated the change and avoided an adverse outcome. The authors note that "enacted [positive] environments can enhance perceived competence and perceived competence can lead to expanded experience."[5]

CHAPTER 29 • High Variability in Surgical Teams

As the surgeon and the new team members move to the OR, there are opportunities to build a team before the first surgical patient is treated. First, they can participate in team-building exercises outside of the OR to learn the communication styles of the individuals and build rapport with other team members. Even if teams vary, a familiar face and prior positive interactions will translate to future collaboration. Next, the surgeon and teams should run through mock elective surgeries and emergencies within the new environment to further their team building and start learning the locations of items within their new workspace. During these processes, if available, observation from outside coaches (OR RNs, surgeons, OR administration) can provide real-time feedback on positive and negative interactions to further enhance the team dynamics. Finally, it is particularly beneficial to ensure that all team members buy in to a common patient outcome-focused mission to provide direction and a singular purpose.

● IMPLEMENTATION OF A SOLUTION

As staff are hired for the new surgical site, lessons learned from the qualitative evaluation of the prior surgical team(s) can be passed on before the site opens and surgery commences. Team-building exercises and mock simulations of surgical cases can help new team members gain knowledge, build social relationships, and understand the goals of the team and institution. As the new surgical site opens, these team-building exercises can transition to the physical space in the new ORs. This can establish the environment in which the teams will work and build knowledge of the local area, supplies, and process flow for patient care. There may be situations where a new member such as a surgeon joins an existing team at a new location or ambulatory surgery center (ASC). Early communication, meet and greets, and team-building exercises break the ice for new, positive relationships before patient care is involved.

Key Steps in Change Management and Potential Pitfalls

Key Steps in Change Management

1. Identify high-functioning, efficient members of the surgical team with quantitative time analysis and qualitative investigation.
2. Interview and understand their methods to succeed at a local environment.
3. Observe known high-functioning surgical teams to develop themes in the local environment.
4. Develop a training curriculum with administration and other OR stakeholders to improve communication, teamwork, and process flow.
5. Pilot the potential solution and solicit feedback from known high-functioning team members.
6. Introduce new hires to this curriculum and include hands-on training during their training and orientation.
7. Evaluate operative time points and patient outcomes to determine if new teams are working well together.
8. Solicit ongoing feedback from new team members which may signal an abnormal signal before quantitative data.
9. When able, recruit and hire OR staff open to change who will embrace teamwork.
10. Request to be involved in the recruitment process.

Potential Pitfalls

1. Assuming that preexisting teamwork themes and personnel can be applied to new situations without modification.
2. A one-size-fits-all approach may not be applicable to OR staff. It is important to consider and acknowledge the diversity of OR staffs' backgrounds and experiences.
3. Failing to continually engage and work with OR staff to build an ongoing positive environment.
4. As the culture changes with OR staff and the institution, failing to adjust the training could lead to outdated or inaccurate training.

SECTION 5 • Ensuring Quality and Safety

These steps are not without challenges. Gathering individualized information from local staff is a time-intensive interview process and may not be completely applicable to the new site or teams. Additional time spent on training the new team is an upfront financial cost and loss of revenue instead of actual surgical procedures. New personnel are likely to be hired after the opening of a new surgical site and would not have access to this training.

● MEASURING OUTCOMES

As the new surgical site comes online, it is important to track patient outcomes after surgery. Time efficiency should not be scrutinized in the initial period as a new physical layout and location may lead to slower times as the team members adjust to the new space. However, as they are established, efficiency metrics should be closely monitored along with qualitative feedback from OR staff. Changes to physical storage, workflow, and patient processes may be modified to a more efficient physical setup in the early stages of a new location. Team members should also be observed and interviewed regarding the team dynamic at the new location. Early adopters may have additional insight that could be disseminated across the staff.

● FOLLOW-UP AND MAINTENANCE

With ongoing changes in health care, it is important to maintain excellent patient outcomes in surgery. This is especially important when expanding an existing location in a previously unknown area. Surgeons, OR staff, and administrators need to acknowledge that the social process of surgery is just as important as the technical aspect. Communication, teamwork, and continual evaluation in a quantitative and qualitative manner will help ensure a healthy social component of the OR, which will help realize excellent patient outcomes.

REFERENCES

1. Oster NV, Skillman SM, Frogner BK. COVID-19's effect on the employment status of health care workers. 2021. Center for Health Workforce Studies, University of Washington.
2. Pattni N, Arzola C, Malavade A, Varmani S, Krimus L, Friedman Z. Challenging authority and speaking up in the operating room environment: a narrative synthesis. *Brit J Anaesth*. 2019;122(2):233–244.
3. Schmutz JB, Meier LL, Manser T. How effective is teamwork really? The relationship between teamwork and performance in healthcare teams: a systematic review and meta-analysis. *BMJ Open*. 2019;9(9):e028280.
4. Gillespie BM, Chaboyer Q, Fairweather N. Factors that influence the expected length of operation: results of a prospective study. *BMJ Qual Saf*. 2012;21(1):3–12.
5. Leach LS, Myrtle RC, Weaver FA, Dasu S. Assessing the performance of surgical teams. *Health Care Manage Rev*. 2009;34(1):29–41.

Provider Burnout Impacting Clinical Care Delivery

30

LIANE S. FELDMAN AND LAWRENCE LEE

Clinical Care Delivery Challenge

You receive a formal report from the operating room manager about unprofessional behavior by an attending surgeon. The reports describe behavior characterized as "belittling" and "rude." The report provides examples of the surgeon "berating the nursing staff when they don't know the next step of the operation" even when the procedure is new, complex, or unusual. The surgeon "throws a tantrum" when they "don't get what they want," such as being able to book an additional case when the operating room is at full capacity. They ignore questions or answer in a sarcastic manner. You had previously received a "heads-up" from the surgical residency program director about this surgeon's interaction with residents. While the residents appreciate the surgeon for their up-to-date knowledge and skills and for "letting them operate," they do not appreciate comments in public like "are you a senior resident or a medical student" and "you are killing me and the patient with that move."

You are dismayed and surprised to receive these reports. The surgeon is newly back on staff within the past 2 years, and you know them very well. They completed general surgery training at your institution and was a "star resident," excelling academically, clinically, and professionally After completing fellowship training at a prestigious program, where they received glowing reviews, you personally recruited them on the surgeon–scientist track. This included a generous start-up package, with the expectation to develop a practice in complex and revisional procedures in their specialty as well as initiate an independent research program. By all conventional metrics they have succeeded: their clinical program is up and running, and they obtained a competitive career development award and published several papers.

When you call the surgeon to let them know about the complaint, they say that "all they want is to take care of patients 'properly'" and that they are "disappointed with the low level of concern for quality in the organization." They then say they "can't take this anymore," feel "burned out," and are "honestly thinking of quitting surgery completely."

● WORKUP

It is important for surgical leaders to address all reports of disrespectful, rude, or unprofessional behavior. High-functioning teams are needed to deliver high-quality surgical care. Unprofessional behaviors interfere with the development of a safety culture that requires communication, respect for all team members, and focus on the complex tasks at hand. Causes and triggers for unprofessional behavior may be grouped into 3 themes including organizational, cultural, and individual factors that all decrease the surgeon's ability to handle conflict.[1] Organizational conditions that increase stress in the high-demand work environment of the OR include production pressures, staff turnover, supply shortages, and perceived inefficiencies and mismanagement, all on top of the inherent stresses of surgical care. Antiquated cultural norms that promoted the "prima donna" surgeon may lead to treating others with a lack of respect. Individual factors include personality traits (eg, Type A personality, narcissism, passive–aggressive tendencies) or underlying conditions such as burnout, depression, substance abuse, and stress. In this case, there has not been a pattern of this type of behavior in the past, the individual cites burnout as a factor and they seem distressed.

195

The first step is to get more information by speaking to the team members reporting the behavior to understand the context, frequency, and impact. However, for a variety of reasons, the affected individuals often wish to remain anonymous, for fear of exacerbating the situation with a surgeon with whom they will continue to work. They may not even feel comfortable talking to you, in which case the information will need to be obtained from trusted managers. The next step is to talk to the surgeon. This meeting should be planned in advance with sufficient time and in a quiet and private environment. This can be an intimidating situation for any young surgeon. The leader should approach this meeting with compassion, humility, and curiosity to create a "safe space" that encourages honest reflection. While it is important for the surgeon to understand that the disruptive behavior must stop and does not meet personal or organizational expectations for high-quality care, the ultimate goal is to help them gain insight into the impact of the negative behavior on team members, colleagues, and trainees. As Maya Angelou said, "… people will forget what you said, people will forget what you did, but people will never forget how you made them feel." As this is the first incidence of this type of behavior, it is important to understand the underlying cause in order to identify solutions and design remediation strategies to prevent recurrence.

The surgeon is encouraged to give their side of the story regarding the specific complaint. They point to systems factors that triggered the incident, including the lack of a dedicated team, difficulty in accessing the OR after hours for emergency cases, and the level of trainees that are allocated to their service. A good question to ask next is whether there may be personal issues that may be interfering or spilling into their professional interactions, especially because this is a change from their previous performance and may be a sign of burnout, psychiatric illness, substance abuse, or stress. After this prompt, the surgeon says they feel "overwhelmed," "exhausted," and "burned out." They are not deriving the sense of accomplishment from their clinical work or research output that they expected they would as they started their career after a decade of training, and feel they are landing short of their own personal expectations. They also had a recent run of complications that they feel ashamed about. They appear in distress and say they are "reaching a breaking point."

● DIFFERENTIAL DIAGNOSIS

Burnout is a term that covers a range of experiences of occupational distress. Although it can occur at any point in the career trajectory, there may be an increased risk in the early years of practice. Burnout is defined by the WHO as a syndrome arising from "chronic workplace stress that has not been successfully managed" that includes 3 main dimensions: (1) emotional exhaustion, (2) increased detachment, negativism or cynicism toward one's job, and (3) feelings of reduced professional effectiveness.[2] Burnout can be associated with disruptive behaviors, interpersonal conflicts, self-reported errors, lower patient satisfaction, and intention to quit, and is a risk factor for depression, substance abuse, anxiety disorders, and relationship problems.[3] Burnout is not a medical diagnosis and while there may be substantial overlap between symptoms of burnout and depression, they are distinct entities.[3] While burnout is associated with suicidal thoughts, this is likely from the confounding effect of coexisting depression.[4] Yet even among surgeons with suicidal thoughts, only a minority seek professional help.

In the research literature, the most common tool used to measure feelings of burnout is the Maslach Burnout Inventory. However, this is typically used to assess groups rather than as an individual diagnostic tool.[5] Even at the group level, there is significant heterogeneity in criteria used to measure burnout leading to wide variability in estimates of its prevalence in physicians, ranging from 0% to 80.5% in a systematic review.[6]

● DIAGNOSIS AND TREATMENT

There is a growing recognition of the importance of surgeon well-being, with consequences to individuals, patients, and organizations. Physician well-being includes dimensions of distress (burnout, fatigue, anxiety, stress) and professional fulfillment (meaning in work, engagement).[7] Evidence supports associations between physician well-being and quality of care, medical errors, patient satisfaction, and self-reported unprofessional behaviors.[8] Therefore, there is a strong imperative to help prevent, identify, and mitigate occupational distress. The responsibility to reduce burnout and promote career satisfaction should be shared between individual physicians and the institutions where they work.[9]

The present case scenario represents a failure at multiple levels that threatens the work environment and may lead to losing a highly qualified and talented individual. One must seek to understand and address this surgeon's issues without stigma and make it clear that the main priority is to reestablish their well-being, in the short term and the long term. A good start is to simply affirm the unique stresses associated with beginning surgical practice, such as dealing with complications and systems issues. Young surgeons in the first years of practice may also have to contend with added pressures of initiating a research program or administrative work. It is also not uncommon for early career attendings to have a life partner going through similar experiences, perhaps with young children as well. All of these tend to occur at the same time in life, making the transition from star trainee to the new attending surgeon a period of particular vulnerability. The young surgeon fears being seen as weak, unprepared, or lacking confidence, and does not realize that many of these feelings and experiences are ubiquitous and related to surgical culture and training that values the suppression of personal needs. Reframing success in a way that emphasizes why we became surgeons and researchers in the first place, that is, it is not actually about the number of papers or presentations but about the sense of purpose to make something better and the connection to patients, students, and to each other. Sharing one's own experience with failure is an important step in changing culture.

Surgical leaders should also know what physician health resources are available and destigmatize access. Depending on the specific environment, this may be through the hospital human resources department, university mentorship programs, or professional organizations. Peer support programs focused on physician well-being can be very helpful in providing confidential advice that is seen as objective and independent. Therapy to address personal issues can also be helpful. Any concern for depressive symptoms or suicidality must trigger a prompt referral to the appropriate mental health professional.

Leaders should also set a good example by having the self-awareness to recognize when they are burning out and exhausted. Practicing and discussing self-care including taking a break to disconnect from work (ie, taking a real vacation) is not a luxury, laziness, or a sign of weakness. Surgical culture has tended to celebrate exhaustion and overwork, so this is an opportunity to be a role model for well-being. Addressing the systems issues that the surgeon brings up is also critical.

● PRINCIPLES AND EVIDENCE

Interest in physician well-being has increased in the past 2 decades, but until recently there has been relatively little literature on the specific contributing factors and effective interventions. Shanafelt summarizes 3 phases of the evolution of the field, beginning with the historic phase, the current state, and what is needed to advance to the next phase (Wellbeing 2.0).[9] In the historic phase, physician distress was largely neglected or ignored. Many aspects of traditional surgical culture accentuated physician burnout. The ability to work without being affected by fatigue, illness, or personal needs was celebrated. There was also the notion that a good surgeon had to be perfect. For example, adverse outcomes were blamed largely on individual decisions or actions at morbidity and mortality conferences, almost with the expectation that surgeons should be able to overcome any systems issues. The long training period leads to an extended period of delayed gratification where personal development is put off sometimes into the future (ie, "when I am a senior resident/fellow/attending, everything will be better"). This culture results can result in a perfectionism mindset where being less than perfect (ie, being human) is seen as being weak.

The current era acknowledges physician stress and burnout, as well as their effects on professional behaviors, functioning, and patient outcomes. The past 15 years have been characterized by a significant change in the way medicine is practiced, measured, and evaluated, as well as important demographic changes. The introduction of many technologies such as electronic medical records (EMRs) was supposed to ease the burden on physicians, but instead increased frustration and burden onto healthcare providers. Physicians also began feeling at odds with healthcare administrators, as the incentives between providers and administrators were often misaligned. Doctors entering the workforce in the past 2 decades also had significant generational and cultural differences that valued life outside of work. There was increasing awareness that these factors contributed to physician distress, but efforts to combat distress during this era largely put the burden onto individual physicians (eg, accessing mental health resources) and cultivating resilience (eg, mindfulness, stress reduction).[9]

Finally, the next phase (Wellbeing 2.0) is represented by shifting the attention away from individual physicians managing burnout to instead focusing on the root causes of distress and burnout. This requires redesigning systems, processes, and teams to promote finding meaning, purpose, and joy in work (ie, the reasons we became surgeons in the first place).

● IMPLEMENTING A SOLUTION

Clinical and administrative leadership will need to work together to address well-being as a shared responsibility and institutional priority, with the same approach, dedication, and resources as used for any other quality improvement initiative.[5] This occurs on several levels (Figure 30.1):

1. Organization: Addressing well-being can seem a daunting task—issues related to staffing levels, EMR, and workload obviously cannot be addressed uniquely at the team, program, division, or departmental levels. While this larger systems-level should be addressed as institutional priorities, ideally through a senior leadership champion (eg, Chief Wellness Officer), there are many issues that can be identified and addressed at the local level. Individual conversations about what matters most in contributing to professional fulfillment and what are impediments (pebbles in the shoe) are a good start. Important promotors of well-being include safety culture, autonomy and choice, camaraderie and teamwork, recognition, professionalism, and flexibility. Safety culture, leadership, and wellness are intertwined. Assessment tools can help identify areas for improvement and track progress at the group level; examples include the Safety Attitudes Questionnaire, Maslach Burnout Inventory, and Mini Z burnout survey. The Mayo Clinic Leadership Dimensions Assessment can be used to evaluate dimensions of effective local or program leadership.
2. Leaders: Dimensions of effective leadership include keeping people informed, seeking their input about how to improve, having career conversations that include personal and life goals, providing mentorship and coaching, recognizing a job well done, supporting teams and community, and inspiring and empowering others to engage in addressing institutional problems. This starts with respect for other people and the diverse life experiences and talents they bring to the organization, understanding the complex needs of individuals and what they need to thrive personally and professionally, and having compassion for others and for themselves. They also nurture collaborative relationships including with administration to find solutions to problems. This has been termed "Wellness Centered Leadership"[10] (Table 30.1).
3. Individuals: Surgeons need to move away from a mindset of perfectionism and self-criticism, which has largely been the hallmark of surgical culture for generations. Instead, an environment where there is support and compassion for setbacks and difficulties should be fostered. Realistic expectations and boundaries should be set that will allow surgeons to focus on personal needs including rest, sleep, breaks, nutrition, and exercise, in addition to clinical service. Surgeons should be encouraged to have a life outside of work and maintain personal relationships, family, friends, hobbies, and physical activity. This mindset of work–life integration needs to start during surgical residency and become a core aspect of professionalism.

Key Steps in Change Management and Potential Pitfalls

Key Steps in Change Management
1. Investigate all reports of disrespectful, rude, or unprofessional behavior.
2. Understand that disruptive behaviors may be a sign of occupational distress.
3. Know what physician health resources are available to address occupational distress and destigmatize access.
4. Create role model for self-care and well-being.
5. Use assessment tools to quantify occupational distress on an annual basis.
6. Adopt and communicate wellness-centered leadership.
7. Work together with administration to make well-being an institutional priority.

Potential Pitfalls
1. Focusing on individuals only, without addressing departmental or institutional root causes.
2. Promoting an outdated surgical culture of "blame and shame" and individual perfectionism.
3. Clinical and administrative leadership working in silos. Lack of an institutional focus on well-being.

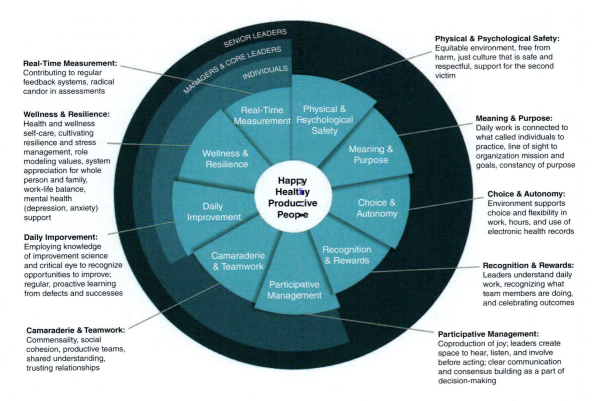

FIGURE 30.1 IHI framework for improving joy at work demonstrating 9 core components and who is responsible for each: senior leaders are responsible for all 9, managers and core leaders for 5, and individuals for 3. Perlo J, Balik B, Swensen S, Kabcenell A, Landsman J, Feeley D. IHI framework for improving joy in work. *IHI White Paper*. Cambridge, MA: Institute for Healthcare Improvement; 2017 (available at ihi.org).[5]

Table 30.1 Summary of the 3 Elements of Wellness Centered Leadership (Care About People Always, Cultivate Relationships, Inspire Change)[10]

Element	Mindset	Behaviors	Outcomes
1. Care about people always	• Recognition that leader's behavior plays important role in professional fulfillment and wellness • Servanthood • Curiosity • Respect • Empathy • Integrity	• Recognize and appreciate individual contributions and talents • Give credit • Openly discuss and role model self-care (sleep, rest, vacations, personal relationships) • Dialogue with active listening to uncover individual needs and gifts • Lead conversations about work–life integration • Provide resources, support, and education on well-being • Recognize and react to signs of distress	• Team members feel valued as people • Team members believe self-care is valued through support for working hours, vacations, breaks • Psychological safety • Team member's help cross-cover each other and support each other's wellness • People openly discuss their well-being
2. Cultivate individual and team relationships	• Respect for people • Each person has unique needs, interests, talents, goals; primary role of leader is to nurture talent • People work best in respectful environments with supportive relationships with colleagues and coworkers • Health care is emotionally demanding and we depend on the support of colleagues • Leader has an important role in keeping the community informed of organizational goals and needs	• Focus colleagues on what they are passionate about—help other reconnect to purpose and what brings them the greatest meaning • Help others develop their careers in the way they want (by asking) • Give respectful feedback and advice to help people manage their reputation • Help team members recognize the importance of providing support to colleagues • Develop and articulate vision and mission and guide process to achieve it • Lead by consensus and empowerment • Tell stories to create shared meaning • Ensure everyone has a voice • Advocate for the needs of the community • Keep community informed • Formal and informal events to allow community to connect, recognize shared experiences, and support each other	• Improved retention and engagement • Leader has formal and informal conversations with team members regularly • There is a culture of teamwork and community • People feel empowered to engage in problem-solving • Improved collaboration • Strong collegiality

Table 30.1	Summary of the 3 Elements of Wellness Centered Leadership (Care About People Always, Cultivate Relationships, Inspire Change)[10] *(Continued)*		
Element	**Mindset**	**Behaviors**	**Outcomes**
3. Inspire change	• Critical job of leader is to motivate teams to achieve meaningful results • Team members know best what is needed to improve the work environment • Providing team members with ability to lead change builds sense of community, meaning, and purpose • Diversity and debate lead to better decisions • Leaders are change agents	• Consistently model desired change • Guide team to identify priorities for change • Delegate tasks that others are capable of performing and interested in doing • Evaluate performance from a growth mindset • Influence others and build consensus • Establish mutual respect • Deliver quick wins that demonstrate commitment to values and vision • Seek advice and input	• Sense of co-owner-ship of the work • Belief that change is possible • Acceptance of (ideally buy-in) of decisions • Improved results—quality, safety, productivity, patient satisfaction • Inspiriting performance that goes beyond expectations

Mindset refers to the attitudes of the leader; behaviors are actions that leaders can take to promote wellness; outcomes are metrics that reflect and promote wellness in groups and organizations.

Adapted with permission from Shanafelt et al.[10]

● FOLLOW-UP AND MAINTENANCE

It is important to schedule regular follow-ups with the surgeon to continue to check in, providing a supportive and caring environment. This should be done in a manner where the junior surgeon does not feel like they are in remediation. The surgeon was told to take time off, and all their clinical and academic responsibilities were reviewed to reset expectations and realign goals. At the next meeting, they report having accessed physician support services, which was very helpful. This provided an outside view to normalize some of the challenges commonly encountered in transition to practice, in contrast to seeing these as a sign of weakness, which they recognize now as a distorted and damaging view. They also began seeing a therapist to help them better understand their thought patterns and motivations. You encourage them to turn down extra work and administrative opportunities that do not further their own goals. You continue regular meetings and they report making steady progress.

The main goal of a leader is to support talented people so that they thrive personally and professionally. Many ingrained aspects of surgical culture may not be compatible with the current work and practice environment and may contribute to burnout. Awareness of physician distress and burnout is only the first step in addressing the problem. The burden of minimizing stressors and other causes of distress should be not left solely to the individual physician. Rather, leaders should promote a culture of well-being in the Department.

In the current case example, you institute several changes in the Department to identify causes of distress and burnout, create solutions to minimize these burdens that "come from the top," and prioritize well-being in the Department. This may include incorporating a well-being screening item in the annual faculty performance evaluation, using the Mayo Leadership Dimensions Assessment to solicit feedback

SECTION 5 • Ensuring Quality and Safety

from faculty about their division chiefs, explicitly inquiring about personal well-being and personal interests in all meetings with individual faculty, approaching professionalism and performance issues through the lens of wellness-centered leadership, speaking about work–life integration and leadership to students and residents, and initiating a surgeon leadership development program. This will also require close collaboration with hospital administration to institute needed changes at the systems level.

REFERENCES

1. Villafranca A, Hamlin C, Enns S, Jacobsohn E. Disruptive behaviour in the perioperative setting: a contemporary review. *Can J Anesth.* 2017;64(2):128–140.
2. World Health Organization. Burn-out an "occupational phenomenon": international classification of diseases. May 28, 2019. Accessed July 19, 2022. https://www.who.int/news/item/28-05-2019-burn-out-an-occupational-phenomenon-international-classification-of-diseases
3. Menon NK, Shanafelt TD, Sinsky CA, et al. Association of physician burnout with suicidal ideation and medical errors. *JAMA Network Open.* 2020;3(12):e2028780.
4. Koutsimani P, Montgomery A, Georganta K. The relationship between burnout, depression, and anxiety: a systematic review and meta-analysis. *Front Psychol.* 2019;10:284. doi: 10.3389/fpsyg.2019.00284
5. Perlo J, Balik B, Swensen S, Kabcenell A, Landsman J, Feeley D. IHI framework for improving joy in work. *IHI White Paper.* Cambridge, MA: Institute for Healthcare Improvement; 2017 (available at ihi.org).
6. Rotenstein LS, Torre M, Ramos MA, et al. Prevalence of burnout among physicians: a systematic review. *JAMA.* 2018;320(11):1131–1150.
7. Karakash S, Solone M, Chavez J, Shanafelt T. Physician work-life integration: challenges and strategies for improvement. *Clin Obstet Gynecol.* 2019;62(3):455–465.
8. Tawfik DS, Scheid A, Profit J, et al. Evidence relating health care provider burnout and quality of care: a systematic review and meta-analysis. *Ann Intern Med.* 2019;171(8):555–567.
9. Shanalfelt TD. Physician well-being 2.0: where are we and where are we going? *Mayo Clin Proc.* 2021;96(10): 2682–2693.
10. Shanafelt T, Trockel M, Rodriguez A, et al. Wellness-centered leadership: equipping health care leaders to cultivate physician well-being and professional fulfillment. *Acad Med.* 2021;96(5):641–651.

SECTION 6

Building Multidisciplinary Service Lines

31 Establishing Service Lines in a Competitive Market
Melissa Pilewskie

32 Efficient, Comprehensive Patient Care for Multidisciplinary Visits
Christopher P. Scally and Christina L. Roland

33 Ensuring Multidisciplinary Access Aligns Across Disciplines
Ashley E. Russo and Alexandra Gangi

Establishing Service Lines in a Competitive Market

31

MELISSA PILEWSKIE

Clinical Delivery Challenge

While breast cancer remains the most common non-skin cancer diagnosis among women in the United States with over 287,000 cases diagnosed annually, a large tertiary care, academic referral center has experienced a decline in the proportion of outpatient breast surgery cases captured in the local market. This has resulted in a decrease in downstream visits to other disciplines including breast imaging, medical oncology, and radiation oncology. The decline has affected hospital profits, reduced the ability to accrue patients to impactful research trials, and reduced the diversity of educational opportunities for trainees. These changes have occurred during a period of minimal change in operational structure, defined by siloed ambulatory care units, inefficient clinical scheduling, lack of care along the breast health continuum, and underutilized patient support services.

Creation of a Breast Oncology Service Line is hypothesized to improve the current clinical situation. However, while historically the primary drivers for service line growth and development have been profit and market differentiation, in the transition to value-based care, new factors are driving service line development. In today's market, service lines must be patient centric and designed to deliver coordinated, evidence-based care.

To compete and succeed in an increasingly competitive healthcare market with declining reimbursements, hospital systems must create and emphasize patient-centered, value-based healthcare delivery. The goal of service line development is to group clinicians and stakeholders involved in the care of similar patients to improve access and efficiency, promote evidence-based, coordinated multidisciplinary care, and ultimately improve clinical outcomes, the patient experience, and the overall value of care.[1-4] This chapter aims to review the establishment or growth of a service line, using breast oncology as an example, in the face of increased competition.

● WORKUP

Prior to putting effort and resources into operational changes, the underlying problems must be fully understood. A decrease in breast surgery visits may be secondary to factors including a lack of surgeon availability, poor access to available visits, a change in clinical practice recommendations, and a change in local referral patterns or insurance coverage. The key to success in improving service line organization is to make decisions based on data and commit to an ongoing review of updated service line analysis to allow improved planning for outcomes-oriented results.[2] In discussion with the clinical team, there have not been clinical advancements in the preceding year that would impact the need for surgical management of breast cancer patients. In this clinical scenario, a review of transparent patient intake metrics, including the number of incoming breast surgery referrals, number of available surgeon clinic slots, time to patient contact, time to provider visit, reason for appointment cancelation, barriers to scheduling, and patient satisfaction with care may help isolate areas in need of improvement. Partnership with the administration is paramount to not only obtain this institutional data but also understand the changes in market share at competing healthcare systems and potential changes in referral patterns.

Given the broad team involved in breast cancer care, involvement of all key stakeholders is necessary for multidisciplinary engagement and coordinated efforts. In this case, stakeholders include all members of the breast oncology care team including physicians, advanced practice providers, and nursing staff involved with surgical oncology, medical oncology, radiation oncology, plastic surgery, and breast imaging, as well as hospital administration, management, and scheduling teams. Each of these members may provide valuable insight into both current barriers and ideas for improvement.

● DIFFERENTIAL DIAGNOSIS

The most likely root cause underlying the issue outlined above is a decline in breast cancer referrals, with an increase in market share noted in competing locations, secondary to decreased patient satisfaction from lack of a patient-centric care model. This could be confirmed by following referral trends in the regional catchment of breast cancer patients. Capturing and reviewing patient satisfaction and reasons for visit cancelation or failure to schedule a new visit would aid in identifying underlying reasons for this change. Programs continuing to rely on a hospital or physician-focused care models, rather than patient-centered care, are at risk of losing market share in the current healthcare market. In breast oncology, providing a coordinated, evidence-based care model with a multidisciplinary care team must replace episodic care. However, notably, oncologic outcomes are no longer the sole determinant for deciding preferences in where to obtain breast cancer care as patients are placing growing emphasis on easy access to solutions and treatment plans as a differentiator in the competitive healthcare marketplace.

● DIAGNOSIS AND TREATMENT

The highest leverage area for improvement for this operational challenge is to create a care model grounded in the patient experience. While this is broad reaching, focusing on areas identified from the data review will highlight initial targets for improvement. In this situation, arming the breast oncology service line with strong leadership is necessary. While a physician leader is crucial, most physicians lack business leadership skills and training to manage a service line with complete independence. Therefore, a dyad model of a physician and administrator working together to share management strategies is often the most successful approach.[2,4] In the current scenario, a motivated physician was appointed as the service line lead; however, there was minimal input from the administration, leading to difficulty in accessing necessary metrics and lack of fluid communication among all disciplines, schedulers, and management. Creating a leadership dyad improved the structure of the service line, data collection and analysis, and visibility across the entire care team.

Second, data review highlighted access to timely new visits was an issue exacerbated by the COVID-19 pandemic. While the breast oncology program historically aimed to schedule patients with a 2-week window from the receipt of a new visit referral, competitor systems were able to schedule patients faster, resulting in canceled appointments from patients who had already established care elsewhere. As true patient-centered care is accessible and timely, this required a restructuring of the new patient scheduling process, evaluation of staffing needs, and creation of competitive scheduling goals, with the aim to schedule a patient on the first call, made within 48 hours of referral placement.

Last, replacing episodic care with coordinated and comprehensive, evidence-based multidisciplinary care improves patient experience, patient outcomes, and the value of care delivered. Working with the breast oncology service line leadership, clinical algorithms were developed to minimize unnecessary care and promote an environment of continual growth.

● SCIENTIFIC PRINCIPLES AND EVIDENCE

Given the ongoing transition from volume to value-based care, there is a shift in factors driving service line development as outlined in Figure 31.1.[1] While historically service lines were grounded within a hospital building, the evolving care model highlights the growing need for improved coordination of the entire continuum of care, including the growing use of outpatient facilities and the need for virtual access to

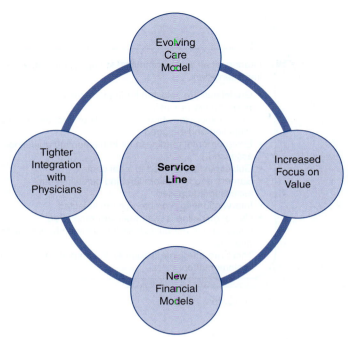

FIGURE 31.1 Factors affecting service lines. Adapted from "Service Lines: Working Toward a Value-Based Future."

meet patients' needs at home. Increasing focus on value means adopting a patient-centered care approach, minimizing care variation, and increasing cost transparency—an area of historic challenge within health care. New financial models are becoming a reality to minimize cost variation in care delivery. Examples may include coverage for care to be provided at the least-intensive setting possible and longitudinal reimbursement for the total cost of care. In Oncology, a pay-for-performance plan is expected, which will require selection and adherence to evidence-based pathways and standardized measurement of patient outcomes. These care-delivery changes will ultimately require a tighter integration with physicians across disciplines. Oncology care is uniquely complex with the involvement of multiple treatment teams and disciplines, emphasizing the importance of structured referral algorithms to promote prompt access to appropriate scheduling and minimization of unnecessary testing and costs. This clinical shift requires physician engagement to implement the outlined components of a service line, including an agreement to minimize clinical variation and help in managing the total cost of care. These strategies aim to improve coordinated, evidence-based care to improve care delivery, value, and patient experience. The International Affairs and Best Practice Guidelines outline strategies to successfully implement patient care guidelines, highlighting that this process requires more than simply awareness and distribution of guidelines, but importantly adaptation of guidelines for each provider, practice, and system to meet local context needs (Figure 31.2).[5]

As noted, the backbone to competing in the competitive healthcare market is providing a patient-centered experience. The Picker Institute and the Commonwealth Fund have identified 8 principles of patient-centered care using data from patient, family, and provider focus groups (Figure 31.3).[6] The creation of a service line requires a critical review of these important patient care factors to assess current strengths and weaknesses and allow for prioritization of strategy implementation. In the breast oncology service line scenario, the review of both quantitative and qualitative data revealed a need to prioritize access to care and continuity and transition through the spectrum of care, an area possibly improved with a nurse navigator. Tan et al. examined studies assessing the impact of navigation for cancer patients and reported emotional and knowledge empowerment of patients exposed to patient navigators through the continuum of cancer care.[7]

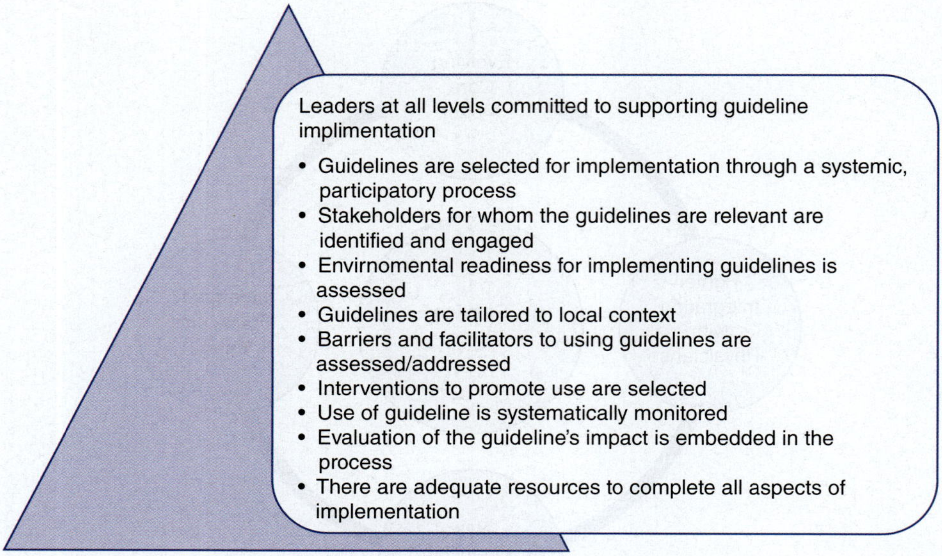

Leaders at all levels committed to supporting guideline implimentation
• Guidelines are selected for implementation through a systemic, participatory process
• Stakeholders for whom the guidelines are relevant are identified and engaged
• Envirnomental readiness for implementing guidelines is assessed
• Guidelines are tailored to local context
• Barriers and facilitators to using guidelines are assessed/addressed
• Interventions to promote use are selected
• Use of guideline is systematically monitored
• Evaluation of the guideline's impact is embedded in the process
• There are adequate resources to complete all aspects of implementation

FIGURE 31.2 Implementation strategies.

Respect for patient's preferences
Coordination and integration of care
Information and education
Physical comfort
Emotional support
Involvement of family and friends
Continuity and transition
Access to care
Patient-Centered Care

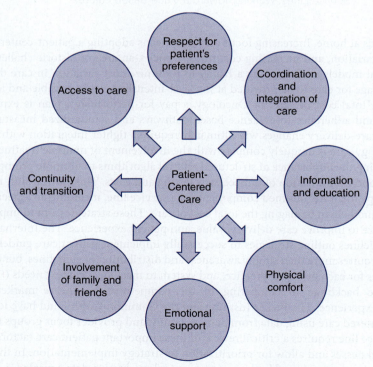

FIGURE 31.3 Picker's 8 principles of patient-centered care.

In addition to ensuring adequate resources and clinic availability for new patient encounters, other strategies are emerging to improve access to care. Vos and colleagues have reported on the benefits of an Enhanced Patient Clinical Streamlining (EPACS) Program in a specialty cancer center to alleviate patient anxiety and wait times. The EPACS Program is designed to have an advanced practice provider contact the patient as a first point of clinical contact, order needed tests or consultations, and begin the clinical coordination. The EPACS program has expedited patient workup, decreased first visit cancelation, and improved the proportion of patients starting treatment at that center. In addition, the program improved clinician satisfaction and reduced anxiety and improved preparedness for patients.[8]

● IMPLEMENTATION OF A SOLUTION

Implementing solutions requires outlining the areas of priority and having service line stakeholder engagement. In this scenario, the areas identified as priorities included building a strong dyad leadership team, improving access to care, and developing breast oncology clinical algorithms to ensure evidence-based, value-driven care by all team members. From a leadership standpoint, the hospital acknowledged the priority to improve the breast oncology service line and committed to assigning an administrative leader to collaborate with the physician lead to move forward with these initiatives. Following leadership, improving access to initial and longitudinal care was identified as the most vital clinical improvement process to enhance the patient experience and address the issue of declining breast surgery catchment. This process was initiated by scheduling a standing meeting with management, scheduling teams, and the leadership dyad to review collected metrics, assess workflow, and address barriers. Based on the data review, 4 issues were identified as directly impacting patient scheduling and satisfaction. These included out-of-date scheduling goals, scheduling team members with minimal breast oncology clinical background, lack of a nurse navigator, and minimal nonphysician involvement in early patient engagement. Prior to regular communication between management and clinical teams, there was disagreement on the expected timeline for new patient scheduling. Additionally, a lack of clinical knowledge on the part of the scheduling team resulted in many patient referrals required triage by busy clinicians, resulting in even longer delays in scheduling. A multitiered approach was implemented to improve these issues. New scheduling metrics were instituted to reflect a competitive position in the market that were approved by all stakeholders. Second, the referral algorithm was updated with the input of the scheduling team members and a standing breast oncology educational series was implemented to educate the nonclinical scheduling team on common terminology, resulting in fewer triage questions. The service line created a position for a nurse navigator who, in addition to promoting continuity of care, also assisted in new patient referral triage to minimize wait time for complex patient referral decisions. Last, the service line instituted an enhanced patient intake program similar to the EPACS program described above where soon after referral patients were scheduled for a telehealth visit with an advanced practice provider for early engagement with the clinical team, a review of care expectations, and ordering of appropriate tests and referrals, for example, to genetic testing or reconstructive surgery, all while minimizing need for an on-site visit. This process has improved satisfaction with the scheduling team, providers, and patients alike. An ongoing review of scheduling metrics is needed to ensure clinician volume and downstream care such as prompt breast imaging and operating room availability is adequate to care for the increasing new patient volume.

Last, development of breast oncology guidelines was recommended to ensure evidence-based, value-driven care by all care team members. Clinical team members met to review evidence-based and value-based care, for example, avoidance of sentinel lymph node biopsy and breast MRI among select patients with invasive breast cancer. These suggested algorithms were then distributed for feedback among all pertinent breast oncology disciplines, including physicians, APPs, nursing staff, and management to ensure a unified message. Utilization of the guidelines was discussed and reviewed on a regular basis when making patient care decisions at multidisciplinary care conferences. This process requires ongoing attention and update as new data emerges to the ensure delivery of current, evidence-based medicine. A pitfall in the

> ## Key Steps in Change Management and Potential Pitfalls
>
> **Key Steps in Change Management**
> 1. Obtain appropriate, granular data to analyze internal metrics and the competitive local market.
> 2. Engage all appropriate stakeholders involved with a service line and elicit ongoing feedback on care-delivery recommendations.
> 3. Understand current barriers to delivering patient-centered care and prioritize areas for improvement.
> 4. Outline key areas for defining value-based care within the service line and measure service line adherence.
> 5. Build a leadership team with both physician and administrative representation.
> 6. Ensure ongoing measurement of data to track progress on developing a service line rooted in patient-centric, value-driven care.
>
> **Potential Pitfalls**
> 1. Failure to obtain adequate leadership support from the administration and relying solely on physician leads.
> 2. Lack of granular data to fully understand the current issues related to poor access to care.
> 3. Emphasizing hospital- or provider-centric care rather than patient-centric care.
> 4. Not planning appropriately for a potential increase in patient volume secondary to patient-centric, service line improvements.
> 5. Assuming provider engagement in adherence to clinical algorithms aimed at improved value-based care.

implementation of service guidelines affecting large service line groups is the potential lack of engagement and unwillingness to change practice without ongoing evaluation of appropriate care-delivery recommendations. This requires thoughtful, ongoing attention from leadership teams and review of data to support the need for progress to value-based care.

● MEASURING OUTCOMES

Following the implementation of these practices, an ongoing review of the metrics is essential. In this clinical scenario, weekly reports were distributed to the leadership dyad outlining the number of incoming referrals, available provider visits, time to first APP and physician visit, and market share. Notably, the improvement and promotion of a breast oncology service line may result in unintended consequences including excess volume growth which may place new barriers to access across disciplines. The measured outcomes therefore need to report on all service line components to ensure ongoing, equal access to prompt care across breast oncology disciplines.

● FOLLOW-UP AND MAINTENANCE

Service line development and maintenance is not a static process and requires ongoing attention from the leadership dyad as well as all stakeholders. As one area of improvement is accomplished, the team should continue to identify additional areas to improve the patient experience as this will continue to define a competitive service line. For example, once access to care and navigation was improved, the leadership team began focusing on patient education materials to reflect updates in breast cancer management strategies and growing the availability of patient services to improve side effect management such as massage therapy and exercise oncology programs. The possible site-specific improvements to promote patient-centered, value-based care require the commitment of the leadership team to continuously assess the local and regional market for new ways to improve the patient experience and the delivery of service line care.

REFERENCES

1. Werner RM, Emanuel EJ, Pham HH, Navathe AS. Service lines: working toward a vale-based future. *Front Health Serv Manage*. 2021;37(3):14–28.
2. Modern Healthcare Insights. Hospital service line organization: innovation in approaches and strategy. 2012. Accessed May 4, 2023. https://www.modernhealthcare.com/assets/pdf/CH81353810.PDF
3. O'Neill M, Sturm M. Service Lines of the Future. Ambulatory Surgery Centers. October 23, 2019.
4. Brown KK. The service line model: a lasting facility trend for operational success. *Healthcare Business Today*. July 9, 2018.
5. Person- and Family-Centered Care [Internet]. Toronto: Registered Nurses' Association of Ontario; 2015 May. Accessed May 4, 2023. http://rnao.ca/sites/rnaoca/files/FINAL_Web_Version_1.pcf
6. Patient- and Family-Centered Care Initiatives in Acute Care Settings: A Review of the Clinical Evidence, Safely and Guidelines [Internet]. Ottawa, ON: Canadian Agency for Drugs and Technologies in Health. August 31, 2015.
7. Tan CH, Wilson S, McConigley R. Experiences of cancer patients in a patient navigation program: a qualitative systemic review. *JBI Database Syst Rev Implement Rep*. 2015;13(2):136–168.
8. Vos EL, Cho JS, Schmeltz J, et al. Enhanced Patient Clinical Streamlining (EPACS): quality Initiative to improve healthcare for new surgical outpatient visits. *Ann Surg Oncol*. 2022;29(3):1789–1796.

Efficient, Comprehensive Patient Care for Multidisciplinary Visits

32

CHRISTOPHER P. SCALLY AND CHRISTINA L. ROLAND

Clinical Delivery Challenge

A 55-year-old woman from a rural area noticed a slowly enlarging mass on her right leg. After several months, she was seen locally by her primary care provider who ordered a CT scan of the affected limb, which demonstrated a 9 cm mass in the anterior compartment of the proximal thigh, followed by an image-guided percutaneous biopsy. The biopsy results showed a high-grade sarcoma. The patient was then referred for specialized care at a comprehensive cancer center. However, the patient lived over 300 miles from the nearest such facility. In this chapter, we will utilize cancer care as an example of coordinated multidisciplinary visits, but these principles apply to other types of multidisciplinary care.

Appropriate workup and management of a complex diagnoses present several challenges for patients and providers. Frequently, this requires a patient to have multiple appointments for testing and visits with specialists from different disciplines. In addition, access to care can be challenging for patients who are geographically remote from tertiary centers. Nonetheless, numerous studies have shown improved patient outcomes when care is delivered in a multidisciplinary fashion. Multidisciplinary clinics have been associated with increases in guideline-concordant care, reduced treatment delays, and improved patient and provider satisfaction.[1–4]

● WORKUP

In this scenario, the patient has a newly diagnosed soft-tissue sarcoma of the extremity. Optimal treatment of this malignancy typically requires the input of multiple specialists and a combined modality approach to treatment. Delivering high-complexity, multidisciplinary care to a patient who faces the issue of a significant travel distance and barriers to access presents a significant healthcare delivery challenge. Access to multidisciplinary care remains a major issue in the United States; for common cancers, such as colorectal cancer, it has been estimated that only half of patients receive access to multidisciplinary care.[5,6]

For a patient with a suspected cancer, initial workup includes tissue biopsy for diagnosis, high-quality imaging of the primary malignancy for treatment planning purposes, as well as complete staging imaging. In the scenario described, the patient has undergone some of these workups previously. To optimize the efficiency of a multidisciplinary visit, providers at the tertiary center need access to these previous studies prior to the patient's arrival to avoid expensive duplicative tests. Despite advances in technology, transferring images still frequently pose a challenge and in some cases require mailing a copy of the imaging on a CD or other portable media. Obtaining these imaging studies and other critical records ahead of the multidisciplinary visit improves efficiency and helps minimize delays in treatment.

● DIFFERENTIAL DIAGNOSIS

One of the more important aspects of care at a comprehensive cancer center is expert pathologic review. Frequently, patients with rare diagnoses, such as soft-tissue sarcoma, will have changes in their diagnosis or tumor subtype/grade after review by a pathologist with specific expertise in this tumor subtype. Pathology review can frequently be delayed as in most cases this requires mailing prepared slides or tissue samples by the facility that performed the biopsy. Arranging for pathologic review in advance of the multidisciplinary visit significantly enhances the quality of recommendations delivered at the time of the patient encounter.

DIAGNOSIS AND TREATMENT

In preparation for the multidisciplinary visit, the specialty surgeon should review the available records and imaging in advance. This helps assure coordinated care and minimize unnecessary patient travel for additional, unanticipated appointments. In some centers, formalized multidisciplinary visits have been developed in which patients are seen by all subspecialists within the same clinic space. In the above patient scenario, given the size and high-grade histology of the tumor, this patient would be seen by a surgical or orthopedic oncologist with expertise in soft-tissue sarcoma, a medical oncologist for the discussion of possible systemic chemotherapy, and a radiation oncologist for the discussion of either pre- or postoperative external beam radiation therapy.

Patients with complex problems also benefit by formal case review in a multidisciplinary conference. Patient history, physical exam findings, and known diagnostic data are presented, including imaging review by radiologist and pathologic review by specialty pathologists. Engaged discussion from specialty providers allows for multiple perspectives from clinicians across the spectrum of care and consensus recommendations to guide treatment, ideally documented in the medical record. Given the travel distances required for this patient, it would be optimal for the medical oncologist at the cancer center to partner with an oncologist locally who can oversee chemotherapy and monitor for safety/toxicities rather than the patient being required to travel for each treatment cycle.

Providers must also be aware of the costs associated with care and travel to a referral center. An important part of a multidisciplinary team is licensed social workers and experienced case managers who can work with patients to identify housing and transportation resources as well as financial assistance programs. Some tertiary centers will designate a patient navigator to help guide patients through the process of establishing and receiving care. However, despite these programs, accessing care remains a significant challenge for patients and can limit the ability of patients to receive care at specialty centers.

SCIENTIFIC PRINCIPLES AND EVIDENCE

Multidisciplinary clinics have become an integral part of patient care at cancer centers, and this approach is being adopted increasingly for nononcologic issues that require comprehensive care from multiple specialties (transplant, inflammatory bowel disease, etc). The importance of these multidisciplinary clinics is highlighted by their adoption as requirements for Commission on Cancer accreditation through the American College of Surgeons.

The core principle of multidisciplinary care is a comprehensive patient-centered approach to care by providers from all medical specialties. Bringing providers from multiple disciplines together in a single patient care encounter allows for efficient workup and improved coordination between teams. Multidisciplinary clinic models have been shown to reduce time to patient evaluation and initiation of cancer treatment, increase use of guideline-concordant cancer care, and increase patient and provider satisfaction. Evaluating the long-term impact of this model of care has proven more challenging; several retrospective studies have attempted to assess the impact of multidisciplinary clinic models on oncologic outcomes, such as the recurrence rate and overall survival, with mixed results and only a minority of studies showing an association between multidisciplinary treatment and improved oncologic outcomes.[7]

IMPLEMENTING SOLUTIONS

Keys steps to successful implementation of multidisciplinary care involves foundational infrastructure for coordination. Utilization of nurse navigators or advanced practice provider-led intake clinics can facilitate the acquisition of provider documentation, previously performed diagnostic image and pathology slide acquisition, ordering and scheduling of missing diagnostic tests, and arranging consultation with appropriate specialists based on anticipated treatment course. Development of intake algorithms can help standardize the process for identifying critical tests needed for optimal new patient evaluation, which can streamline and assist in coordination prior to the patient commencing travel (Figure 32.1).

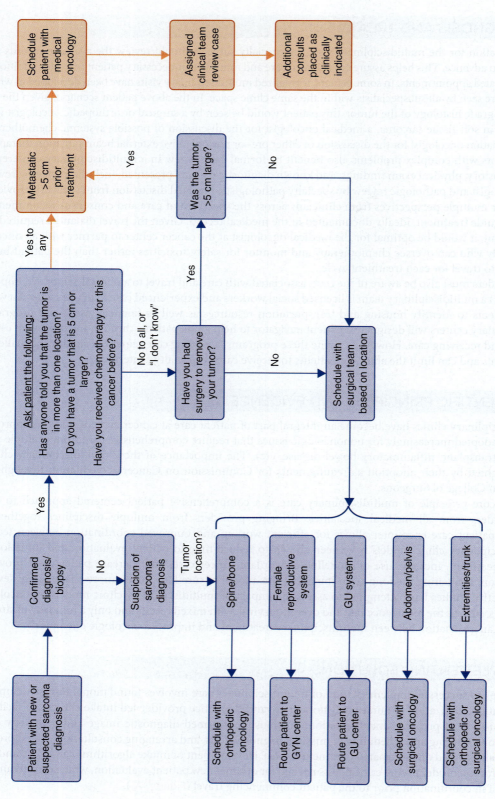

FIGURE 32.1 Algorithm to help standardize the process for scheduling complex patients for multi-disciplinary care.

Key Steps in Change Management and Potential Pitfalls

Key Steps in Change Management

1. Identify a clear problem with a measurable outcome of multidisciplinary care.
2. Understand the process leading up to patient traveling to a tertiary referral center.
3. Spend time on the front line (eg, intake center) with key stakeholders involved, including residents, surgeons, schedulers, administrators, and patients.
4. Identify sources of quantitative data (eg, electronic medical record timestamps) to bring measurable outcomes to understand your potential sources of uncoordinated visits.
5. Introduce possible solutions to key stakeholders to test face validity (ie, do they think that is a problem?) and refine based on feedback.
6. Pilot the potential solution (eg, scheduling algorithm, intake clinic) in a high-yield area and have regular opportunities to solicit feedback. Make sure that you can track a measurable outcome (ideally what you identified in #1).

Potential Pitfalls

1. Jumping straight to a solution (eg, we need more schedulers) without testing alternatives.
2. Lack of a clear conceptual model for the process from a new patient call to the initial visit.
3. Not engaging enough with the correct stakeholders.
4. Forgetting to monitor unintended consequences of your solution.
5. Broadly implementing your solution (eg, intake clinic) across the whole department, without pilot testing it within one division or section first.

As discussed previously, patient access to the multidisciplinary clinic remains a challenge and a key issue in healthcare delivery across the United States. The COVID-19 pandemic has also added to this challenge; however, the pandemic has rapidly sped up the development of telehealth or virtual appointments, and improvements in the legislature and medical licensing process have allowed for expanded reach of cancer centers and multidisciplinary clinics. Consideration of virtual new patient/consult/second opinion appointments can increase outreach and patient access.[8–10]

● MEASURING OUTCOMES

Key metrics for optimal multidisciplinary visits include time from initial call to new patient visit, number of tests or consultations ordered after primary appointment, duration of patient appointments or stay, and time to initiation of treatment. Monitoring and continuous tracking of these metrics helps optimize the efficiency of a multidisciplinary clinic and ensure high-quality patient care.

● FOLLOW-UP AND MAINTENANCE

A challenge of a multidisciplinary clinic model is that over time the enthusiasm of the initial effort wanes. To maintain efficient and high-quality patient care, stakeholders in the multidisciplinary clinic need to continually monitor for provider engagement and upholding the high standards of the multidisciplinary clinic model. Tracking of key metrics as outlined above can assist in this; engaging in discussions with providers and leadership at regular intervals can help identify ways to maintain and improve upon the multidisciplinary care model.

REFERENCES

1. Meguid C, Schulick RD, Schefter TE, et al. The multidisciplinary approach to GI cancer results in change of diagnosis and management of patients: multidisciplinary care impacts diagnosis and management of patients. *Ann Surg Oncol.* 2016;23(12):3986–3990.
2. Levine RA, Chawla B, Bergeron S, Wasvary H. Multidisciplinary management of colorectal cancer enhances access to multimodal therapy and compliance with National Comprehensive Cancer Network (NCCN) guidelines. *Int J Colorectal Dis.* 2012;27(11):1531–1538.
3. Kozak VN, Khorana AA, Amarnath S, Glass KE, Kalady MF. Multidisciplinary clinics for colorectal cancer care reduces treatment time. *Clin Colorectal Cancer.* 2017;16(4):366–371.
4. Korman H, Lanni T Jr, Shah C, et al. Impact of a prostate multidisciplinary clinic program on patient treatment decisions and on adherence to NCCN guidelines: the William Beaumont Hospital experience. *Am J Clin Oncol.* 2013;36(2):121–125.
5. Morris AM, Billingsley KG, Hayanga AJ, Matthews B, Baldwin LM, Birkmeyer JD. Residual treatment disparities after oncology referral for rectal cancer. *J Natl Cancer Inst.* 2008;100(10):738–744.
6. Vu JV, Morris AM, Maguire LH, et al. Development and characteristics of a multidisciplinary colorectal cancer clinic. *Am J Surg.* 2021;221(4):826–831.
7. Pillay B, Wootten AC, Crowe H, et al. The impact of multidisciplinary team meetings on patient assessment, management and outcomes in oncology settings: a systematic review of the literature. *Cancer Treat Rev.* 2016;42: 56–72. doi: 10.1016/j.ctrv.2015.11.007
8. Aghedo BO, Svoboda S, Holmes L, et al. Telehealth adaptation for multidisciplinary colorectal cancer clinic during the COVID-19 pandemic. *Cureus.* 2021;13(9):e17848. doi: 10.7759/cureus.17848
9. Cathcart P, Smith S, Clayton G. Strengths and limitations of video-conference multidisciplinary management of breast disease during the COVID-19 pandemic. *Br J Surg.* 2021;108(1):e20–e21.
10. Uppal A, Kothari AN, Scally CP, et al. D3CODE Team: adoption of telemedicine for postoperative follow-up after inpatient cancer-related surgery. *JCO Oncol Pract.* 2022;18(7):e1091–e1099. doi: 10.1200/OP.21.00819

Ensuring Multidisciplinary Access Aligns Across Disciplines

33

ASHLEY E. RUSSO AND ALEXANDRA GANGI

Clinical Delivery Challenge

A 69-year-old woman with a past medical history of hyperlipidemia presented to her local emergency department with right upper quadrant pain, jaundice, dark urine, and a several-month history of unintentional weight loss. Blood work revealed a total bilirubin of 9.4 mg/dL, alkaline phosphatase of 312 U/L, aspartate transaminase of 443 U/L, alanine transaminase of 267 U/L, and albumin of 1.9 g/dL. A magnetic resonance cholangiopancreatography was done which revealed moderate intrahepatic and extrahepatic biliary ductal dilatation and diffuse dilation of the main pancreatic duct concerning for an ampullary neoplasm. A triple-phase computerized tomography (CT) scan of the abdomen was then performed which demonstrated a mass in the head of the pancreas measuring at least 2.5 cm in diameter, with a tumor-portal vein interface > 180°. Following imaging, an endoscopic retrograde cholangiopancreatography and endoscopic ultrasound were then done, during which tissue was obtained via biopsy confirming the diagnosis of invasive poorly differentiated adenocarcinoma of the head of the pancreas. During this procedure, a sphincterotomy was performed and a metal stent was placed to relieve the patient's biliary obstruction. Following discharge, the patient was referred to the closest Comprehensive Cancer Center for specialized care, which is over 300 miles from where the patient lives. In this chapter, we will utilize cancer care as an example of coordinated multidisciplinary visits and will discuss principles that can be applied broadly to all types of multidisciplinary care.

Multidisciplinary care is particularly important in the management of cancer patients, especially in the time immediately following diagnosis. The unique clinical needs of cancer patients can span from multi-modality cancer treatments to pain management, nutritional support, and psychosocial support. Multidisciplinary collaboration and coordination are critical in not only ensuring that the needs of cancer patients are appropriately managed but also facilitating the timely creation of a treatment plan and initiation of therapy. While multidisciplinary care coordination seems intuitive in theory, it is not always easily achieved in practice. Effective coordination of care requires the buy-in from several stakeholders, adequate resources, and a commitment to communication. When done effectively, however, the outcome is the delivery of high-quality patient care.

Multidisciplinary collaboration is critical to providing comprehensive patient care. While each specialty provider has a specific skill set and unique knowledge, it is the coordination of a group of providers that allows for the delivery of high-quality and effective care. Multidisciplinary care coordination not only benefits the patient, but when done effectively can benefit providers as well. For patients, effective coordination of care can result in more efficient workup and treatment, decrease in duplication of services, and ultimately time and cost savings. For providers, care coordination and multidisciplinary collaboration can lead to improved provider education through multidisciplinary conferences and other educational opportunities, enhanced efficiency in the clinic through information sharing, and ultimately improvement in physician burnout.

● WORKUP

To understand the quality and effectiveness of multidisciplinary collaboration in any given medical system, you first need to understand what attempts are being made to achieve effective care coordination. If this is done in an informal setting, that is, person-to-person coordination for a single patient or on a case-to-case basis, it is likely neither the most effective way to achieve coordination of care nor is it the most effective use of resources. Practicing multidisciplinary collaboration in a more formal setting, like in a multidisciplinary tumor board or conference setting, is a superior way to facilitate the effective delivery of care. Understanding which of these care coordination models exist within a healthcare system will allow for an assessment of the quality of the framework and will help to identify areas in which improvement could be achieved.

To evaluate the success of any multidisciplinary team effort, it is important to be able to collect primary data on which to judge the efforts. This, however, can be challenging because the efficacy of teamwork is not entirely objective and can be a difficult metric to measure. Effective collaboration requires a commitment to communication, conflict resolution, information sharing, education, and a dedication to providing high-quality patient care. Beyond the interpersonal skills, intellectual competency, and effective provider relationships that are required to ensure effective collaboration, multidisciplinary collaboration requires a tremendous contribution of time and a commitment to the coordination of time between several different stakeholders. Metrics by which to measure the success of collaborative efforts can include the number of patients discussed, the attendance of providers and key stakeholders, the time to consensus on a treatment plan, and the time to initiation of said plan. In the long run, being able to measure the time from diagnosis to initiation of treatment with and without the utilization of highly effective multidisciplinary care teams may be used to provide evidence for the true clinical benefit of care coordination. It also may be possible to measure patient-based metrics to demonstrate the benefit of streamlined multidisciplinary care coordination by evaluating things such as the number of days patients come to the hospital/clinic for consultations, the number of missed days of work, and the total miles and cost of travel. In theory, the delivery of streamlined care through the utilization of multidisciplinary coordination should result in a decrease in all these patient-based metrics, the importance of which should not be underestimated.

In the situation of coordination of cancer care, one of the most widely used and most effective ways to achieve multidisciplinary care coordination is in the utilization of tumor boards and multidisciplinary case conferences. In these settings, providers can present their patients to a panel of experts who can all weigh in on the management of a patient based on their unique knowledge set and experience. It is in these conferences that providers can learn of clinical trial opportunities and different therapeutic options for their patients in which they may not have previously been well versed. The scope of these conferences goes beyond just a discussion of the medical treatment options for patients, as other key participants include case management, genetic counselors, registered dieticians, and supportive care. It is through the collaboration of all these providers that a comprehensive treatment plan can be made that not only prioritizes the patient's primary cancer diagnosis but also makes sure to address the significant psychosocial needs of cancer patients and their support systems. Additionally, in specific health systems, patient care is coordinated in such a way that patients are seen in a multidisciplinary clinic where both the patient and the providers have access to individuals from all treatment teams. This allows for an even higher level of efficiency but requires health system buy-in and collaboration from the providers to be available.

● DIFFERENTIAL DIAGNOSIS

There are several inherent challenges to ensuring effective teamwork, and multidisciplinary care coordination is no exception. For one, multidisciplinary care coordination requires a significant time commitment and coordinating the schedules of several providers can be extremely challenging. Second, it is essential to have 1 or 2 key stakeholders who oversee gathering the information for the patients to be discussed so that different providers can adequately prepare prior to multidisciplinary conferences so that the time spent in a multidisciplinary discussion can be used efficiently and effectively. Lack of organization can lead to a complete dissolution of multidisciplinary efforts. Third, effective teamwork requires an alignment of goals, which should be centered around a commitment to delivering high-quality patient care. While the end goal may be shared, the path to achieve this goal can be disrupted by differences in professional values, approach to problem-solving, communication styles, and perceived provider hierarchy. It is essential to keep these

DIAGNOSIS AND TREATMENT

Once the current multidisciplinary efforts have been evaluated, areas for improvement can be identified. There are 3 main levels at which improvements can be achieved: the institutional level, the provider level, and the patient level.

At the institutional level, it is important that there is a commitment from the leadership. If institutional leadership can see the clinical benefit and improvement in the delivery of high-quality patient care as a direct result of effective multidisciplinary collaboration, then they will place value on care coordination and will be more likely to support institutional efforts by contributing resources to ensure that patients have access to multidisciplinary care. It is therefore the responsibility of the multidisciplinary team to track evaluable outcomes and patient measures to demonstrate the impact and benefit of care coordination so that this data can be presented in a convincing and meaningful manner to institutional leadership.

At the provider level, it is important to track the ways in which care coordination and resource sharing lead to benefits for the provider. The benefits for providers are many, from improving clinical efficiency to decreasing physician burnout. It may be useful to track metrics of clinical efficiency and care delivery by tracking the amount of time spent gathering and reviewing outside records, time obtaining potential insurance authorizations, the amount of provider-to-provider communication occurring during provider "down-time" and change in provider perception of the quality of care delivered to patients before and after the implementation of formal multidisciplinary efforts. In theory, having official multidisciplinary meetings should streamline these efforts and improve these metrics.

At the patient level, there are several areas to target for improvement. Understanding a patient's perception of the quality of care they are receiving is a critical aspect of making sure that multidisciplinary efforts are worthwhile. If patients do not feel as though they are receiving adequate information, unified messages, or appropriate attention, then it is likely that the multidisciplinary efforts are not functioning effectively. In the case of cancer care, patients are typically informed that they will be discussed at multidisciplinary tumor boards. This provides them with a certain level of comfort that their case will be evaluated by several different experts and the confidence that the most appropriate treatment course will be offered based on consensus opinion. It is critical that the decision of the tumor board is then shared with the patient as well so that they can make the most informed decisions moving forward. This is also an excellent way for providers who have not yet seen the patient to learn about the patient in a concise and comprehensive manner so that if they eventually do see the patient in the future, they will already be well informed of the specifics of the patient's case. Another area in which patients may benefit is by having dedicated nurse navigators who help patients through the complex and, at times, confusing medical system.

SCIENTIFIC PRINCIPLES AND EVIDENCE

The American Commission on Cancer (COC) has made it a requirement that multidisciplinary cancer conferences be part of the patient treatment planning process in order to receive COC accreditation.[1] Based on this requirement, there have been several studies that have evaluated the role of effective multidisciplinary care coordination in the quality of care delivered to cancer patients. A randomized controlled trial by Wagner et al. in 2014 evaluated whether or not the utilization of nurse navigators improves the quality of life and patient experience for patients with a recent diagnosis of breast, colorectal, or lung cancer.[2] In this study, patients were randomized to either enhanced usual care or nurse navigator support for 4 months. Patient-reported measures were gathered using several validated assessment tools and were assessed at baseline, 4 months, and 12 months. One of the important findings of this study was the identification of 3 major challenges faced by cancer patients and their caregivers. These challenges were identified as delays in and a lack of coordination of care, a lack of information relevant to their diagnosis, and inadequate attention to patients' emotional and social problems. Ultimately, this study found that while there were no differences in patient-reported quality of life, there was a significant improvement in patient experience and a reduction in problems with care coordination and information delivery in the patients who were randomized to nurse navigator support.

There are other studies that have evaluated whether multidisciplinary care coordination improves patient outcomes. In the thoracic malignancy literature, there is evidence to demonstrate that multidisciplinary conferences lead to an increased percentage of patients being appropriately staged, receiving appropriate multidisciplinary evaluation, and improved adherence to standard of care guidelines in addition to resulting in a significant decrease in the time from diagnosis to initiation of treatment.[3] This has also been shown to be true in the breast cancer literature, with the demonstration of a significant reduction in the interval between diagnosis to treatment from 42.2 days to 29.6 days ($p < 0.0008$) for patients treated for breast cancer before and after the implementation of a multidisciplinary breast cancer clinic.[4] Several studies have also shown that multidisciplinary cancer conferences have led to an improvement in patient selection for certain cancer treatments. For example, in the colorectal cancer literature, there is evidence that shows that discussion of potentially resectable patients with complete radiographic review during multidisciplinary cancer conferences significantly decreased the rate of positive circumferential resection margins from 26% to 6% in patients discussed during these conferences.[5] Studies such as this not only demonstrate an improvement in patient selection but also provide objective clinical evidence that multidisciplinary care coordination can significantly improve the quality of care provided to cancer patients. As such, there are now COC-accredited rectal cancer centers of excellence where at least 50% of patients with a new diagnosis of rectal cancer must be discussed prior to definitive therapy.

Another proposed benefit of multidisciplinary cancer care is an increase in the enrollment of patients in appropriate clinical trials. A study done by the gynecology oncology department at Brown University demonstrated an increase in the enrollment in clinical trials by 2.5 times for patients discussed during tumor board, highlighting the importance of multidisciplinary discussion to identify patients who meet trial eligibility and support trial accrual, which can often times be a rate-limiting step for the timely completion of practice-changing clinical trials.[6] Finally, there have also been studies to evaluate whether or not multidisciplinary cancer care has had an effect on improved clinical outcomes. A study by Yopp et al. evaluated median overall survival (OS) in patients with newly diagnosed hepatocellular carcinoma (HCC) before and after the implementation of a multidisciplinary HCC clinic. The study demonstrated that the median OS improved to 13.2 months from 4.8 months ($p = 0.005$) after the implementation of the multidisciplinary clinic.[7] The ability to achieve improved OS is perhaps the most compelling argument for the formation of formal multidisciplinary cancer clinics, particularly those which focus on a specific disease type.

Patient-centered benefits are not the only outcomes measured by studies evaluating the impact of multidisciplinary cancer care, as provider-centered outcomes have also been an area of great interest. A study published in the *British Medical Journal* in 2010 revealed the findings of a group out of the United Kingdom who performed a nationwide survey of providers regarding their perception of working in a multidisciplinary cancer care model. They found that 90% of participants found working in multidisciplinary teams to be beneficial and over 80% responded that working in multidisciplinary teams improved job satisfaction.[8] Other studies have outlined the findings after observing different multidisciplinary case conferences, which have demonstrated an improvement in awareness of current literature, appropriate care delivery, improvement in continuity of care, and a perception of improved patient satisfaction with treatment plans.[9]

● IMPLEMENTING A SOLUTION

Ensuring effective multidisciplinary care first requires an assessment of the status of multidisciplinary efforts. Next, it is critical to evaluate the effectiveness and efficiency of these efforts to identify areas for process improvement with the goal of improving the delivery of high-quality patient care. Understanding the degree of institutional support as well as identifying the key stakeholders and participants in multidisciplinary care

Key Steps in Change Management and Potential Pitfalls

Key Steps in Change Management

1. Assess the state of current multidisciplinary efforts
2. Understand the degree of institutional support.
3. Identify key stakeholders in multidisciplinary care coordination.
4. Schedule recurring multidisciplinary conferences with clear and reasonable attendance requirements.
5. Select measurable outcomes and collect objective data (including patient- and provider-reported outcomes) to track the progress and effectiveness of multidisciplinary efforts.

Potential Pitfalls

1. Failure to ensure appropriate infrastructure and resources exist prior to establishing multidisciplinary efforts will likely lead to unsuccessful outcomes.
2. Setting too strict of attendance policies and not allowing for shared responsibility among similar providers could lead to physician burnout.
3. Failing to track measurable outcomes will not allow for an accurate assessment of the progress of multidisciplinary efforts.

coordination is also critical to ensure that the necessary providers have a voice and presence at multidisciplinary care conferences.

As stated previously, the implementation of dedicated multidisciplinary care coordination requires a significant time commitment by both the coordinators and the participants. The goal of these conferences is to result in care delivery improvements for both the patients and the providers, therefore it is important that the implementation of formal multidisciplinary care coordination does not lead to the unintended consequence of increasing provider or patient burden. There are several ways in which this can be addressed. First, selecting a dedicated time each week or month to discuss patients in a multidisciplinary setting will allow providers to arrange their schedules such that they do not have other clinical responsibilities during this time. It also allows providers to inform patients of when these multidisciplinary discussions will take place and to set appropriate expectations for patients with regard to when a consensus decision about treatment options will be made. This also gives patients the time to obtain second opinions if they so desire before deciding on providers and/or treatment pathways. It is also possible that providers of the same specialty may share the responsibility of being the specialty representative during multidisciplinary conferences or clinics. For example, in our institution's multidisciplinary pancreatic cancer clinic, providers from each of the participating services (surgical oncology, medical oncology, radiation oncology, interventional gastroenterology, pathology, supportive care medicine, genetics, and nutrition) rotate on a bimonthly basis and the consensus decision of the multidisciplinary conference discussion is shared with the patient's primary referring provider, even if that provider was not the provider assigned to that week's clinic. This allows for shared responsibility among different providers which hopefully results in less provider burnout and less disruption to a provider's usual clinical schedule. Finally, it is important to collect objective data to track the progress and effectiveness of multidisciplinary efforts.

● MEASURING OUTCOMES

To ensure effective multidisciplinary efforts and make improvements when indicated, it is important to objectively measure outcomes. Important information to collect includes subjective data points such as patient- and provider-reported outcomes as well as objective data points such as measuring time from diagnosis to treatment, rate of clinical trial enrollment, and survival outcomes. It is also important to constantly assess the structure and organization of these multidisciplinary meetings so that process improvement can take place when deficits in efficiency or effectiveness are identified.

● FOLLOW-UP AND MAINTENANCE

Like most areas of medicine, the delivery of patient care must be constantly evaluated and improved to ensure the delivery of the highest-quality patient care as the field of medicine evolves. One of the ways in which to ensure that our patient management keeps up with changing treatment paradigms, which is particularly important in the care of cancer patients, is to have formal multidisciplinary conferences and discussions during which treatment options are discussed. This not only identifies the most contemporary and appropriate treatment pathways for patients, but it also allows for the most comprehensive patient care by prioritizing not only the medical management of patient diagnosis but also the evolving psychosocial needs that accompany a new diagnosis. Tracking both patient- and provider-reported outcomes and objective measures of treatment improvements as a direct result of multidisciplinary care coordination is a critical aspect of ensuring efficient and effective care coordination and providing evidence to institutional leadership so that they may provide the necessary support of multidisciplinary efforts.

REFERENCES

1. Cancer, A.C.o.S.C.o. Ensuring patient-centered care, in *American College of Surgeons*. 2012. https://www.facs.org/media/t5spw4jo/2016-coc-standardsmanual_interactive-pdf.pdf to reference.
2. Wagner EH, Ludman EJ, Bowles EJA, et al. Nurse navigators in early cancer care: a randomized, controlled trial. *J Clin Oncol.* 2014;32(1):12–18.
3. Freeman RK, Van Woerkom JM, Vyverberg A, Ascioti AJ. The effect of a multidisciplinary thoracic malignancy conference on the treatment of patients with esophageal cancer. *Ann Thorac Surg.* 2011;92(4):1239–1242.
4. Gabel M, Hilton NE, Nathanson SD. Multidisciplinary breast cancer clinics. Do they work? *Cancer.* 1997; 79(12):2380–2384.
5. Burton S, Brown G, Daniels IR, Norman AR, Mason B, Cunningham D. MRI directed multidisciplinary team preoperative treatment strategy: the way to eliminate positive circumferential margins? *Br J Cancer.* 2006;94(3):351–357.
6. Kuroki L, Stuckey A, Hirway P, et al. Addressing clinical trials: can the multidisciplinary Tumor Board improve participation? A study from an academic women's cancer program. *Gynecol Oncol.* 2010;116(3):295–300.
7. Yopp AC, Mansour JC, Beg MS, et al. Establishment of a multidisciplinary hepatocellular carcinoma clinic is associated with improved clinical outcome. *Ann Surg Oncol.* 2014;21(4):1287–1295.
8. Taylor C, Munro AJ, Glynne-Jones R, et al. Multidisciplinary team working in cancer: what is the evidence? *BMJ.* 2010;340:c951.
9. Gagliardi AR, Wright FC, Anderson MA, Davis D. The role of collegial interaction in continuing professional development. *J Contin Educ Health Prof.* 2007;27(4):214–219.

SECTION 7

Healthcare Equity

34 "Top" Hospital Is Bypassed or Avoided by Minorities in the Community Who Feel More Comfortable at Other Hospitals: Distrust of Medical System and Minority Health Care

Kakra Hughes and John H. Stewart V

35 Inadequate Diversity in Hospital Committees Charged With Review of Clinical Operations and Quality

Shukri H.A. Dualeh, Vanessa S. Niba, and Erika A. Newman

36 Dismantling Capacity Management Policies That Prioritize Highly Reimbursed Specialty Surgery Over Caring for Uninsured Patients

Sidra N. Bonner and Christopher J. Sonnenday

SECTION 7

Healthcare Equity

34. "Top" Hospital Is Bypassed or Avoided by Minorities in the Community Who Feel More Comfortable at Other Hospitals: Distrust of Medical System and Minority Health Care
Kara Hughes and John H. Stewart IV

35. Inadequate Diversity in Hospital Committees Charged With Review of Clinical Operations and Quality
Shikha A. Huilgol, Marissa S. Cantu, and Erika A. Newman

36. Diminishing Capacity Management Policies That Ethically Prioritize Highly Reimbursed Specialty Surgery Over Caring for Uninsured Patients
Sara N. Horst and Christopher J. Sonnenday

"Top" Hospital Is Bypassed or Avoided by Minorities in the Community Who Feel More Comfortable at Other Hospitals: Distrust of Medical System and Minority Health Care

34

KAKRA HUGHES AND JOHN H. STEWART IV

Clinical Delivery Challenge

A 72-year-old Black man presents to an emergency department at a major tertiary academic medical center, by ambulance, with a 4-month history of a right great toe gangrenous ulcer. He has a history of hypertension, diabetes mellitus, and a 40-pack year smoking history (and continues to smoke half a pack per day). He reports that he has been getting treatment at a local wound care center at his community hospital without any significant relief. His visiting daughter called the ambulance when she noted the toe had turned black. On physical examination, he has a strong femoral pulse on the right, and absent distal pulses with monophasic popliteal, posterior tibial, and dorsalis pedis signals. On the left, he has strong pulses on the femoral, popliteal, posterior tibial, and dorsalis pedis arteries. His right great toe has dry gangrene up to the metatarsophalangeal joint. A diagnosis of chronic limb-threatening ischemia is made, and he is given an appointment to follow up in the Vascular Surgery Limb Salvage Clinic the following week for planned revascularization followed by toe amputation. The patient, however, chooses to go to his local community hospital where, unfortunately, vascular surgical expertise is unavailable. He undergoes a toe amputation which does not heal and subsequently ends up with a below-knee amputation 4 months later.

When given referrals for specialized care at tertiary academic medical centers, some minority patients choose to bypass these sites in favor of an alternate site of care where necessary expertise is unavailable. This phenomenon of minority patients bypassing care at hospitals that may have advanced resources is a situation that continues to contribute to health disparities in this county. A major root cause of this problem is distrust of the medical system by many minorities and difficulty in accessing complex academic settings which can be viewed as exclusive.

● WORKUP

In evaluating this challenge, determining the availability of expertise to address the patient's problem is necessary operational data. This may be obtained by determining how many vascular surgeons and/or vascular interventionalists practice at his local hospital versus at the academic medical center; how many revascularization procedures—open and/or endovascular are performed at his local community hospital; and how the outcomes compare to the academic medical center. Statewide inpatient and outpatient databases and administrative claims databases may be utilized to obtain this information.

Furthermore, to better understand this problem, it will be essential to talk to patients in the local community who have undergone amputation. Questions to explore would include where they received treatment and if they received any attempt at revascularization. It will also be helpful to explore with amputation patients how and why they chose to go to the site where they ultimately received treatment. A qualitative approach, such as using structured interviews, will be helpful to identify underlying themes impacting patients' decision-making. In addition to patients, other key stakeholders in the community include wound care specialists, primary care physicians, endocrinologists, and podiatrists.

● DIFFERENTIAL DIAGNOSIS

That many racial and ethnic minority populations in the US distrust medical research and the healthcare system in general is well documented. Two unfortunate historical occurrences serve to undergird this mistrust. First is the **Tuskegee Syphilis Study** which was conducted by the US Public Health Service with the goal of understanding the natural history and complications of syphilis. Six hundred poor, Black sharecroppers were recruited for this study, and of these, 399 had syphilis. They were all told that they were being treated for "Bad Blood." This study continued from 1932 until 1972. Even though penicillin was discovered, and established as an effective treatment for syphilis by 1945, these study participants were denied treatment leading to several participants' deaths and multiple complications as well as several spousal deaths.[1] Following whistleblower activities, the study was eventually ended in 1972. Unfortunately, it was not until decades later, in the late 1990s, that an official national apology was issued by President Clinton.

A second episode fueling many Black patients' distrust of the healthcare system relates to the treatment of several Black slaves for vagino- and vesico-colonic fistulae by Dr. Sims. James Marion Sims, who is occasionally referred to as the "Father of Modern Gynecology," performed operations on several young Black women in Montgomery, Alabama, in the 1840s without anesthesia. At the time, the thinking was that Blacks did not experience pain in the same way as Whites. Following these operations, he administered opium for pain. While this may have been a common practice at that time, it is also clear that these patients—who were considered property—could almost certainly not have given consent for these operations. In another case, he described an 18-year-old named Lucy who screamed uncontrollably while he conducted an operation with no fewer than 12 men observing. Dr. Sims records that it took him 4 years to perfect his technique of treating vagino- and vesico-colonic fistulae. He subsequently relocated to Manhattan, New York, in the 1850s where he performed these operations, using his now-perfected technique, on White women while routinely using anesthesia.[2] Stories such as these are commonly circulated in the Black community, and this serves to fuel general mistrust of the healthcare system.

Another cause for minorities bypassing excellent hospitals is a failure of our healthcare systems—and often, major academic medical centers—in effectively reaching out to and cultivating relationships with minority populations. Lack of effective community outreach often leads to a situation where minority patients are uncomfortable accessing care at the tertiary–quaternary academic medical center, and rather choose to obtain care at a smaller community hospital often with more limited expertise and resources.

● DIAGNOSIS AND TREATMENT

Rebuilding trust with minority populations will require recognition and acknowledgment of past failures, including past research misconduct. Not surprisingly, when these stories of past research misconduct are reported, they are often mistakenly portrayed as being even worse than they were (eg, many believe the government infused the Tuskegee participants with the syphilis virus and few realize that penicillin did not exist when the study began). Beginning conversations with an attempt to correct such inaccuracies could suggest that these atrocities were not as bad as some make them out to be, further alienating minority patients and communities. Instead, to rebuild trust, we suggest the following:

1. Inviting minority populations into our research programs as true partners.[3] The National Institutes of Health's (NIH) Community-Based Participatory Research Programs are designed to do just that. Another example is the University of Maryland's Center for Health Equity's Health Advocates In-Reach and Research (HAIR) Program where the Black community is engaged as research partners in barbershops and hair salons.
2. As a nation, we would need to enact clear policy efforts to eliminate racial and ethnic health disparities. Dr. Jones in her Cliff of Good Health Analogy indicates that Minorities and the socioeconomically disadvantaged are in grave danger of falling off the "cliff of good health" with no safety net once they fall.[4] Programs utilizing social determinants of health focus would create a much-needed safety net. These programs would be particularly helpful not only to health care for minorities but would also demonstrate to these populations that the medical and research community cares about their overall well-being.[5,6]

● SCIENTIFIC PRINCIPLES AND EVIDENCE

Principles of implementation science will be helpful in addressing this health equity challenge. As defined by the NIH, implementation science is the "study of methods to promote the adoption and integration of evidence-based practices, interventions, and policies into routine health care and public health settings to improve the impact on population health." Healthcare inequities can be exacerbated when available treatments are underutilized in minority communities often due to poor access. In addition to patient and clinician factors, structural and systemic considerations significantly contribute to these disparities. Implementation science frameworks are typically categorized into determinant (establishing relevant factors), process (confronting determinants), and evaluation (assessing implementation outcomes). Determinants typically include innovation, recipients, context, and process. In their proposed Health Equity Implementation Framework (Figure 34.1), Woodward

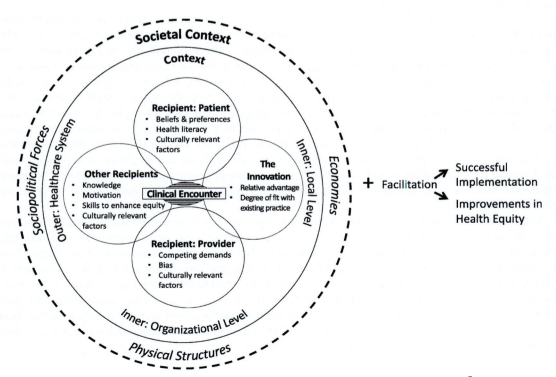

FIGURE 34.1 Health Equity Implementation Framework. Reprinted from Woodward et al.[7]

and colleagues incorporate the domains of culturally relevant factors (such as patient mistrust of the healthcare system), clinical encounter (physician–patient interaction), and societal context (social determinants of health).

● IMPLEMENTATION OF A SOLUTION

Specific implementation science research frameworks may be harnessed to address health equity research to address this problem. This approach allows one to utilize familiar research methods to rigorously test disparity-reducing implementation strategies. One such useful framework is the Consolidated Framework for Implementation Research (CFIR).[8] This framework describes 5 domains (along with 39 sub-domains), namely intervention characteristics, outer setting, inner setting, characteristics of individuals involved in the implementation, and the implementation process. *Intervention Characteristics* refer to key attributes of a clinical intervention that are known to influence the success of implementation. In this case, this would include the ease of obtaining an appointment with the academic tertiary medical center's Vascular Surgery Limb-Salvage Clinic, the ease of navigating around the academic medical center, and whether the practice accepts Medicaid insurance or not.[9] *Outer Setting* includes the larger societal context within which an organization operates, that is, has this organization historically been considered a minority-friendly organization? Is this institution perceived to want to take care of minority patients or is this perceived as a hospital primarily for the "rich White folk"? *Inner Setting* describes aspects of an organization's culture, climate, and structure that impact the implementation process. Is the process streamlined or does it involve excessive paperwork and multiple visits? Is there flexibility in scheduling recognizing many minority patients need to work during normal business hours? *Characteristics of individuals* describe the attitudes of clinicians and others that influence the adoption and implementation process. When necessary, will physicians and surgeons be accommodating to minority patients many of whom come from lower socioeconomic status? The *implementation process* itself often involves a host of strategies that typically require proactive action.

The first key management step is to ensure access. The hospital must engage in a comprehensive community engagement campaign to vigorously ***invite*** minority communities into the academic medical center. This will involve visiting primary care physicians' offices, dialysis access centers, wound care centers, churches and other houses of worship, barbershops, hair salons, and grocery stores. Employing and utilizing individuals who are from and live in the community will go a long way toward credibly engaging with the minority community and establishing rapport with potential future patients. Hospitals should implement strategies emphasizing a single point of contact or phone number to access appointments and ensure the calls are promptly answered by a courteous staff member. While access to online scheduling for appointments should be readily provided, this should not be the only option. Evening and Saturday appointments should be offered for working adults. Once new patients visit the practice, they should be welcomed warmly and generously and treated with the utmost courtesy. Paperwork must be kept to a minimum and assistance in filling out paperwork should be provided when necessary.

While these academic tertiary hospitals may have greater expertise and resources to offer, a potential, perhaps fatal, pitfall will be in coming across as arrogant or superior to where these patients may already be receiving their care. It will be helpful to remember these patients have established relationships and attempts to characterize their current physician and hospital as inferior will be counterproductive. Patients referred by primary care practitioners should be returned to their referring physician, nurse practitioner, or physician assistant, and not be provided with a new primary care physician at the academic medical center. The campaign ought to be one of building relationships and partnering with the local community hospitals, other local sites of service, and local physicians as a willing supportive partner eager to serve and available to support in whatever way is needed.

Key Steps in Change Management and Potential Pitfalls

Key Steps in Change Management

1. Engage in a vigorous community-wide invitation of the minority community to the tertiary academic medical center.
2. Partner with community hospitals and health facilities.
3. Partner with community physicians/clinicians presenting the vascular surgery/limb-salvage center as a resource for the community.
4. Visit wound care centers and dialysis access sites.
5. Welcome new minority patients coming to the limb-salvage center.
6. Obtain a short survey about patients' experiences.

Potential Pitfalls

1. Belittling patients' current hospital and/or physician/clinician.
2. Failure to greet new patients warmly and make them feel welcome.
3. Cumbersome, scheduling processes with excessive paperwork.
4. Failure to send patients back to their referring physicians/clinicians, that is, "stealing patients."
5. Failure to send correspondence back to the referring physicians/clinicians and facilities.

● MEASURING OUTCOMES

After implementing possible solutions, several outcome metrics should be measured. These include the following:

1. The proportion of minority patients with chronic limb-threatening ischemia who are treated at the academic medical center versus at a hospital without these capabilities.
2. The proportion of minority patients with chronic limb-threatening ischemia who continue to be seen at the tertiary academic medical center following their initial visit.
3. The proportion of minority patients with chronic limb-threatening ischemia in the community who undergo an attempted revascularization versus primary amputation.
4. The proportion of minority patients with chronic limb-threatening ischemia who are successfully revascularized and, therefore, avoid amputation.
5. The short surveys that are filled out by minority patients describe their experiences at the academic medical center.

● FOLLOW-UP AND MAINTENANCE

Follow-up will require continued engagement of, and a continual show of appreciation for, the community by the academic medical center. It will be necessary to have academic medical center personnel be visible in the community, attend health fairs, visit local primary care offices and other sites of care, send correspondence, and continually engage the community so that the community can eventually see this as "a hospital for us too."

REFERENCES

1. Belmont Report, Original Version, September 1978. U.S. Health & Human Services Website.
2. Wall LL. The medical ethics of Dr J Marion Sims: a fresh look at the historical record. *J Med Ethics*. 2006;32(6):346–350.
3. Stewart BA, Stewart JH 4th. Disparities in clinical trial participation: multilevel opportunities for improvement. *Surg Oncol Clin N Am*. 2022;31(1):55–64.

4. Jones CP, Jones CY, Perry GS, Barclay G, Jones CA. Addressing the social determinants of children's health: a cliff analogy. *J Health Care Poor Underserved.* 2009;20(4 Suppl):1–12.
5. Thomas SB, Quinn SC, Butler J, Fryer CS, Garza MA. Toward a fourth generation of disparities research to achieve health equity. *Annual Rev Public Health.* 2011;32:399–416.
6. Thornton RL, Glover CM, Cené CW, Glik DC, Henderson JA, Williams DR. Evaluating strategies for reducing health disparities by addressing the social determinants of health. *Health Aff (Millwood).* 2016;35(8):1416–1423.
7. Woodward EN, Singh RS, Ndebele-Ngwenya P, et al. A more practical guide to incorporating health equity domains in implementation determinant frameworks. *Implement Sci Commun.* 2021;2(1):61. http://creativecommons.org/licenses/by/4.0/
8. Chinman M, Woodward EN, Curran GM, Hausmann LRM. Harnessing implementation science to increase the impact of health equity research. *Med Care.* 2017;55 (Suppl 9: 2):S16–S23.
9. Hughes K, Mota L, Nunez M, Sehgal N, Ortega G. The effect of income and insurance on the likelihood of major leg amputation. *J Vasc Surg.* 2019;70(2):580–587.

Inadequate Diversity in Hospital Committees Charged With Review of Clinical Operations and Quality

35

SHUKRI H.A. DUALEH, VANESSA S. NIBA, AND ERIKA A. NEWMAN

Clinical Delivery Challenge

A 36-year-old Black woman with no known past medical history presented to the emergency department (ED) for the third time in 3 weeks demanding pain medication for chest pain. Her workup had included normal cardiac labs, a normal chest x-ray, and a normal EKG. Her clinical care notes described multiple neck and arm tattoos and noted her interactions with the staff were "rough." The clinical notes also mentioned drug-seeking behaviors, references to homelessness, and a lack of social support at home. She was discharged from the ED for the third time without further workup and collapsed the next day in the subway station. The postmortem autopsy revealed a large straddle pulmonary embolism. The hospital's clinical quality and safety committees assigned to perform the root cause analysis review found the care provided by the ED to be reasonable and did not outline areas for improvement. One committee member noted the patient could have been observed overnight but that nothing would have changed the outcome.

As health disparities persist and the U.S. population becomes increasingly diverse, there is an urgent need to ensure that healthcare operational systems and decision-making administrative committees are representatives of the communities they serve. Representation is important because the impact of race on patient outcomes is multifactorial and includes healthcare provider bias and physician–patient communication barriers. Teams with diverse abilities, perspectives, backgrounds, and education have increased capacity for complex problem-solving and cultural humility.

● WORKUP

To understand if the hospital safety and quality committee provided adequate care oversight, the adequacy of diversity in hospital committees charged with clinical operations safety and quality must be examined. When considering the makeup of the committee, there are 3 major areas to probe: (1) the level of racial/ethnic representation on the committee in relation to the patient communities, perspectives, and experiences served; (2) the committee member appointment processes; and (3) the quality of cultural competency, antiracism, and bias training provided to committee members. Performing this in-depth analysis will aid in collecting pertinent data to evaluate the current state of diversity in these committees, identify key stakeholders, and target key areas of interventions.

● DIFFERENTIAL DIAGNOSIS

While many medical schools have made significant steps toward diversifying student classes, diversity diminishes in advanced specialty training and in academic advancement in rank. Deans, academic

231

departmental chair, and executive leadership positions remain persistently and severely underrepresented by race, ethnicity, and gender. For example, in 2019, over 90% of division chiefs were male, 4% were Black and 2.5% were Hispanic.[1] This pattern was similar for the program director and chair positions.[1] Furthermore, according to the American College of Healthcare Executives, in 2019, 89% of United States Hospital Chief Executive Officers were White.[2] This underrepresentation in the healthcare workforce has led to a lack of diversity within clinical and administrative operational teams and committees with decision-making capacity and influence priorities.

● SCIENTIFIC PRINCIPLES AND EVIDENCE

Those who hold higher academic ranks are an integral part of healthcare operational systems and are typically selected to join executive committees. In recent years, countless studies and books have described the benefits of diverse teams, though there has not been a focus on how a lack of diversity in healthcare teams and clinical committees impacts patient health outcomes and quality of care. Parity may be beyond reach without targeted attention and strategic initiatives toward leadership advancement and assuring diversity in executive teams and clinical committees tasked with the daily operations of healthcare systems.

Representation is important because of the impact of race on patient outcomes.[3] Recent evidence demonstrates that healthy Black children with low preoperative surgical risk have worse postoperative outcomes compared to their white counterparts. This risk includes 30-day mortality, that is, 3.5 times that of White patients.[4] To evaluate and address the root causes of alarming disparities such as these, health systems require leadership teams with diverse clinical operational and quality committees that can provide oversight and analyses, set inclusive priorities, and implement strategic change through a health equity lens.

Teams with diverse abilities, perspectives, backgrounds, and education have increased capacity for complex problem-solving and cultural humility. Cultural humility is important to provide equitable care to patients from all backgrounds.[3] Individuals or families undergoing medical treatment may experience and interpret illness and their care differently compared to patients with different cultural backgrounds. If health care is not informed by cultural differences, the patient's experiences and subsequent interactions within the health care system can be negatively impacted. Patient–physician racial concordance has been shown to significantly improve morbidity and mortality, and increase trust for adults and children.[5] Many studies such as this have detailed the importance of representation and equity in clinical care and highlight the need for strategies to increase diversity in healthcare system clinical and quality committees.

● DIAGNOSIS AND TREATMENT

This case study demonstrates the hazardous outcome of unconscious or conscious bias being perpetuated at the bedside. When it came time for a critical review of a poor outcome, the committee in place did not comprehensively assess the impact that this patient's race, appearance, and multiple ED visits had on her care. It is vital that members in the committee tasked with evaluating quality of care be critical of the processes and systems-based discrimination that affects a patient's care.

● IMPLEMENTATION OF A SOLUTION

We will introduce 4 ways hospitals and departments can combat inadequate diversity in committees charged with clinical operations and quality of care: implementing a cultural complications curriculum, increasing diversity through clinician recruitment, establishing a system-wide anti-racism mission, and utilizing third-party assessors as a part of a health equity consulting service.

Cultural Complications Curriculum

One way to approach evaluation and analysis of complex clinical safety challenges that may augment committee structures is open discussion and analysis of matters that relate to diversity and culture in real time. In the Department of Surgery at the University of Michigan, a curriculum titled "Cultural Complications" was implemented, in which the structure and design of a morbidity and mortality conference are utilized to bring issues related to culture and environment to the forefront.[6] This novel approach continues to be a part of the learning curriculum.[5] The morbidity and mortality conference is a core practice of resident and attending physician education and provides an environment for the in-depth assessment of surgical complications and deaths. It is a regular opportunity to humbly assess what could have been done better with the goal of applying these lessons to future cases. For the cultural complications curriculum, the same structure and principles are applied to a case where there is a breakdown in culturally inclusive communication or when an event that is not aligned with an ideal work culture has occurred. The morbidity and mortality conference is highly regarded and willingness to prioritize the department-wide discussions demonstrates knowledge of the importance of culture to surgical quality. The conference has also been critical in fostering an environment that prioritizes improving the daily lived experiences of individuals from traditionally marginalized groups. Using the setting of a formal conference well attended in most surgical departments allows for engaged discussions and open problem-solving. A main takeaway from the success of this curriculum is providing evidence-based data on why addressing cultural complications is vital to create an open and inclusive culture.

Clinician Recruitment

With more published data demonstrating greater diversity is associated with improved patient outcomes, there has been a push to increase workforce diversity.[5,7] At our institution, we implemented a holistic interview system led by a faculty recruitment committee, which consists of faculty and resident members from across the department. After a detailed review of applications, a panel interview is conducted by the committee using standardized questions, then the team utilizes objective scoring criteria to come to a consensus on the top candidate. The faculty recruitment committee is empowered by the Department Chair and the Division Chiefs to influence the selection of the best candidate. We recommend a holistic interview process with the inclusion of tailored attribute-based questions including the key value areas of diversity, equity, and inclusion (DEI). While developed in an academic setting for faculty recruitment, these key best recruitment capacities can be tailored to the local setting of nonacademic clinicians. Recruiting diverse teams is not the only step. We recommend providing education and leadership training to diverse team members so that they may progress through the leadership ladder successfully. As we become more effective and successful in diverse recruitment and hiring, we will have a greater impact on the pool of potential hospital committee membership at every level.

System-Wide Anti-Racism Oversight Committee

At our institution, a system-wide Anti-Racism Oversight Committee (ARCC) was formed in 2020 as a response to the nation's racially charged events. This committee is comprised of multiple members including executive and leadership sponsors and works intimately with the Office of Health Equity and Inclusion (https://ohei.med.umich.edu/anti-racism-oversight-committee). Together multiple diverse committees work to foster an inclusive culture, create sustainable opportunities for anti-racist conversations, include an anti-racist curriculum within the medical school curriculum, and continue to work toward diversifying the composition of our workforce. Increasing diversity within these committees provides the opportunity to approach problems with multiple perspectives and offer solutions that can have a wide impact.

Health Equity Consulting Service

In cases of mistreatment or large communication breakdown within care team members or across multidisciplinary care teams, our institution has implemented a consulting service, the Healthcare Equity Consult Service (HECS), to provide expertise through a health equity lens (https://www.uofmhealth.org/healthcare-equity-consult-service). The team consists of expert clinicians, social workers, and spiritual care services tailored to patients who may have been affected by conscious or unconscious bias at some point in their medical care process. Any care provider, patient, family member, or friend may request a consult. The HECS team also connects with the medical team members if the consult was not made anonymously. This is a novel way of using existing resources and incorporating a system-based approach to form an independent review by a third party to address issues around bias and concern for health inequities in real time.

Key Steps in Change Management and Potential Pitfalls

Key Steps in Change Management

1. Engage in a hospital-wide invitation of underrepresented minority members to the relevant quality committees.
2. Review committee appointment processes to ensure diverse and inclusive representation.
3. Provide training to committee members on topics of cultural competency, anti-racism, and bias.
4. Consider implementation of a cultural competency or cultural complications curriculum to systematically review quality through a health equity lens.

Potential Pitfalls

1. Lack of diverse team members to serve on committees prior to changes in recruitment practices.
2. Overburdening a select few diverse team members to serve in diversity, equity, and inclusion roles (ie, "the minority tax").

● MEASURING OUTCOMES

Diversifying committees charged with the review of clinical operations and quality is an essential task that hospital systems should prioritize. It is important to first start by evaluating the current state and demographics of decision-making committees and identifying key stakeholders that will prioritize enhancing committee diversity. This outcome can be tracked over time. It is equally critical to bring intentional focus to open and inclusive faculty recruitment and hiring clinicians that prioritize DEI initiatives. Implementing segment-wide solutions, such as starting a cultural complications curriculum, and creating system-wide programs, such as the AROC and HECS, are other ways to usher in change.

● FOLLOW-UP AND MAINTENANCE

The goal of increasing diversity within executive committees is only a starting point. Including DEI efforts as a metric for promotion can aid in the continued prioritization of diversity within clinical operational and executive committees. This will ensure that those who incorporate DEI solutions to multiple aspects of their career are able to be promoted and may inspire more clinicians to participate in DEI work. This may also incentivize faculty to gain more cultural humility and participate in anti-racist endeavors with the goal of positively impacting health system decision-making, quality, and safety, and ultimately improving healthcare outcomes.

REFERENCES

1. Kassam AF, Taylor M, Cortez AR, Winer LK, Quillin RC 3rd. Gender and ethnic diversity in academic general surgery department leadership. *Am J Surg.* 2021;221(2):363–368. doi: 10.1016/j.amjsurg.2020.11.046. Epub 2020 Nov 25.
2. "Increasing and Sustaining Racial Diversity in Healthcare Leadership." *Increasing and Sustaining Racial Diversity in Healthcare Leadership | American College of Healthcare Executives*, https://www.ache.org/about-ache/our-story/our-commitments/policy-statements/increasing-and-sustaining-racial-diversity-in-healthcare-management
3. Salsberg E, Richwine C, Westergaard S, et al. Estimation and comparison of current and future racial/ethnic representation in the US health care workforce. *JAMA Netw Open.* 2021;4(3):e213789. doi: 10.1001/jamanetworkopen.2021.3789
4. Nafiu OO, Mpody C, Kim SS, Uffman JC, Tobias JD. Race, postoperative complications, and death in apparently healthy children. *Pediatrics.* 2020;146(2):e20194113. doi: 10.1542/peds.2019-4113. Epub 2020 Jul 20.

5. Greenwood BN, Hardeman RR, Huang L, Sojourner A. Physician-patient racial concordance and disparities in birthing mortality for newborns. *Proc Natl Acad Sci U S A*. 2020;117(35):21194–21200. doi: 10.1073/pnas.1913405117. Epub 2020 Aug 17.
6. Harris CA, Dimick JB, Dossett LA. Cultural complications: a novel strategy to build a more inclusive culture. *Ann Surg*. 2021;273(3):e97–e99. doi: 10.1097/SLA.0000000000004219
7. Capers Q, McDougle L, Clinchot DM. Strategies for achieving diversity through medical school admissions. *J Health Care Poor Underserved*. 2018;29(1):9–18. doi: 10.1353/hpu.2018.0002

Dismantling Capacity Management Policies That Prioritize Highly Reimbursed Specialty Surgery Over Caring for Uninsured Patients

36

SIDRA N. BONNER AND CHRISTOPHER J. SONNENDAY

Clinical Delivery Challenge

A 57-year-old woman from a city has had persistent worsening shortness of breath and lower extremity edema over the last month. She is currently uninsured after losing her job 6 months ago due to layoffs. Her last primary care appointment was 6 months ago, when she was insured, where her PCP at the time recommended that the patient undergo a workup for new hypervolemia potentially due to cardiac, renal, or hepatic dysfunction. Unfortunately, she was unable to complete this work up due to her loss of insurance. She now presents to the emergency department with preliminary work up concerning for heart failure with reduced ejection fraction. However, upon request for an admission bed, the emergency room physician is told by the bed capacity manager that they are holding the last remaining beds for multiple elective hip replacements overnight.

In this chapter, we will discuss how capacity management policies prioritize highly reimbursed specialty surgery over providing care for uninsured patients.

Hospital capacity management remains central to delivering safe, high quality, and efficient healthcare to patients in an environment with perpetual fluctuating demand for healthcare services.[1,2] Historically, the key components of hospital capacity management strategy have been the acquisition and allocation of facilities and hospital beds, workforce staffing, and availability of specific equipment and expertise.[1,2] In the face of evolving healthcare policy, financial pressures within the healthcare landscape, and individual and population healthcare needs, hospitals and healthcare systems may create policies that delineate the allocation of resources. In addition, hospitals may have strategic growth initiatives and business plans aimed at expanding procedure-based care that optimize revenue and reimbursement. Such capacity management policies and strategies serve to balance the demand of healthcare services with the financial realities and pressures of the healthcare organization.[1-3] Given these 2 interdependent and at times conflicting priorities, hospitals and healthcare systems may disproportionately prioritize the allocation of hospital facilities and resources for highly reimbursed surgical service lines, particularly for patients with private insurance.

● WORKUP

Understanding how individual hospital or healthcare system's capacity management policies lead to the unintended consequence of prioritizing highly reimbursed specialty surgery over care for uninsured patients involves collecting key data and identifying stakeholders. Specific data elements that should be collected include hospital bed occupancy rate, total inpatient hospitalization days, total operations performed by specialty, admissions from the emergency department, and interfacility transfers. Data fields of scheduled operations and trends in bed allocation should be completed for certain highly reimbursed specialties such as orthopedics, cardiac surgery, and solid organ transplantation. For uninsured patients, there should be an assessment of baseline admission rates, emergency cases and emergency department trends, and length of stay. These data can be primarily collected from the electronic health records and routine collection of data from hospital or healthcare system transfer centers. Once these all data are collected, they should be routinely stratified by insurance payer: Private, Medicare, Medicaid, Uninsured. This allows for routine assessment of variation and potential disparities in care by insurance status in addition to provide healthcare systems with a baseline of the proportion of uninsured patients requiring in-patient services. Examples include assessment of in-patient admissions from the emergency department for specific disease conditions or initiated or accepted interfacility transfers evaluated by insurance payer. These routine assessments could highlight the need to change admission or transfer policies that consider insurance status.

In addition to these internal health system data, appropriate assessment of the impact of capacity management policies should include some assessment of the needs of the population served (or potentially served) by the health system. Population health statistics regarding leading diagnoses accounting for hospital admission, and the relative distribution of patients by demographics, insurance status, and admission diagnosis are essential to understand the distribution of healthcare supply and demand in the catchment area served by the health system. Local referral patterns and clustering of marginalized populations may serve to perpetuate inequities in access to highly specialized care. For example, well-resourced tertiary and quaternary care centers may provide a preponderance of highly reimbursed specialty surgery, whereas critical access hospitals divert most of their resources to care for medically complex and uninsured populations.

Beyond routine data collection, healthcare leaders interested in centering health equity in hospital capacity management policies will need to seek out the perspectives and expertise of key hospitals, health systems, and community stakeholders. The health system stakeholders to be involved can be categorized within the domains of finance, clinical operations and clinical strategy. The primary goal of finance departments is acquiring and managing funds within the organizations as well as planning for expenditures for resources. Therefore, given the financial implications of shifting bed capacity strategies from highly reimbursed surgical services to care delivery for uninsured patients, it is important to involve members within the domain of finance to identify targets, goals, and offsetting strategies. Leaders in clinical operations maintain the planning and evaluation of the daily operations of a hospital or healthcare system. Clinical operations teams set policies for optimal patient flow, bed capacity management, hospital transfer, and inpatient admissions. Stakeholders from this group are necessary to identify current practices and to build new systems for the allocation of hospital or system resources toward the care of uninsured patients. In addition, a review of all current transfer and admission policies is necessary to understand if there exist barriers to admission for uninsured patients. Community stakeholders should be engaged to help identify barriers to access that may not be readily apparent to hospitals. Referral patterns and patient preferences for specific hospitals and health systems may be driven by a multitude of factors not apparent to hospital leaders, including access to affordable transportation, systemic biases or historic behaviors of certain hospitals towards marginalized communities, and the preferences of local primary care providers and referring physicians.

● DIFFERENTIAL DIAGNOSIS

Directing capacity management policies towards increasing care for uninsured patient populations requires analysis of current bed allocation policies, institutional financial status, and community needs and preferences. Assessment of the assignment of beds, and the financial implications of that assignment, for highly reimbursed procedures versus inpatient admission demand for beds by uninsured patients should be identified. This information can be gathered from systems admissions and bed capacity management teams. Additionally, trends in surgical scheduling and necessary beds for highly reimbursed surgical services should be assessed. Understanding how the capacity management behaviors of the hospital compare to the needs of the community and the capacity management behaviors of surrounding hospitals will help inform a comprehensive view of how the health system meets (or does not meet) the healthcare needs of the community.

SCIENTIFIC PRINCIPLES AND EVIDENCE

Surgical care delivery remains central to the financial status of hospitals and therefore optimization of surgical services is an important component of hospital capacity management decisions.[4–6] The Agency for Healthcare Research and Quality (AHRQ) has previously found that inpatient hospitalizations with operations performed account for nearly a third of hospitalizations but half of hospital cost.[4] Furthermore, it has been well documented that elective procedures, particularly orthopedic and cardiac surgical procedures, are key drivers of hospital revenue.[4] Furthermore, among inpatient hospitalizations involving a surgical operation, the most common payer is private insurance (41%) followed by Medicare (34%).[4] This is particularly important given that current hospital price discrimination demonstrates that private insurance plans pay on average 200% of Medicare rates.[7,8] The overall cost of elective procedures and price discrimination between insurance payers create financial incentives for hospitals to prioritize surgical care to privately insured patients.[7,8] Unfortunately, given the limited resources within a given hospital or healthcare system, policies prioritizing highly reimbursed specialty surgery may have a disparate impact on patients who are uninsured given that policies may be in place to maximize highly reimbursed services to insured patients.[4–10]

DIAGNOSIS AND TREATMENT

Transitioning the health system towards optimized bed capacity and equitable care will require key changes in current hospital practices. First, there should be clear identification of current transfer and admissions policies that include insurance authorization. These policies may disproportionately affect uninsured patients in terms of their ability to be transferred to systems for higher levels of care. These policies may also be associated with higher inter-facility transfer or discharge of uninsured patients from the emergency department. Once these policies are identified and data is collected to identify the overall trends in demand for beds for uninsured patients, simulation models to understand the impact of removing these policies should be performed. This would provide data regarding the expected changes to demand for beds and financial implications in terms of expected costs, uncompensated care, and change in relative value units to a given healthcare system.

IMPLEMENTING A SOLUTION

In addition to dismantling current policies that potentially limit the inpatient hospitalization of uninsured patients, there will need to be a concordant change in operative scheduling, bed optimization, and staffing to account for increased admissions bed utilization for uninsured patients admitted for surgical and medical diagnoses. Potential system strategies to facilitate improved efficiency and equity include the development of clear admission and discharge criteria without insurance consideration and real-time data analytics to improve match capacity for patient demand and patient flow. The overall solutions required to change practice to include a more equity-based approach to bed capacity management is included in the Key Steps in Change Management and Potential Pitfalls table.

Further policy level interventions to aid healthcare systems in seeking more equitable capacity management practices will require ongoing policy changes to limit price discrimination that is, "the fact that hospitals and healthcare systems charge different payers different amounts for the same services at the same point in time."[8] This is necessary to disrupt the current financial incentives leading to healthcare systems prioritizing highly reimbursed surgical care for populations with private insurance. Finally, in an ideal state local hospitals will collaborate to meet the needs of the community, particularly those of high-risk or marginalized populations. Expecting critical access hospitals to absorb most of the medical care for uninsured and medically vulnerable populations is not sustainable, as was exposed in the first surge of the COVID-19 pandemic in early 2020. Collaborative quality initiatives and state health agencies can play roles in helping to optimize the distribution of care among populations and regions.

CHAPTER 36 • Dismantling Capacity Management Policies

Key Steps in Change Management and Potential Pitfalls

Key Steps in Change Management

1. Identify disparities in admissions and transfer of uninsured medical and surgical patients, relative to insured patients.
2. Understand the process and steps leading up to a patient's insurance status being used for inter-facility transfer or admission.
3. Analyze and interpret current data regarding emergency department admissions, transfers, and current bed demand and allocation stratified by medical or surgical service and insurance payer.
4. Health system leaders must spend time on the front line (eg, Gemba Walks) with key stakeholders involved including admission and transfer centers, finance departments, clinical operations leads, and providers.
5. Identify current policies that require documentation of insurance status for admissions and transfers.
6. Introduce possible solutions to key stakeholders to test face validity and refine based on feedback.
7. Pilot the potential solution (eg, removal of insurance pre-authorization policies for admission and transfer) in a high-yield area and have regular opportunities to solicit feedback. Make sure you can track a measurable outcome (ideally an impact on the disparities identified in #1).

Potential Pitfalls

1. Jumping straight to a solution without understanding changes to overall bed capacity and changes to hospital financial status.
2. Lack of a clear conceptual model for how insurance status is used for admission decisions.
3. Not engaging enough of the correct stakeholders and spending time with them, in their space, whereas their work is in action. Specifically, representatives from the finance department, admission and transfer management, and bed capacity management.
4. Lack of community involvement, and/or lack of an understanding of the epidemiology of local care delivery. Addressing the needs of uninsured patients requires healthcare systems leaders to understand local rates of uninsured patients in order to inform estimates for bed capacity required for uninsured patients.
5. Forgetting to monitor to unintended consequences of your solution.
6. Broadly implementing your solution across a healthcare system without pilot testing it within one division or section first.

● MEASURING OUTCOMES

The process of dismantling of capacity management policies that either limit the admission of uninsured patients or prioritize highly reimbursed surgical care will need to have clear measurable goals. Measuring changes in patient payer-mix for services or departments that remove policies requiring insurance authorization prior to admission or transfer should be obtained. Other key metrics to be obtained would be changes in emergency department admissions and approvals of transfers stratified by insurance payer. Measurable impacts such as reduced patient flow inefficiencies, longer lengths of stay, or increases in uncompensated care should also be measured, as they may impact both local care delivery as well as health system's financial status.

● FOLLOW-UP AND MAINTENANCE

Ultimately, decisions to increase access to care for uninsured and underinsured patients relative to more well-reimbursed specialty surgery care will require health system level prioritization decisions to value providing care to vulnerable populations. Sustainability of such practices will likely require both careful management of resources by health systems, and systemic policy change to reduce both the number of uninsured patients and the increased cost of urgent care relative to preventative medical care.

REFERENCES

1. Ravaghi H, Alidoost S, Mannion R, et al. Models and methods for determining the optimal number of beds in hospitals and regions: a systematic scoping review. *BMC Health Serv Res.* 2020;20(1):186.
2. Green LV. Capacity Planning and Management in Hospitals. In: Brandeau ML, Sainfort F, Pierskalla WP eds. Operations Research and Health Care. International Series in Operations Research & Management Science, vol 70. Boston, MA: Springer, 2005.
3. Li L, Benton WC. Hospital capacity management decisions: emphasis on cost control and quality enhancement. *Eur J Oper Res.* 2003;146(3):596–614.
4. McDermott KW (IBM Watson Health), Liang L (AHRQ). Overview of Operating Room Procedures During Inpatient Stays in U.S. Hospitals, 2018. HCUP Statistical Brief #281. August 2021. Agency for Healthcare Research and Quality, Rockville, MD. www.hcup-us.ahrq.gov/reports/statbriefs/sb281-Operating-Room-Procedures-During-Hospitalization-2018.pdf.
5. Hoskins NN, Cunicelli MA, Hopper W, Zeller R, Cheng N, Lindsey T. The value surgical services bring to critical access hospitals. *Cureus.* 2021;13(4):e14367. doi: 10.7759/cureus.14367
6. Resnick AS, Corrigan D, Mullen JL, Kaiser LR. Surgeon contribution to hospital bottom line: not all are created equal. *Ann Surg.* 2005;242(4):530–539. doi: 10.1097/01.sla.0000184693.61680.24
7. Whaley CM, Briscombe B, Kerber R, O'Neill B, Kofner A. Prices Paid to Hospitals by Private Health Plans: Findings from Round 4 of an Employer-Led Transparency Initiative. Santa Monica, CA: RAND Corporation, 2022. https://www.rand.org/pubs/research_reports/RRA1144-1.html.
8. Kaplan A, O'Neil D. Hospital price discrimination is deepening racial health inequity. *NEJM Catalyst.* 2020. doi: 10.1056/CAT.20.0593
9. Venkatesh AK, Chou SC, Li SX, et al. Association between insurance status and access to hospital care in emergency department disposition. *JAMA Intern Med.* 2019;179(5):686–693. doi: 10.1001/jamainternmed.2019.0037
10. Kindermann DR, Mutter RL, Cartwright-Smith L, Rosenbaum S, Pines JM. Admit or transfer? The role of insurance in high-transfer-rate medical conditions in the emergency department. *Ann Emerg Med.* 2014;63(5):561–571.e8. doi: 10.1016/j.annemergmed.2013.11.019

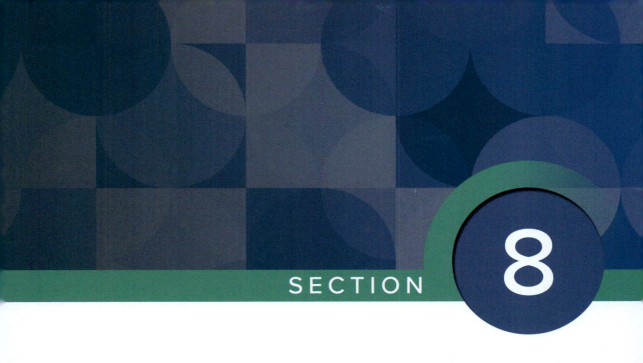

Policy-Responsive Leadership

37 Enrolling in Voluntary Bundled Payment Programs in Surgery
Nicholas L. Berlin and Scott E. Regenbogen

38 Considerations in Accountable Care Organizations (ACOs)
Ian Berger, Robert S. Saunders, Devdutta Sangvai, and Deborah R. Kaye

39 Out-of-Network Billing: The Surgical Leader's Perspective
Karan R. Chhabra, Mihir S. Dekhne, and Sunil Eappen

Enrolling in Voluntary Bundled Payment Programs in Surgery

37

NICHOLAS L. BERLIN AND SCOTT E. REGENBOGEN

Clinical Delivery Challenge

Surgical care has been an important focus for payment reform. Both its episodic nature and established variations in spending and clinical outcomes suggest opportunities to reduce clinically unwarranted spending and improve outcomes. Since the 1970s, prospective payment for hospitalization (eg, diagnosis related groups) incentivized reductions in length of stay, but did not address spending on care after discharge.[1-3] Amidst the growing pressure to control inpatient costs, hospitals expedited discharges, and post-acute care services proliferated.[2] Episode-based bundled payment models were thus conceived as a mechanism to incentivize hospitals and providers to consider the efficiency of care for both during the index hospitalization and after discharge, for selected surgical conditions (eg, major lower extremity joint replacement, coronary artery bypass grafting). Although these models were initially piloted and disseminated for federally-insured patients, there are emerging examples of episode-based, bundled reimbursement programs in the private sector.[4,5]

In bundled payment programs, hospitals and providers will receive fixed payment for services received by a patient across all care settings, either during a pre-defined time period around a discrete event (eg, inpatient surgery) or throughout the course of a defined clinical condition (eg, a course of chemotherapy) (Figure 37.1).[6] Hospitals and providers gain revenue through shared savings if spending is less than risk-adjusted benchmarks (often called "target prices") during the episode. On the contrary, hospitals may also lose revenue if overall spending is higher than benchmarks. In some models, the bundled payment is made prospectively, and the primary recipient is then responsible for reconciling payments with other providers involved in the episode. In other models, overall episode spending is assessed retrospectively, compared with target benchmarks, and the primary provider is either afforded bonus payments for net savings, or required to make reconciliation payments to the payor for excess spending. Although there have been examples of mandatory bundled payment programs, such as the federal Comprehensive Care for Joint Replacement Model, participation in most bundled payment programs has been voluntary. Therefore, hospitals and providers must weigh decisions to participate episode-based incentive programs, considering the likelihood of gaining revenue through shared savings against the possibility of financial losses.

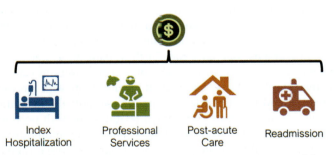

FIGURE 37.1 Conceptual overview of major components of the bundled payment for surgical conditions.

Imagine that a hospital is eligible to participate in an episode-based bundled payment model for inpatient surgery, including major joint replacement of the lower extremity, coronary artery bypass grafting, and/or major bowel surgery. Institutional leaders are asked to determine whether they should participate and to design and oversee an operational strategy for the hospital to be successful in one or more of the models.

● WORKUP

To understand whether the hospital can be successful in a surgical episode-based bundled payment model, hospital leaders must first thoroughly understand the structure of the model in consideration. The arrangements of bundled payment models differ in important ways that may impact the hospital's likelihood of success. For instance, they must understand the duration of clinical episodes (30 days, 60 days, 90 days, etc.), the methodology for calculating the target price (including approaches to risk adjustment), whether the model includes downside risks (ie, potential financial penalties for over-spending, versus only bonuses for shared savings), and whether there are case volume minimums for eligibility.

Next, hospital leaders need a detailed understanding of overall spending, both during and after hospitalization, for their patients in each of these surgical episodes. Unfortunately, many hospitals lack comprehensive data on post-discharge spending and care utilization that occurs outside of their walls. In some programs, the payor may provide hospitals with their historical episode spending data, helping to enable informed decisions about participation. However, administrative claims data are often subjected to significant processing and analysis delays and thus past performance may not necessarily reflect the current state at the time of decision-making for participation. Facing these analytic challenges, many hospitals have turned to private consulting groups to guide participation decisions and to craft improvement strategies for spending reduction in clinical episodes.[7] Uniquely, in the state of Michigan, hospitals can obtain comprehensive spending data around surgical episodes through a Blue Cross Blue Shield of Michigan-funded initiative, the Michigan Value Collaborative. This voluntary statewide hospital collaborative enables access to both private and federal insurance claims data for the vast majority of patients treated in the state.[8–11] These data are cleaned and analyzed with risk adjustment to highlight variation in episode spending, and identify the key actionable sources of spending variations for more than 30 medical and surgical conditions. Regardless of their setting, however, hospitals considering participation in a voluntary bundled payment program must evaluate their pre-participation spending patterns, and understand their relationships to comparators and target prices.

With an understanding of the hospital's range of care patterns and spending, leaders should then consider grouping patient-level data into higher and lower spending quantiles, to gain an improved understanding of variation in episode spending between patients treated at their hospital. The leaders can compare care utilization between high and low cost patients, evaluating common potential sources of savings, which for surgical conditions often include readmissions and post-acute care.

Finally, the leaders will need to identify key stakeholders, both within the hospital and among external care providers commonly involved in their patients' post-discharge care. These stakeholders will inform decisions on participation in specific clinical episodes and comprise strategic partnerships during the implementation of the model. Key stakeholders for surgical bundles may range from clinicians and surgeons with experience delivering surgical and perioperative care for these patients, as well as nursing leadership, case managers, physical therapists, and social workers who play critical roles in care coordination following discharge from the inpatient stay. It will also be essential to collaborate with individuals in administrative leadership to secure financial and non-financial resources to support the institutional effort to succeed in the model. Finally, it will be important to strengthen relationships with post-acute care facilities and home health and therapy providers, consider shared staffing models, communicate with facilities to provide continued assurance of referrals, and negotiate how financial gains and responsibilities from participation may be shared among them.

DIFFERENTIAL DIAGNOSIS

It is essential to understand the sources of spending variations within the hospital and the specific differences in modifiable spending for each surgical condition.[12] For instance, the majority of savings in bundled payment models for major joint replacement are attributed to reducing utilization and intensity of post-acute care services.[13-15] The inpatient stay and readmissions are a more important source of spending variations for coronary artery bypass grafting and major bowel surgery.[10,12] For colectomy, there is some evidence that the surgical approach (eg, laparoscopic versus open) may also account for variation in episode spending.[16] Therefore, it is critical to have detailed understanding of length of stay, readmissions, utilization, and discharge disposition (ie, rehab versus skilled nursing facility) for the surgical condition, and, as explained earlier, to be aware of historical performance relative to peer hospitals and target prices benchmarks.

For major joint replacement surgery, one of the major initial strategies may be to estimate how much inpatient rehabilitation and post-acute care can be eliminated without compromising the quality of care delivered. Next, evaluate whether it is possible to reduce the intensity of post-acute care, either by reducing length of stay in institutional post-acute care or by substituting extended care facility services (eg, skilled nursing facility, or inpatient rehabilitation) with lower-cost non-institutional care settings (eg, home health care, outpatient rehabilitation).[17]

Readmissions are another important source of potentially avoidable spending, especially in the case of coronary artery bypass grafting or major bowel surgery. Thus if readmission rates are higher than expected, it will be essential to determine modifiable causes that may be amenable to improvement during participation in the model. For example, strategies to reduce avoidable postoperative complications, improve care coordination and care transitions, and streamline communication may be effective in many settings.

When making the final decision about participation in these episode-based bundled payment models, the leaders will need to estimate the potential reduction in spending that may be achievable during the "performance period" of the model and compare with expected target prices. It may be possible to evaluate expected gains based on simple comparisons of baseline performance against expected payments, even without significant changes in practice. It is then important to consider the internal financial and personnel resources that would be required to implement comprehensive strategies to reduce episode spending further, as well as the opportunity costs of other initiatives they might forgo. These estimates will largely depend on each hospital's unique circumstances, and conservative estimates are generally appropriate because significant cost-reducing practice changes can be challenging to achieve. Some hospitals may consider voluntary payment programs in the context of other initiatives already in progress, as there may be opportunities for synergy between multiple ongoing efforts to improve quality, safety, and cost.

DIAGNOSIS AND TREATMENT

Based upon the initial quantitative investigation, the leaders should aim to identify several strategic targets to reduce spending for patients who undergo each of these surgical procedures in their institution. It is important to understand that there may more than one key source of reducible spending and the drivers of this spending may not be immediately obvious from the initial quantitative analyses. For this reason, the leaders should leverage the identified stakeholders to perform a more detailed investigations into the causes of spending variation. These analyses may involve focus groups, or individual interviews with stakeholders, modeled after the hospital's quality improvement efforts (eg, lean approaches). The results should be organized and shared with individuals involved in developing the strategy to reduce spending for each surgical episode individually.

After performing both quantitative and qualitative investigations into drivers of episode spending variation within the hospital, the leaders may determine that there are potential levers in all aspects of the perioperative care process to reduce unnecessary spending and improve patient outcomes. In this case, perhaps there was no standardized approach to optimizing preoperative comorbidities known to contribute to postoperative complications (eg, uncontrolled diabetes mellitus and hypertension). During the preoperative period and the initial inpatient stay, interviews with nursing leadership and other providers identify opportunities to improve communication with patients about postoperative expectations for the recovery process and to implement an enhanced recovery after surgery protocol that includes a multi-modal strategy for pain control. The care managers and clinic staff find limited real-time understanding of patient progress towards therapy goals among those patients who had been discharged to subacute nursing facilities (SNF) and potential communication challenges with providers at those facilities. The quantitative investigation into intensity of post-acute care use can determine whether certain outlier SNFs comprise the majority of cases with prolonged length of stay among eligible joint replacement patients treated at your hospital. These discrete, potentially remediable, sources of excess spending could then be a focus for spending reduction initiatives, and may suggest opportunities for success in the bundled payment program under consideration.

● SCIENTIFIC PRINCIPLES AND EVIDENCE

Bundled payments are an increasingly common alternative payment model, aiming to reduce spending for some surgical conditions.[13–15,18–20] Optimistically, these programs have been shown to reduce spending by ~1% to 3% through decreased use of post-acute care and other hospital resources without affecting access or quality of care.[13–15,18–20] The majority of evidence supporting their efficacy has come from the Comprehensive Care for Joint Replacement Model, a nationwide, mandatory trial of bundled payments for major lower extremity joint replacement procedures in selected geographic areas. However, recent studies of newer bundled payment models have been promising for other conditions as well,[13,20] leading the Centers for Medicare and Medicaid Services and private payors continue to test and expand similar payment models to a broad range of surgical conditions, including 13 surgical conditions in the bundled payments for care improvement advanced.

There are several examples of hospitals' successful participation within voluntary bundled payment programs that leaders may use to guide implementation of a strategy within their own institutions. The hospital for special surgery has described the clinical, operational, and financial components of their successful bundled payment program for lower extremity total joint replacement.[21] The authors designed and implemented a comprehensive approach to program development, including a rehabilitation care pathways program, strategies to determine the appropriateness of inpatient rehabilitation, a home health agency program, strategies to optimize the use of postoperative telehealth, and development of a preoperative optimization program. Another case study from Baptist Health System highlighted use of behavioral economics principles to leverage sustained success in a bundled payment model for orthopedic surgery.[22] In this article, the authors describe how governance methods and payout design may increase physician commitment and participation in bundled payment models. For instance, their strategy of individual- and cohort-level incentives maximized behavior change within their organization, and data transparency was essential to create a culture of improvement that extended even beyond the performance period of the model.

● IMPLEMENTING A SOLUTION

Success in bundled payments requires a deep understanding of payment model characteristics and incentives, clinical workflow for surgical conditions, and operational strategies for effective interventions to reduce episode spending while preserving the quality of care. Key steps in change management and potential pitfalls for enrollment in voluntary bundled payment models in surgery are shown below. Since the primary sources of savings may often be from care delivered outside the index hospitalization, the strategy implemented by the hospital will need to address the communication and data challenges that occur throughout the full episode of care. Establishing a plan for data and analytics, in addition to internal and external stakeholder engagement is critical.

Effective strategies will also require buy-in from multiple levels of clinical and administrative leadership. After identifying key focus areas for spending reduction, financial and non-financial incentives should be defined clearly and early in the planning stages to gain engagement from departmental leadership, nursing staff, and other stakeholders. Consider including representatives from these stakeholder groups in the

Key Steps in Change Management and Potential Pitfalls

Key Change Management Steps

1. Data Access and Management	Obtain total episode spending data for patients undergoing the surgical procedure at the hospital. Plan for data analysis before, during, and following participation in the model. Identify data sources for out-of-hospital spending and utilization.
2. Stakeholder Engagement	Identify and engage all relevant stakeholders within and outside of hospital, for the entire episode of care, including them in work up, design, and implementation of the operational strategy.
3. Quantitative Investigation	Perform rigorous quantitative analysis to characterize potentially remediable sources of unnecessary spending.
4. Qualitative Investigation	Perform stakeholder inquiries using quality improvement methodologies (eg, lean processes) to understand sources of excessive spending, identify opportunities and clarify potential barriers to implementation of an operational strategy.
5. Operational Strategy	Design a comprehensive operational strategy, reflecting the findings of quantitative and qualitative investigations, with engagement from stakeholders, including clinical and administrative leadership.
6. Outcome Measurement	Formulate plan for measuring relevant outcomes beyond health spending, including quality and equity metrics that are relevant to the surgical episode.
7. Audit and Feedback	Engage with stakeholders to overcome challenges during the implementation of the model and leverage experience from participation for other alternative payment models in the future.

Potential Pitfalls

1. Inadequate Work-up	A superficial understanding of episode spending within and (especially) outside of the hospital may lead to flawed decision-making about participation in the model and targets to reduce spending in the operational strategy.
2. Operational Barriers	Without an appreciation for the administrative and clinical barriers to the implementation of the strategy, the likelihood of success is limited.
3. Lack of Buy-in	A lack of support from administrative and clinical stakeholders will limit hospital resources allocated to the effort and the overall effectiveness of the strategy.
4. Data Mismanagement	Inadequate data and analytic support will limit the ability to make strategic changes in real time and monitor progress.
5. No Incentives for Stakeholders	Without financial and non-financial incentives, stakeholders may not be motivated to participate or prioritize other projects ahead of this one.

decision-making process for designing and implementing the operational strategy to improve transparency and set reasonable, timely objectives as key change management steps. Potential pitfalls to avoid include inadequate understanding of the sources of excess spending, an underappreciation for the barriers to effect change, a lack of support from administrative and clinical leadership, a poorly designed plan for data monitoring and analysis, and limited or no incentives for change agents to implement solutions.

● MEASURING OUTCOMES

The most important metric to assess effectiveness of hospital strategy will be trends in average episode spending and between-patient variation. Early attention to the key contributors to variation (eg, post-acute care spending, readmissions) will provide insights into leading indicators of success in the program overall. Depending on the reconciliation model, hospitals may not fully recognize the balance of gains or losses until well into their period of participation. In fact, they may be called upon to decide future years' enrollment before the first year's performance has been adjudicated. Ultimately, shared savings bonus, if earned, will then be weighed against the financial and other resources consumed in the design and implementation of their hospital's strategy for participation. At the same time, it will be critical to pay attention to the possibility of adverse trends in clinical outcomes such as postoperative complications and unplanned readmissions, as well as patient-reported outcomes such as satisfaction and functional recovery, if measured. The clinical case-mix of patients who undergo surgery in the hospital needs also to be monitored closely, both by the hospital and by the payor to identify any unintended consequences, such as adverse selection against high risk patients, that could exacerbate access to surgery, especially for underserved populations.

● FOLLOW-UP AND MAINTENANCE

The experience gained from participation in a novel episode-based bundled payment incentive program will likely have significant spillover in programmatic infrastructure and expertise that will serve hospitals well in other initiatives. The strategies and interventions critical to success may thus translate to successful participation in other surgical episodes in future bundled payment models. The care pathways and perioperative optimization programs likely drive reduced postoperative length of stay, which can improve contribution margins for inpatient surgery across the institution. The financial opportunities presented by other voluntary bundled payment models will continue to incentivize administrative support for participation and ultimately improve care more broadly throughout the hospital. By continuing to leverage new technologies and care strategies, leaders can drive ongoing improvement in care delivery as new opportunities arise.

REFERENCES

1. Ackerly DC, Grabowski DC. Post-acute care reform–beyond the ACA. *N Engl J Med.* 2014;370(8):689–691.
2. Buntin MB, Colla CH, Escarce JJ. Effects of payment changes on trends in post-acute care. *Health Serv Res.* 2009;44(4):1188–1210.
3. Davis C, Rhodes DJ. The impact of DRGs on the cost and quality of health care in the United States. *Health Policy.* 1988;9(2):117–131.
4. Rastogi A, Mohr BA, Williams JO, et al. Prometheus payment model: application to hip and knee replacement surgery. *Clin Orthop Relat Res.* 2009;467(10):2587–2597.
5. Spinks T, Guzman A, Beadle BM, et al. Development and feasibility of bundled payments for the multidisciplinary treatment of head and neck cancer: a pilot program. *J Oncol Pract.* 2018;14(2):e103–e112.
6. Ryan AM. Medicare bundled payment programs for joint replacement: anatomy of a successful payment reform. *JAMA.* 2018;320(9):877–879.
7. Berlin NL, Peterson TA, Chopra Z, et al. Hospital participation decisions in medicare bundled payment program were influenced by third-party conveners. *Health Aff (Millwood).* 2021;40(8):1286–1293.
8. Regenbogen SE, Cain-Nielsen AH, Syrjamaki JD, et al. Spending on postacute care after hospitalization in commercial insurance and medicare around age sixty-five. *Health Aff (Millwood).* 2019;38(9):1505–1513.
9. Thompson MP, Yost ML, Syrjamaki JD, et al. Sources of hospital variation in postacute care spending after cardiac surgery. *Circ Cardiovasc Qual Outcomes.* 2020;13(11):e006449.

10. Vu JV, Li J, Likosky DS, et al. Achieving the high-value colectomy: preventing complications or improving efficiency. *Dis Colon Rectum*. 2020;63(1):84–92.
11. Ellimoottil C, Ryan AM, Hou H, et al. Medicare's new bundled payment for joint replacement may penalize hospitals that treat medically complex patients. *Health Aff (Millwood)*. 2016;35(9):1651–1657.
12. Miller DC, Gust C, Dimick JB, et al. Large variations in medicare payments for surgery highlight savings potential from bundled payment programs. *Health Aff (Millwood)*. 2011;30(11):2107–2115.
13. Barnett ML, Wilcock A, McWilliams JM, et al. Two-Year evaluation of mandatory bundled payments for joint replacement. *N Engl J Med*. 2019;380(3):252–262.
14. Agarwal R, Liao JM, Gupta A, et al. The impact of bundled payment on health care spending, utilization, and quality: a systematic review. *Health Aff (Millwood)*. 2020;39(1):50–57.
15. Dummit LA, Kahvecioglu D, Marrufo G, et al. Association between hospital participation in a medicare bundled payment initiative and payments and quality outcomes for lower extremity joint replacement episodes. *JAMA*. 2016;316(12):1267–1278.
16. Sheetz KH, Dimick JB, Regenbogen SE. How patient complexity and surgical approach influence episode-based payment models for colectomy. *Dis Colon Rectum*. 2019;62(6):739–746.
17. Chen LM, Norton EC, Banerjee M, et al. Spending on care after surgery driven by choice of care settings instead of intensity of services. *Health Aff (Millwood)*. 2017;36(1):83–90.
18. Chopra Z, Gulseren B, Chhabra KR, et al. Bundled Payments for Care Improvement (BPCI) efficacy across three common operations. *Ann Surg*. 2021; doi: 10.1097/SLA.0000000000004869
19. Finkelstein A, Ji Y, Mahoney N, et al. Mandatory medicare bundled payment program for lower extremity joint replacement and discharge to institutional postacute care: interim analysis of the first year of a 5-year randomized trial. *JAMA*. 2018;320(9):892–900.
20. Joynt Maddox KE, Orav EJ, Zheng J, et al. Year 1 of the bundled payments for care improvement-advanced model. *N Engl J Med*. 2021;385(7):618–627.
21. MacLean C, Titmuss M, Lee J, Russell L, Padgett D, et al. The clinical, operational, and financial components of a successful bundled payment program for lower extremity total joint replacement. *NEJM Catalyst*. 2021;2(10). doi: 10.1056/CAT.21.0240
22. Liao JM, Holdofski A, Whittington GL, et al. Baptist health system: succeeding in bundled payments through behavioral principles. *Healthc (Amst)*. 2017;5(3):136–140.

Considerations in Accountable Care Organizations (ACOs)

38

IAN BERGER, ROBERT S. SAUNDERS, DEVDUTTA SANGVAI, AND DEBORAH R. KAYE

Clinical Delivery Challenge

Accountable care organizations (ACOs) are one of the most common value-based payment models, with over 35 million people covered by some type of Accountable care organization (ACO) in 2021. Evidence suggests that ACOs will continue to grow; the Center for Medicare and Medicaid Innovation has indicated that accountable care is a key part of their strategy and commercial payers have recently introduced ACO products. While ACO programs have significant heterogeneity in their design and implementation, they are united in their focus on accountability for spending and quality for a predetermined set of patients. ACO programs often allow participating organizations to share in savings if spending is reduced below a predetermined benchmark (determined by historical spending, regional spending patterns, or some other approach), with more advanced programs having ACOs share in losses if spending rises above that benchmark. ACO programs also incorporate quality into their accountability, with most programs preventing ACOs from sharing in savings if they do not meet certain quality metric scores.

ACOs have demonstrated limited improvements in cost and quality.[1] One barrier to high-level performance in early ACOs is the lack of specialist engagement. While ACO programs are generally designed with patients attributed based on their primary care utilization, most ACOs are responsible for the total cost of care, including surgical care. Specialty physicians, including surgeons, are often unaware of their participation and/or the objectives of the ACO, they frequently do not share the risk that the organization faces, and their incentives often do not align with the goals of the ACO.

In this chapter, we describe the perspective of an integrated health system with a defined set of contracted surgeons. Three years into our ACO implementation, we have made investments in our technological infrastructure and have increased care coordination between our primary care providers and specialists. In the introductory period, our ACO predominately had upside shared savings with minimal risk of loss, however, we will be transitioning to a two-sided track with both shared savings and increased risk of losses. During the transition to additional risk, our ACO has identified surgical care as an area to improve cost-effectiveness.

ACOs theoretically provide an important avenue to improve care coordination and health outcomes. However, many ACOs have limited surgeon engagement, despite surgical care comprising a critical component of overall healthcare costs and quality.[2] In this chapter, we describe strategies to improve surgeon engagement in ACOs.

● WORKUP

To improve the performance of our ACO, we must first understand the current operational state. Since shared savings are often based on improvements over historical benchmarks, a good place to start is by comparing our current surgical spending per beneficiary to past time points. While surgical spending centers on an operation, many costs occur after this event. Thus, we evaluate surgical episodes of care, including the day of surgery and 30 days postoperatively, as a key operational variable for calculating cost.

We must also understand surgeon participation within our ACO. A survey of surgeon awareness about ACO operations and his/her role within the ACO would reveal any knowledge gaps that require intervention. Focus groups on surgeon values, burdens, and the financial and nonfinancial incentives that would

CHAPTER 38 • Considerations in Accountable Care Organizations (ACOs)

promote practice change can lay the foundation for our future resource allocation. Identifying individual surgeons to participate in multidisciplinary ACO administrative teams is critical for ACO integration and success. These stakeholder surgeons can provide knowledge of clinical processes, areas for improvement, concerns with ACO structure and requirements, and can assist with educating their surgical colleagues. Knowledge of the current compensation packages could be used to improve financial incentives.

Understanding current health outcomes and care patterns within our ACO will also be critical to improve cost and quality. Targets for improvement include process variations that result in similar outcomes despite varying costs (ie, the use of low value surgical services or discharges to low quality post-acute care facilities) and/or those that result in differing outcomes with similar costs. We must also identify our ACO beneficiaries that obtain surgical care, including post-acute services, outside of our ACO. This referral leakage can occur through physicians or via self-referral. While we do not control the quantity or quality of care delivered at other institutions, these metrics still affect our savings or losses.

Our evaluation indicates that since becoming an ACO, surgical cost and quality has remained stagnant, despite improvements in nonsurgical areas. However, almost 90% of our surgical staff are either uninformed that we are an ACO or do not know that his/her care contributed to the performance of the organization. Similarly, they are unaware that decreasing costs could lead to shared savings. Our surgeons are compensated predominately for quantity of care and do not receive benefits if our ACO performs well; and when asked about the financial and nonfinancial incentives that would drive them to improve quality and decrease costs, most were so unclear about the idea of the ACO that they could not respond to the question. Furthermore, while outcomes are similar across surgeons, costs vary substantially. High-quality post-acute services are only utilized for approximately 50% of patients and teams lack resources to identify these high-quality, low-cost facilities. Approximately 15% of beneficiaries obtain surgical care outside of our ACO.

● DIFFERENTIAL DIAGNOSIS

Based on our data, surgeons within our ACO lack engagement and are either unaware or not incentivized to align themselves with the goals of our ACO. Surgeons further do not face any downside to using low value services. Our teams lack the resources to identify and utilize high value care. Many beneficiaries obtain surgical care outside of the ACO.

● DIAGNOSIS AND TREATMENT

Driver diagrams for our organization (Figure 38.1) demonstrate that improving cost and quality of surgical care for our beneficiaries requires a multifaceted approach. Motivation for change should come from surgeon-led interdisciplinary teams who develop ACO awareness, instill ideals, and share best practices throughout all levels of care. However, they must be supported by the ACO which provides resources and infrastructure to promote improvement. When approaching department leadership, ACO appeal may come from presenting a business case where the organization offsets startup costs of ACO initiatives and provides an expedited return on investment through shared savings. Leadership awareness of ACO goals potentially allows for prioritization of initiatives that improve ACO-aligned care. Third, successful, early ACOs have identified physician liaisons or champions who communicate ACO values with their colleagues and staff.[3] We must identify these representatives and provide them with dedicated time for ACO activities, recognition, and/or additional compensation.

To facilitate engagement, surgeons should be incentivized to provide high value care which aligns with the ACO mission. Most specialists across the country are compensated based on productivity. While little data are known about specialist compensation within ACOs, anecdotal evidence suggests most ACO surgeon compensation follows this trend, and very few receive financial incentives that are tied to ACO performance. While several categories of financial packages exist, a final solution would incorporate multiple strategies. The organization must ensure the metrics used to distribute incentives are fair and support behavior that improves value-based care without unintended consequences.

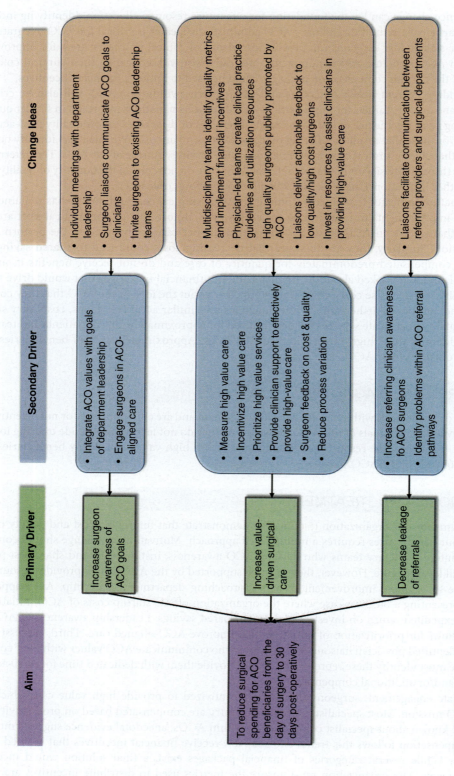

FIGURE 38.1 Driver diagram to reduce surgical costs for our ACO beneficiaries.

CHAPTER 38 • Considerations in Accountable Care Organizations (ACOs) **253**

Finally, knowledge of referral pathways is critical to reducing leakage to outside organizations. ACO beneficiaries may have long wait times to appointments and/or surgery within the ACO. Alternatively, ACO referring clinicians may have greater trust in the quality of outside surgeons. Open communication with referring clinicians would reveal these challenges; changes could be made accordingly to promote the quality of surgeons within the ACO. Importantly, this process represents a continuous feedback loop, so as the ACO structure changes, new referral challenges can be quickly addressed.

● SCIENTIFIC PRINCIPLES AND EVIDENCE

Nationwide, surgeon awareness and participation in ACOs are low; likely due to a lack of prioritization of surgical care within the ACO model.[4-6] While prior work demonstrates that increased ACO awareness is associated with a perceived ability to avoid low value care, the evidence surrounding specialist awareness and engagement in ACOs is nascent and often based on anecdotal experience.[6] The Centers for Medicare and Medicaid Services (CMS) published a provider engagement toolkit based on examples from early successful ACOs that addresses the introduction of ACO values to an organization.[3] Their examples utilize organizational leadership to promote a shift in culture while employing clinician liaisons and written communication to disseminate information to their colleagues.

Surgeon engagement may take a variety of forms. While surgeons that participate in ACOs should receive financial benefits, it unlikely that the shared savings alone will be enough to change behavior.[4,7] Representatives across the organization need to be involved in identifying and improving both financial and nonfinancial incentives. As most metrics captured by CMS are not directly applicable to surgical care, novel quality measures could be developed and tied to shared savings for the ACO. Both measures of utilization (ie, care costs or use of low value services) and quality (ie, complication rates) are useful for designing incentives. Graded cutoffs, such as 25%, 50%, and 75% of the maximum incentive, reward effort while also encouraging future performance. Evidence suggests that surgeons are responsive to feedback which can also be leveraged to reduce cost and improve quality.[8] However, this feedback must be provided in an actionable framework. Furthermore, these measures must be accurately risk-adjusted and physicians must not be overburdened with ACO requirements.

Quality improvement frequently results in standardization through identification and promotion of value-driven pathways. In particular, Intermountain Health System in Utah has used this approach since the 1980s with protocols that save millions of dollars each year.[9] Physician led multidisciplinary teams meet monthly to identify areas of improvement. Clinical practice guidelines are developed to influence care in these areas and undergo a series of updates based on provider input. Some of Intermountain's guidelines undergo over a hundred updates within the first year. Guidelines around management of acute conditions, postoperative care, and utilization of post-acute care services can be instituted to decrease variation.

● IMPLEMENTING A SOLUTION

Experience from early ACOs demonstrates that single solutions do not result in significant savings or quality improvement. Thus, our approach is multifactorial: increase ACO awareness among surgeons, engage these clinicians in high value care, and decrease the leakage of referrals.

To start our evaluation, we survey our surgeons about their awareness of our ACO, their knowledge of how clinical care contributes to its performance, possible drivers to improve clinical practice, and resources that our ACO can provide in support. Concurrently, we gather data from our financial office about our ACO beneficiary surgical spending over the last 3 years in a 30 day window around the date of surgery. Following this evaluation, we invite surgeons to our multidisciplinary ACO transformation teams to allow them the opportunity to shape the future of the ACO. We also make a business case for ACO aligned care to departmental leadership, including a discussion of the department's quality and costs. We further work with leadership to conceptualize areas for improvement, financial and nonfinancial incentives that would drive behavior change, and to identify clinician concerns. These meetings may serve to identify ACO liaisons who communicate the ACO structure, values, and benefits of participation with their colleagues and relay apprehension from their colleagues back to ACO leadership.

Once our surgeons have more ACO awareness, we work to engage them in value-driven care. Each department is expected to contribute a representative to a multidisciplinary panel that is responsible for developing quality measures and evaluating reimbursement incentives. Given that our quality measures may differ from those mandated by CMS, our ACO's early investment in technological infrastructure is important to track these metrics. Using data from our financial office, physician-led multidisciplinary teams identify areas of high surgical cost and low quality with process variation and meet to devise and implement clinical guidelines. These guidelines may require multiple updates in the months after implementation based on feedback from clinical staff. The organization must support surgeons with resources (eg, additional clinical support staff and/or a list of high value preferred post-acute care facilities) to promote high value care without undue burden and increased fatigue/burnout. Surgical spending is monitored by the financial office and incentives distributed regularly. Surgeons are provided with actionable feedback through the liaison on how their quality and spending compares to individual, local, and national levels along with suggestions on how to improve their performance. Surgeon engagement and satisfaction with ACO participation is monitored with regular surveys and acted upon accordingly. The liaison also communicates concerns and opportunities for improvement back to the ACO leadership. High value surgeons are publicly promoted, both external and internal to the ACO, which allows them an opportunity to increase their productivity while improving value-driven care for ACO beneficiaries. The liaison directs interventions for low value surgeons. Finally, the liaison develops avenues of communication with major referring groups to identify barriers to referrals and discuss the high value care being delivered by the department.

Key Steps in Change Management and Potential Pitfalls

Key Steps in Change Management

1. Evaluate surgeon awareness of ACO goals, knowledge of how their clinical care contributes to its performance, and potential drivers of practice change through survey and focus groups.
2. Measure historical surgical spending over the last 3 years using a 30 day window after surgery.
3. Provide surgical department leaders with a business case for the benefits of ACO engagement; discuss departmental healthcare quality and costs, areas for improvement, financial, and nonfinancial incentives to drive behavior change, and concerns for ACO aligned care.
4. Identify surgeons to serve as liaisons. Liaisons introduce ACO-aligned care into their departments and meet with referring providers to identify problems that contribute to referral leakage.
5. Actively invite surgeons to join the existing ACO leadership team. Create a multidisciplinary panel to develop fair quality measures and evaluate incentives for reimbursement.
6. Using surgeon-led multidisciplinary teams, create clinical practice guidelines to reduce process variation and provide resources to assist with high value utilization.
7. Provide individual actionable feedback to surgeons on spending and quality. Publicly promote high value surgeons both internal and external to the ACO.
8. Monitor surgical spending, quality, surgeon engagement, and surgeon satisfaction with ACO participation. Liaison continues communication between surgical teams, department leadership, and referring providers.

Potential Pitfalls

1. Failure to understand surgeon knowledge about the ACO and his/her contribution to its success.
2. Failure to identify multifactorial influences on surgeon clinical practice.
3. Inability to overcome the incentives related to delivery of quantity of care.
4. Quality metrics fail to engage surgeons and are not adequately risk-adjusted. They may be viewed as unfair or require excessive administrative burden. Alternatively, they may be too easily achieved.
5. Increased physician burnout related to ACO participation.

Our efforts to engage surgeons will fail if we do not fully understand clinician awareness of the ACO and its values, if we fail to recognize the many influences on clinical decisions, or if we don't include surgeons as integral leaders of the organization. Furthermore, quality metrics must be carefully developed and risk-adjusted. Metrics or administrative ACO tasks perceived as unfair or burdensome will lose surgeon support and may contribute to clinician burnout. Alternatively, metrics that are too easily achieved may not encourage higher performance.

● MEASURING OUTCOMES

The ultimate measure of our program's success is a reduction in the total cost of surgical care and improved quality. However, we can track our progress with process measures such as survey data on surgeon engagement and satisfaction in ACO participation, implementation of surgical quality improvement initiatives, and number of surgeons in ACO leadership roles. Over time, we should see departments reaching higher quality metrics. We must be wary of unintended consequences of implementation. Surgeons who are unhappy with their ACO participation may suffer additional burnout and/or leave the health system. We may not see immediate return on investment as quality improvement is not always successful and may require several rounds of revision to create an effective intervention.

● FOLLOW-UP AND MAINTENANCE

Surgeon engagement requires a continuous cycle of communication, improvement, and feedback. The liaison should set regular meetings with their department to continue to engage surgeons, review performance, improvement projects, and clinician concerns about the ACO. They should also communicate with referring physicians about potential barriers to referrals and/or solutions to overcome those barriers. Quality metrics should be a moving target and receive feedback from the multidisciplinary committee. Once they are achieved, raising the bar can promote innovation within the organization. Incentives that do not result in ACO savings and/or those that have unintended consequences should be discontinued.

REFERENCES

1. Zhu M, Saunders RS, Muhlestein D, et al. The Medicare Shared Savings Program in 2020: positive movement (and uncertainty) during a pandemic. *Health Affairs Blog* 2021. Accessed 2 May 2022. https://www.healthaffairs.org/do/10.1377/forefront. 20211008.785640/
2. Kaye DR, Luckenbaugh AN, Oerline M, et al. Understanding the costs associated with surgical care delivery in the medicare population. *Ann Surg.* 2020;271(1):23–28.
3. Centers for Medicare and Medicaid Services. Provider engagement toolkit. 2020. Accessed 7 April 2022. https://innovation.cms.gov/media/document/2020-provider-engagement-toolkit
4. Dupree JM, Patel K, Singer SJ, et al. Attention to surgeons and surgical care is largely missing from early medicare accountable care Organizations. *Health Aff (Millwood)*. 2014;33(6):972–979.
5. Markovitz AA, Ryan AM, Peterson TA, et al. ACO Awareness and perceptions among specialists versus primary care physicians: a survey of a large medicare shared savings program. *J Gen Intern Med.* 2022;37(2):492–494.
6. Markovitz AA, Rozier MD, Ryan AM, et al. Low-value care and clinician engagement in a large medicare shared savings program ACO: a survey of frontline clinicians. *J Gen Intern Med.* 2020;35(1):133–141.
7. Berenson RA, Kaye DR. Grading a physician's value: the misapplication of performance measurement. *N Engl J Med.* 2013;369(22):2079–2081.
8. Maruthappu M, Trehan A, Barnett-Vanes A, et al. The impact of feedback of surgical outcome data on surgical performance: a systematic review. *World J Surg.* 2015 39(4): 879–889.
9. James BC, Savitz LA. How intermountain trimmed health care costs through robust quality improvement efforts. *Health Aff (Millwood)* 2011;30(6):1185–1191.

Out-of-Network Billing: The Surgical Leader's Perspective

39

KARAN R. CHHABRA, MIHIR S. DEKHNE, AND SUNIL EAPPEN

Clinical Delivery Challenge

A surprise medical bill is a charge from an out-of-network clinician that was not foreseen by the patient at the time of service and is not covered by the patient's insurance plan. These bills occur when patients choose physicians and hospitals that participate in their insurance network but receive additional bills from physicians who participated in the patient's care, but do not participate in their insurance network. In elective surgery, patients can usually choose in-network surgeons and facilities, but many other providers' involvement is beyond their control (eg, anesthesiologists, surgical assistants, pathologists, etc).[1] In emergency surgery, patients cannot choose the surgeon and an out-of-network surgical bill is still possible. These situations are more common when physicians are not employed by the hospital or don't belong to a closely aligned physicians' organization.

Out-of-network physicians typically charge a "usual and customary" rate which can be many times higher than what an insurance plan would pay them if in-network. Insurance plans are not legally obligated to pay these rates in full. If the insurance plan pays less than what the out-of-network provider charges, the out-of-network provider may send the patient a "balance bill" for the difference. These bills can amount to thousands of dollars, without the usual limits on out-of-pocket obligations. By going out-of-network with the major payers in the region, Anesthesia Associates of Ann Arbor (A4) would be able to send out-of-network bills to patients undergoing procedures at Trinity Health. This could harm the reputation of Trinity Health, drive patients and surgeons elsewhere, and attract negative attention from insurers and regulators.

A4, the exclusive provider for 6 Trinity Health System hospitals in Michigan, terminated contracts with multiple payers due to rate disputes, Trinity was left with a shortage of in-network anesthesia providers. Leadership at Trinity Health feared that A4s actions would drive patients to other hospitals to seek surgical care, leading to either millions of dollars of lost revenue and/or leaving patients with unexpected and exorbitant out-of-pocket costs. Trinity sued A4 claiming violation of state and federal antitrust laws and attempted to directly employ A4s anesthesiologists. A4 countersued alleging Trinity ignored its exclusive contract obligations and noncompete agreements. Meanwhile, payers were unable to reach an agreement regarding reimbursement rates for A4.[2]

Surgical leaders are likely to encounter situations in which physicians do not participate in all patients' insurance plans. Although health system leadership may not have a direct role in negotiations between these specialists and the insurance plans, as this scenario illustrates, these discussions can directly affect high-margin service lines for the health system. Failed rate negotiations are a setup for "surprise" out of network bills, a healthcare delivery challenge that surgical leaders must understand (Table 39.1).

Table 39.1 Specialties Involved With Out-of-Network Billing in Surgical Episodes

	% of Out of Network Bills Involving Specialty	Mean Potential Balance Bill From Specialty, $ (95% CI)
Surgical assistant	37	3,633 (3,384–3,883)
Anesthesiologist	37	1,219 (1,049–1,388)
Pathologist	22	284 (257–311)
Radiologist	7	321 (103–539)
Medical consultants	3	708 (599–816)
Other	13	754 (673–835)

Adapted with permission from Chhabra et al.[1] Copyright © 2020 American Medical Association. All rights reserved.

● WORKUP

For a health system with key providers going out-of-network with the region's major payers, it is essential to understand those providers' reimbursement and compensation as well as the health system's ability to recruit new staff. Key terms and data points are as follows:

- **Charges:** The "usual and customary" rate requested by the provider. Insurance plans are typically not required to pay these charges in full if the provider is out-of-network. In anesthesia, physician charges average 5.8 times Medicare's payment.[3]
- **Out-of-Network Allowed Amounts:** The actual amount paid to the out-of-network provider by the insurance plan. Insurance plans sometimes have a specific amount that is allowed for out-of-network payment, and this may be higher than their in-network allowed amount. On the other hand, insurance plans without out-of-network coverage (eg, HMOs or EPOs) may have zero coverage when patients leave their network for care, leaving the patient responsible for the entire charged amount.
- **Balance Bill:** The out-of-network charges less the out-of-network allowed amount represents the highest possible balance bill. Not all providers send patients balance bills, and even if they do, it may not be for this entire amount. The actual amount of the balance bill is often known only to the patient, thus in research using claims data they are often referred to as "potential" balance bills or "potential" surprise bills. One study of out-of-network bills at in-network ambulatory surgery centers found that the insurance plan paid full out-of-network charges in 24% of cases, meaning that patients could be vulnerable to a balance bill in the remaining 76% of cases.[4]
- **Mean In-Network RVU Conversion Factor:** For providers in a specific specialty at a specific health system, the average factor by which RVUs are multiplied to arrive at the in-network allowed amount.
- **Regional Benchmark RVU Conversion Factor:** The regional average of the conversion factor above, across competing health systems and surgical centers (holding constant the provider specialty, eg, anesthesia).
- **Total Provider Collections:** The total clinical revenue of the providers in question, ideally while they were in-network with major insurance plans.
- **Total Provider Wages:** The gross pay of the providers in question (will differ from total collections due to overheads, profit margin, and shareholder distributions, stipends, profit sharing, etc).

● DIFFERENTIAL DIAGNOSIS

Going out-of-network can be a legitimate way to contest below-market reimbursement rates, but sometimes it is a profit-maximizing tactic used to extract above-market reimbursements from patients and insurance plans. The key questions in this scenario are *(1) whether the providers going out-of-network intend to balance bill patients, (2) whether the providers have a reasonable complaint about their rates relative to the market, and (3) whether the health system ought to develop an alternative contracting model for these specialty services.*

● DIAGNOSIS AND TREATMENT

With the above definitions and questions in mind, the health system can determine whether the providers in question intend to charge more than the expected allowed amount, and whether they intend to send balance bills if they are paid less than they charge. These will determine whether their out-of-network status has a financial impact on patients. The institutional and regional RVU conversion factors will help determine whether the providers in question are currently being paid below-market rates, or if their in-network compensation is in fact a fair reflection of current market conditions. The difference between provider collections and wages will also help determine how much of the providers' clinical revenue is going toward their wages versus to the practice or a holding company.

Arising from widespread discontent with surprise billing, *the No Surprises Act* (passed December 27, 2020) placed tight restrictions on out-of-network billing at hospitals and surgical centers across the United States. Effective January 1, 2022, patients receiving out-of-network services at in-network facilities may be billed only the amount they would have owed an in-network provider—taking patients "out of the middle" of billing disputes. If out-of-network providers and insurers disagree on a fair payment rate, they have 30 days to negotiate on payment before invoking a *binding arbitration* process that will determine the ultimate payment rate. In this process, both parties will submit "final offers" for a fair payment, and a neutral arbitrator will choose from the two, incorporating the regional median in-network payment rate, prior contracted rates between the 2 parties, and specific information about the patient's illness and provider's expertise. Prior experience with surprise billing laws in New York and New Jersey suggests that clinicians may win the majority of payment disputes, but that arbitrators are heavily influenced by the benchmark payment (ie, the median in-network payment) provided in the decision-making process.[5] This legislation will free patients from balance bills, potentially averting the reputational harm to hospitals and health systems discussed earlier. However, it has become legally contentious, prompting multiple federal lawsuits challenging the centrality of the median in-network payment as its payment benchmark. (In fact, one of these lawsuits was brought by an acute care surgery group whose billing is 78% out-of-network.[6]) Thus there is a possibility that this payment benchmark—or the surprise billing prohibition altogether—may be invalidated by the courts in the coming years. Even if the No Surprises Act remains unchanged, out-of-network billing remains possible; the law creates a process for handling these without burdening patients but does not eliminate out-of-network bills altogether.

● SCIENTIFIC PRINCIPLES AND EVIDENCE

Surprise billing relies on a practice model in which the healthcare provider is not directly chosen by the patient. For elective surgeons, primary care providers, and even hospitals, being out-of-network with common insurance plans means that these providers will see fewer patients—patients will generally seek out and choose in-network providers when possible due to their financial incentive to do so. These physicians often decide that it is worth accepting a lower payment from insurance providers (the in-network price) in exchange for the higher volume that they will receive by being in-network. On the other hand, emergency surgeons, surgical assistants, and hospital-based specialists (anesthesiology, emergency medicine, radiology, pathology) do not face this tradeoff when they are not chosen by the patient. Since patients are generally unable to anticipate when their anesthesiologist or radiologist is out-of-network, these hospital-based specialists do not face the same price-volume tradeoff as other providers. This may have led over time to reimbursements that are significantly higher (relative to Medicare prices) than reimbursements for other specialties. For instance, commercial payments for anesthesiologists exceed 360% of Medicare, whereas orthopedic surgeons performing knee replacements are typically paid 164% of the Medicare price.[7]

Among patients undergoing elective surgery, surgical assistants and anesthesiologists are the providers most frequently responsible for out-of-network charges, according to a recent paper.[1] One in five patients undergoing elective surgery with an in-network surgeon and facility received an out-of-network bill, and out-of-network anesthesiologists and surgical assistants were each responsible for 37% of those out-of-network bills. Out-of-network surgical assistant charges were on average $3,633 higher than the typical in-network payment, thus the typical patient could be balance billed up to this amount. Out-of-network anesthesiology charges were, on average, $1,219 more than the typical in-network payment.[1] Out of network pathologists, radiologists, and other medical consultants contributed smaller shares of out-of-network bills, in that order.

● IMPLEMENTING A SOLUTION

Going out-of-network is often one in a series of steps for providers in negotiating payment rates with an insurance plan. It is useful to know whether the provider group intends to balance bill patients (though this may not be transparent), because this will determine whether patients could suffer financial harm and/or whether the health system could suffer reputational harm. As mentioned earlier, some provider practices may have legitimate concerns that they are being paid less than a fair market rate, whereas others may simply be trying to extract more out of an already generous payment rate; benchmarking their reimbursement rates helps disentangle these possibilities. In the former scenario, binding arbitration processes (explained above) offer a formal mechanism for these grievances to be discussed before an impartial arbitrator. In the latter scenario of unnecessarily aggressive negotiation, the health system would be wise to pursue alternative provider contracts.

Finally, if providers are collecting significantly more than they were being paid in network, this may suggest that either that the specific specialty provider is being underpaid or that the provider is utilizing out-of-network rates in order to siphon away a larger share of collections. Understanding current regional benchmarks will help sort out this issue. Regardless, the health system should consider bringing these services in-house or contract with a different provider group. If the practice's collections are close to paid wages, but the service enables additional high-margin revenue streams for the hospital (eg, anesthesiology), the health system should consider subsidizing wages for this specialty in order to entice them to remain in-network. Most hospitals already make substantial direct payments to their anesthesiology groups to supplement their third-party reimbursements in order to keep anesthesiologists in their workforce, due to their relative undersupply.[8]

Key Steps in Change Management and Potential Pitfalls

Key Steps in Change Management

1. Obtain data on in-network and out-of-network payments, out-of-network billing practices, and institutional as well as regional RVU conversion factors and compensation benchmarks.
2. Analyze finances and goals of the practice going out-of-network.
3. Understand the process and steps leading up to the patient getting their procedure.
4. If practice currently being paid below-market rates while in-network, propose binding arbitration as a method to approach fair market payment. If practice being paid above-market and trying to raise rates further, consider that they may be exploiting the process, and explore alternate provider contracts.
5. If practice underpays clinicians (relative to their billing), consider employing this specialty in-house and retaining their margin.
6. If specialty is underpaid (relative to value to health system), consider adding or increasing subsidy.
7. Monitor out-of-network billing practices before and after any intervention.

Potential Pitfalls

1. Assuming exploitative negotiation tactics when providers' compensation is below market.
2. Violating noncompete agreements when employing physicians.
3. Contracting with provider groups that have a record of predatory billing or contracting.

● MEASURING OUTCOMES

The key outcome for patients, in this case, is, *of all encounters in which the patient is in-network with the health system, what percent of encounters contain out-of-network charges from other providers.* Other outcomes of interest to patients include: the sources of these out-of-network charges, the size of these out-of-network charges, and the amount of balance bills and/or financial complaints made by patients. For physician groups, the key outcomes are the RVU conversion factor when in- and out-of-network with each major payer. For health systems, the key outcomes are the cost of adequate provider contracts for the specialties in question.

● FOLLOW-UP AND MAINTENANCE

A onetime solution to rate disputes does not guarantee a future free of similar problems. Some physician groups, especially those backed by several large private equity firms, use out-of-network billing systematically and routinely to push reimbursements above market rates.[9] Thus if the provider group has a pattern of similar behavior at other times and in other locations, the health system should strongly consider contracting with other providers of the same services. A more durable solution may be to employ the specialists in-house, though this is sometimes not economically sustainable without a substantial subsidy.

In the example scenario discussed here, Trinity Health asserted that A4s out-of-network status violated their contract with the health system. Trinity Health attempted to recruit and directly employ A4s anesthesiologists; however, this violated the anesthesiologists' noncompete agreements and led to a temporary restraining order prohibiting Trinity Health from further contacting A4s anesthesia providers.[10] Ultimately, both parties reached a compromise in which anesthesiologists at certain locations were released from their noncompete agreements, and another group practice was engaged to take over anesthesia services at other system hospitals.[11] Antitrust litigation between A4 and Blue Cross Blue Shield of Michigan is ongoing.

REFERENCES

1. Chhabra KR, Sheetz KH, Nuliyalu U, et al. Out-of-network bills for privately insured patients undergoing elective surgery with in-network primary surgeons and facilities. *JAMA.* 2020;323(6):538–547. doi: 10.1001/jama.2019.21463
2. Kacik, A. Trinity health sues anesthesiology group amid insurer rate disputes. Modern Healthcare. Published July 24, 2019. Accessed March 18, 2020. https://www.modernhealthcare.com/law-regulation/trinity-health-sues-anesthesiology-group-amid-insurer-rate-disputes
3. Bai G, Anderson GF. Variation in the ratio of physician charges to medicare payments by specialty and region. *JAMA.* 2017;317(3):315–318. doi: 10.1001/jama.2016.16230
4. Duffy EL, Adler L, Ginsburg PB, Trish E. Prevalence and characteristics of surprise out-of-network bills from professionals in ambulatory surgery centers. *Health Aff (Millwood).* Published online April 15, 2020:10.1377/hlthaff.2019.01138. doi: 10.1377/hlthaff.2019.01138
5. Chhabra KR, Fuse Brown E, Ryan AM. No more surprises: new legislation on out-of-network billing. *N Engl J Med.* Published online March 17, 2021. doi: 10.1056/NEJMp2035905
6. Herman B. The doctor who is trying to bring back surprise billing. *STAT.* https://www.statnews.com/2022/04/27/the-doctor-who-is-trying-to-bring-back-balance-billing/. Published April 27, 2022. Accessed May 16, 2022.
7. Cooper Z, Nguyen H, Shekita N, Morton FS. Out-of-network billing and negotiated payments for hospital-based physicians. *Health Aff (Millwood).* 2019; Epublished ahead of print.
8. Kheterpal S, Tremper KK, Shanks A, Morris M. Workforce and finances of the United States anesthesiology training programs: 2009–2010. *Anesth Analg.* 2011;112(6):1480–1486. doi: 10.1213/ANE.0b013e3182135a3a
9. Cooper Z, Morton FS, Shekita N. Surprise! Out-of-network billing for emergency care in the United States. *Natl Bur Econ Res Work Pap Ser.* 2019; No. 23623. doi: 10.3386/w23623
10. Anesthesia Group Relationship with Trinity Health Devolves into a Flurry of Lawsuits. Enhance Healthcare Consulting. Published August 27, 2019. Accessed May 16, 2022. https://enhancehc.com/anesthesia-group-lawsuit-with-trinity-health/
11. Greene J. Trinity Health, Anesthesia Associates Reach Settlement on Lawsuits, Non-competes. Modern Healthcare. Published September 5, 2019. Accessed May 16, 2022. https://www.modernhealthcare.com/legal/trinity-health-anesthesia-associates-reach-settlement-lawsuits-non-competes

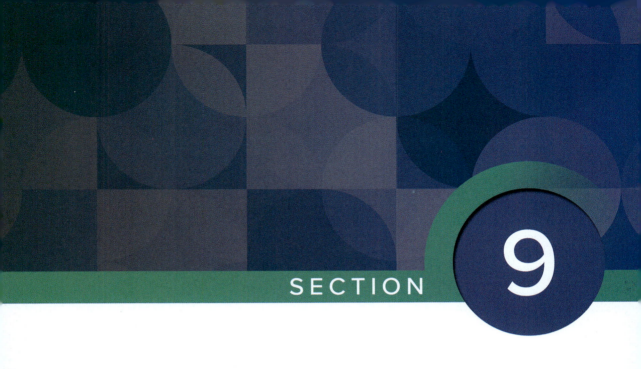

SECTION 9

Improving Value of Care

40 **Overuse of Preoperative Testing in Low-Risk Patients**
Nicholas L. Berlin and Erika D. Sears

41 **Incorporating New Technology That Is Not Reimbursed**
Abhishek Satishchandran and Allison R. Schulman

42 **Consolidating OR Supply Chain to a Single Vendor**
Mariam Maksutova, Janet Abbruzzese, and Chandu Vemuri

43 **When Healthcare Systems Become Their Own Insurer**
Sean Michael O'Neill and Steven R. Crain

SECTION 6

Improving Value of Care

40. Overuse of Preoperative Testing in Low-Risk Patients
    Nicholas L. Berlin and Erika L. Sears

41. Incorporating New Technology That is Not Reimbursed
    Achilleas Saharidan and Alison B. Schulman

42. Consolidating OR Supply Chain to a Single Vendor
    Marina Mikhuriva, Janet Andrews, and Christa Martin

43. When Healthcare Systems Become Their Own Insurer
    Sean Michael Chaki and Steven R. Crain

Overuse of Preoperative Testing in Low-Risk Patients

40

NICHOLAS L. BERLIN AND ERIKA D. SEARS

Clinical Delivery Challenge

Recognizing an opportunity to improve care and reduce waste in the healthcare system, the Choosing Wisely® campaign initiated an international movement to reduce low-value care over the past decade.[1,2] Through this campaign, professional medical societies have submitted more than 600 recommendations to avoid tests and treatments that provide limited or no benefit to patients, as determined by clinical trials or expert opinion. One of the most common clinical settings targeted by Choosing Wisely is the preoperative setting, with an emphasis on eliminating routine preoperative testing (eg, baseline diagnostic cardiac testing, laboratory studies, chest radiography) in patients undergoing low-risk surgery.

Eliminating routine preoperative testing for these patients is a focus of this campaign, because testing does not prevent adverse events and can lead to dangerous care cascades involving risky interventional diagnostic studies (eg, heart catherization) with unclear benefit for patients. In a study of Medicare beneficiaries undergoing cardiac testing prior to cataract surgery, those tested incurred an additional $1,707 in expenditures during a 90-day period and 25% underwent at least 4 additional "cascade events" (eg, follow-up tests, treatments, visits, hospitalizations, and new diagnoses).[3] Reducing unnecessary preoperative testing also presents an opportunity to improve access to surgical care. Testing often requires additional travel, missed days of work, and unnecessary out-of-pocket expenses that can be burdensome to patients. Furthermore, testing may lead to delays in access to timely surgical care for marginalized groups and those with less financial and employment flexibility.

Eliminating this low-value care has proven to be more elusive than originally anticipated.[4,5] In a study of Medicare beneficiaries undergoing non-cardiac procedures, 45% of patients underwent unnecessary preoperative cardiac testing.[4] Similarly, approximately 47% of patients undergoing carpal tunnel release procedures in the Veteran's Affairs system underwent at least one low-value preoperative test.[6] These data confirm that guidelines alone are unlikely to change practice patterns within the United States' healthcare system. Instead, abandonment of unproven and entrenched medical practices is a complex and poorly understood process involving knowledge acquisition, behavior change, and coordination of key stakeholder groups.[7]

Imagine that a hospital is interested in decreasing overuse of preoperative testing for low-risk patients undergoing surgery. This initiative is part of a larger effort to improve delivery of efficient, high-value surgical, and perioperative care. Institutional leaders are asked to oversee the design and implementation of an operational strategy to reduce testing for these patients.

● WORKUP

In our hypothetical scenario, prior to designing an operational strategy to reduce preoperative testing for low-risk surgery patients, the healthcare leader must first gain a better understanding of the current prevalence and patterns of testing within the hospital. The leader should assemble a list of high-volume, low-risk surgical procedures and a list of common preoperative tests (see Tables 40.1 and 40.2 for suggestions). Using patient-level data, the proportion of patients who receive at least one preoperative test during a specified time interval (eg, year, quarter, month) should be calculated for each surgical procedure. It is

SECTION 9 • Improving Value of Care

Table 40.1 Example List of Low-Risk Surgical Procedures

Surgical Specialty	Procedure	CPT Code
Ophthalmology	Cataract surgery	66982
	Lid ptosis repair	67904
General Surgery	Lumpectomy	19301
	Laparoscopic cholecystectomy	47562
	Laparoscopic appendectomy	44970
	Laparoscopy inguinal hernia repair	49650
Plastic Surgery	Breast reduction	19318
Otolaryngology	Septoplasty	30520
	Tonsillectomy	42826
Vascular Surgery	Endovenous ablation of vein	36475
Hand Surgery	Carpal tunnel release	64721
	Trigger finger release	26055
Dermatology	Mohs surgery of the head, neck, hands, feet, genitalia	17311
	Mohs surgery of the trunk, arms, or legs	17313

CPT, Current Procedural Terminology.

also helpful to calculate the proportion of patients receiving each type of test for all procedures together and individually. Department- or provider-specific data may be helpful (if available) to determine the need for intervention at the individual-level, systems-level, or both. In addition to understanding the scope and severity of this low-value care, this approach will also highlight procedures where testing is routinely performed and others where it is not.

Table 40.2 List of Preoperative Testing CPT Billing Codes

Description	CPT Code
Electrocardiography	93000, 93005, 93010, 93040, 93041, 93042
Trans-thoracic echocardiography	93303, 93304, 93306, 93307, 93308, 93320, 93321, 93325
Cardiac stress tests	78451, 78452, 93015-18, 93350-52
Chest X-ray	71010, 71020-22, 71030, 71034, 71035
Urinalysis	81000-3, 81005, 81007, 81015, 81020, 81099
Complete blood count	85025, 85027
Basic metabolic panel	80047, 80048
Coagulation tests	85345, 85347, 85348
Pulmonary function tests	82803, 94010, 94016, 94060, 94070, 94200, 94375, 94620, 94621, 94664, 94726, 94727, 94729, 94760, 94761, 95070, 95071

CPT, Current Procedural Terminology.

Next, the healthcare leader should identify and engage key stakeholders who are involved in the decision-making process for preoperative testing. This includes surgeons, anesthesiologists, mid-level providers, preoperative clinic leadership and staff, primary care physicians, clinic nurses, preoperative nurses, and patients. From an administrative standpoint, the quality department may also be a key stakeholder and source of financial and non-financial support for this initiative. Payers are another stakeholder because they provide financial compensation for overused preoperative tests and may be a partner in this effort. Gaining the trust and support of stakeholders is critical to understanding the modifiable drivers of testing, as well as the potential barriers and facilitators to implementation of an operational strategy that changes practice patterns.

● DIFFERENTIAL DIAGNOSIS

Given the multitude of stakeholders in perioperative care, the drivers of preoperative testing may be complex and multi-dimensional. There are provider, procedure, patient, guideline, organizational and practice environment, and health system-level factors that may play a role in driving overuse of testing. For example, a lack of communication or accountability for testing between provider groups, a limited understanding of current evidence, a lack of a risk stratification protocol for testing, outdated automated EMR-based prompts and algorithms, surgeon or anesthesiologist preferences, a lack of standardization, or a general perception that overuse of testing is not an important problem may be driving the testing patterns within the hospital. Many of these factors suggest a need for systems-level processes that engage all stakeholders to reduce routine testing for these patients.

● DIAGNOSIS AND TREATMENT

Through a combination of quantitative and qualitative approaches, the leader will gain a deeper understanding of preoperative testing for low-risk patients within the hospital and modifiable drivers of these practices. Depending on how siloed different surgical subspecialties are at the hospital, it may be helpful to conduct subspecialty-specific interviews (eg, focusing on high-volume low-risk ophthalmology or hand procedures). The interviews should be conducted using a semi-structured approach based in conceptual models from implementation science (eg, Theoretical Domains Framework, Consolidated Framework for Implementation Research), or the iterative quality improvement processes within the hospital (eg, lean thinking). An investigation should also be performed into whether there are protocols, electronic medical record (EMR)-based decision tools, or institutional bylaws that guide preoperative testing for surgery. Ideally, there will be systems-wide patient-centered solutions that leverage stakeholder input and evidence-based guidelines. This may be embedded within the EMR or standardized into a preoperative clinic.

In our hypothetical scenario, the healthcare leader identifies several procedures for which patients undergo high rates of preoperative cardiac testing (eg, electrocardiography (EKG)) and lab studies (eg, complete blood count and basic metabolic panel). For cataract surgery, which is a high-volume, low-risk, ambulatory surgical procedure, the healthcare leader discovers that approximately 90% of older adults undergo preoperative EKG at their hospital. For patients undergoing lumpectomy, nearly 50% of patients undergo laboratory studies and there appears to be wide variation in practice patterns depending on surgeon preferences. Qualitative interviews with mid-level providers in clinic identify an internal protocol for cataract surgery that encourages ordering preoperative EKGs, but this does not reflect evidence-based guidelines. Furthermore, interviews with surgeons, anesthesiologists, and other providers indicates that there is no centralized process to guide preoperative testing that considers both patient and procedural risk, which has led to variable testing rates based upon the presumed preferences of the surgeon and anesthesia teams for patients undergoing lumpectomy.

● SCIENTIFIC PRINCIPLES AND EVIDENCE

Unnecessary tests and treatments represent 2 major sources of excess spending and preventable harm to patients in the United States.[1] Overtreatment and low-value care are estimated to contribute at least 100 billion dollars of wasteful healthcare spending in the United States annually.[1] Numerous societies including the American Society of Anesthesiologists, the Society of General Internal Medicine, the American College of Surgeons, and the American Society for Clinical Pathology have targeted routine preoperative testing (eg, complete blood counts or coagulation studies, EKGs, cardiac stress tests, or chest radiographs) for patients undergoing low-risk surgery (eg, cataract surgery, breast surgery, ambulatory procedures). However, eliminating unnecessary, low-value preoperative testing has proven to be more elusive than originally anticipated.

Although frameworks for the implementation of evidence-based practices into clinical settings are well described, there is a growing recognition that "deimplementation" of non-evidence-based practices may require different considerations. Experts in implementation science suggest that a multi-level understanding of the de-implementation of low-value care (eg, system, hospital, provider, patient) is needed.[7-9] With regard to preoperative testing for low-risk surgery patients, there are ongoing trials leveraging the Theoretical Domains Framework to understand the drivers of this practice in healthcare settings. However, the literature has only recently moved beyond describing patterns and potential drivers of preoperative testing from claims data to qualitative or mixed-methods investigations and systems-level interventions.

With the literature of strategies to reduce this form of testing still in its nascency, the healthcare leader in our hypothetical scenario should design an operational strategy to reduce testing based upon conceptual models from implementation science or the iterative quality improvement processes within the hospital. These frameworks describe multi-level drivers of this practice which consider patient, provider, and system-level factors.

● IMPLEMENTING A SOLUTION

To identify potential solutions to eliminate routine low-value testing, healthcare leaders should have a solid understanding of who orders and why they are ordering tests, who follows up on the test results, whether patients are involved in this decision-making process and if the decision-making process is guided by institutional protocols, EMR-based decision tools, or institutional bylaws. Potential solutions may include provider education, implementation of evidence-based protocols, or decision support tools embedded within the EMR. Implementing a solution will require stakeholder buy-in and assurance that patients who need testing may be able to undergo these services prior to their procedure. Surgeons will likely be motivated to reduce preoperative testing if it can be shown to reduce the time to surgery. Therefore, a data management plan to monitor for improved efficiencies in access will be helpful for selected surgical procedures. Futhermore, the data management plan should also include monitoring for negative consequences related to policy changes which can be helpful for stakeholder buy-in, including whether the change is associated with more frequent same-day cancellations, unplanned readmissions, or perioperative complications. Potential pitfalls during the implementation phase include limited engagement with stakeholders and a lack of institutional support for this inititiative, a poorly designed plan for data management and monitoring, limited alignment with the results of the quantitative and qualitative investigations, and a lack of consideration for financial and non-financial incentives to motivate behavior change. Key steps in change management and potential pitfalls for the de-implementation of low-value preoperative testing are shown below.

It may also be possible to collaborate with payers to implement a policy-level solution that leverages financial incentives to reduce preoperative testing for low-risk surgery patients. In the state of Michigan, there is a voluntary statewide hospital collaborative called the Michigan Value Collaborative (MVC) that enables access to both private and federal insurance claims data for the vast majority of patients treated in the state.[10] This Blue Cross Blue Shield of Michigan-funded collaborative is currently developing and implementing a pay-for-performance measure related to preoperative testing that leverages risk-adjusted hospital-specific preoperative testing benchmarks and financial incentives. Hospitals that participate in MVC currently receive reports detailing hospital- and procedure-specific rates of preoperative testing for patients undergoing common low-risk surgeries, including peer benchmarking with similar hospitals across the state.

Key Steps in Change Management and Potential Pitfalls

Key Steps in Change Management

1. Data Access and Management	Establish clear plan for data access and analysis during the planning stages and throughout implementation of an operational strategy.
2. Stakeholder Engagement	Identify and engage all relevant stakeholders and include them in work-up, design, and implementation of the operational strategy.
3. Quantitative Investigation	Perform rigorous quantitative analysis to characterize scope and severity of low-value preoperative testing within the hospital.
4. Qualitative Investigation	Perform stakeholder inquiries using quality improvement methodologies to understand drivers of preoperative testing before low-risk surgery and to identify potential facilitators and barriers to implementation of an operational strategy.
5. Operational Strategy	Design an operational strategy that is comprehensive, reflecting the findings of quantitative and qualitative investigations, with engagement from stakeholders, including clinical and administrative leadership.
6. Outcome Measurement	Measure key outcomes related to preoperative testing (ie, rate of testing) and unintended consequences (eg, perioperative complications and same day cancellations).

Potential Pitfalls

1. Inadequate Work-up	A superficial understanding of drivers of low-value testing will lead to ineffective solutions.
2. Operational Barriers	Without an appreciation for the administrative and clinical barriers to implementation of the strategy, the likelihood of success is limited.
3. Lack of Buy-in	A lack of support from administrative and clinical stakeholders will limit hospital resources allocated to the effort and the overall effectiveness of the strategy.
4. Data Mismanagement	Inadequate data and analytic support will limit the ability to make strategic changes in real time and monitor progress.
5. No Incentives for Stakeholders	Without financial and non-financial incentives, stakeholders may not be motivated to participate or may prioritize other projects ahead of this one.

● MEASURING OUTCOMES

The most important metric to assess effectiveness of the operational strategy is rates of preoperative testing before specific procedures, within a specialty, and among all patients undergoing low-risk surgery at the hospital. The rates of testing can be compared before and after the intervention using interrupted time series analysis and should be adjusted for patient comorbidities. Furthermore, the healthcare leader may find it helpful to measure time to surgery from the initial surgical consultation date to understand whether reducing preoperative testing improves access to surgical care and the efficiency of surgical care delivery at the hospital. The healthcare leader should also plan to monitor for unintended consequences from interventions to reduce preoperative testing, including more frequent same-day cancellations, unplanned readmissions, or perioperative complications. The results of these investigations should be carefully reviewed and discussed with a multidisciplinary team to assess the effectiveness and impact of interventions on a routine basis.

● FOLLOW-UP AND MAINTENANCE

The experience gained from designing and implementing an operational strategy to reduce preoperative testing for low-risk patients may have spillover effects on other procedures as well, especially if a systems-level approach is standardized within the electronic medical record or through the preoperative clinic. Hospitals and health systems may be incentivized by payment models in the near future to reduce low-value preoperative care as a means to improve financial margins. By continuing to leverage the experience and strategies from this initiative, leaders can drive improved efficiencies in perioperative care delivery more broadly and be more successful in value-based care models in the future.

REFERENCES

1. Shrank WH, Rogstad TL, Parekh N. Waste in the US health care system: estimated costs and potential for savings. *JAMA*. 2019;322(15):1501–1509.
2. Choosing Wisely: An initiative of the ABIM foundation: clinician lsts. 2019. https://www.choosingwisely.org/clinicianlists/
3. Ganguli I, Simpkin AL, Lupo C, et al. Cascades of care after incidental findings in a US National Survey of Physicians. *JAMA Netw Open*. 2019;2(10):e1913325.
4. Colla CH, Morden NE, Sequist TD, et al. Choosing wisely: prevalence and correlates of low-value health care services in the United States. *J Gen Intern Med*. 2015;30(2):221–228.
5. Berlin NL, Yost ML, Cheng B, et al. Patterns and determinants of low-value preoperative testing in Michigan. *JAMA Intern Med*. 2021;181(8):1115–1118.
6. Harris AHS, Meerwijk EL, Kamal RN, et al. Variability and costs of low-value preoperative testing for carpal tunnel release surgery. *Anesth Analg*. 2019;129(3):804–811.
7. Norton WE, Chambers DA. Unpacking the complexities of de-implementing inappropriate health interventions. *Implement Sci*. 2020;15(1):2.
8. Berlin NL, Skolarus TA, Kerr EA, et al. Too much surgery: overcoming barriers to deimplementation of low-value surgery. *Ann Surg*. 2020;271(6):1020–1022.
9. Grimshaw JM, Patey AM, Kirkham KR, et al. De-implementing wisely: developing the evidence base to reduce low-value care. *BMJ Qual Saf*. 2020;29(5):409–417.
10. Regenbogen SE, Cain-Nielsen AH, Syrjamaki JD, et al. Spending on postacute care after hospitalization in commercial insurance and medicare around age sixty-five. *Health Aff (Millwood)*. 2019;38(9):1505–1513.

Incorporating New Technology That Is Not Reimbursed

41

ABHISHEK SATISHCHANDRAN AND ALLISON R. SCHULMAN

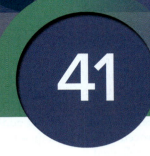

> ### Clinical Delivery Challenge
> Implementation of a new procedure or technology in the medical field faces a multitude of clinical delivery challenges. These challenges include, but are not limited to, infrastructure issues, training of physicians and staff, establishment of referral networks, and most importantly, reimbursement. While the endoscopic suturing device used in TORe has been cleared by the Food and Drug Administration (FDA) for soft tissue approximation, the narrow scope of approval, despite substantial data, has not led to the designation of a specific CPT code. As a result, insurance coverage varies drastically, requiring patients to pay out-of-pocket or health systems to incur a financial loss when these procedures are performed. The creation of large data registries is also hindered given the lack of consistent coding for these procedures.

Roux-en-Y Gastric Bypass (RYGB) has traditionally been the mainstay for surgical management of obesity with rapid weight loss and excellent metabolic outcomes. Weight regain, however, affects a significant portion of patients. The mechanism of weight regain is multifactorial and includes neurohormonal, behavioral, and anatomic factors. One significant culprit is dilation or enlargement of the gastro-jejunostomy (GJA), with the diameter correlating linearly with weight recidivism.[1] Surgical revision of the gastric bypass is technically challenging and carries a high rate of morbidity.[2] Endoscopic revision, a procedure known as transoral outlet reduction endoscopy (TORe), is an incisionless minimally invasive option with encouraging results. This procedure is performed using an endoscopic suturing device (OverStitch; Apollo Endosurgery, Austin, Tex, USA) to reduce the diameter of the GJA and reestablish restriction (Figure 41.1). Various suture patterns have been reported, with a purse-string approach demonstrating the most encouraging short- and long-term results.[3–6] At most centers, this procedure is performed on an outpatient basis, unlike surgical revision, which requires hospitalization.

Despite numerous studies demonstrating the safety and efficacy of this procedure, widespread adoption of TORe has been largely hampered by lack of a Current Procedural Terminology (CPT) code resulting in variable insurance coverage and restricting its availability to large medical centers and patients who can afford out-of-pocket costs. These challenges are pervasive in medical innovation. In this chapter, we will use TORe as an example of a new technology that is not reimbursed and highlight the challenges faced in medical innovation.

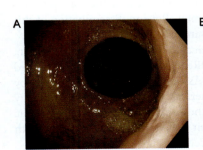
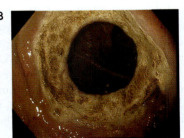
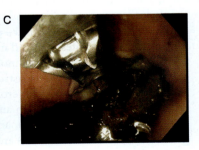

FIGURE 41.1 Dilated gastrojejunal anastomosis (**A**) followed by mucosal ablation (**B**) and endoscopic transoral outlet reduction (TORe) (**C**).

SECTION 9 • Improving Value of Care

● WORKUP

Surgical revision of gastric bypass anatomy has historically been the most effective treatment for weight recidivism. While the operative approach varies between institutions, all require a laparoscopic, robotic, or open technique which are more challenging and carry a burden of increased morbidity and mortality than the original surgery.[2] To understand where TORe fits into this existing treatment paradigm, metabolic outcomes, in addition to data on morbidity, mortality, adverse event rates, length of stay, procedure cost, and quality adjusted life years, for both surgical and endoscopic approaches, needs to be collected.

Currently, level 1 evidence for TORe exists based on the RESTORe trial, a sham-controlled trial including 77 patients who were randomized to TORe or demonstrating a 3.5 percent total weight loss (%TWL) versus 0.4% in the treatment vs. sham groups, respectively.[7] Follow-up studies have demonstrated long term efficacy and safety of this technique at 3 and 5 years.[5] While these results are encouraging, the creation of larger patient registries may aid in tracking patient outcomes, wider dissemination of the procedure, and more consistent insurance coverage. At present, no such centralized database exists. Gastrointestinal and surgical societal efforts to create such a database are underway. Furthermore, surgical programs participating in the Metabolic and Bariatric Surgery Accreditation and Quality Improvement Program (MBSAQIP) may also track endoscopic weight loss interventions.

There are several key stakeholders necessary for the adoption and integration of new medical technology into practice. It is imperative that these stakeholders believe that the innovation either increases efficiency or decreases cost than existing interventions. This need is specifically highlighted in the management of obesity and weight regain following bariatric surgery. Treatment of patients who have undergone RYGB complicated by weight regain requires the collaboration of multiple specialists including, but not limited to, primary care physicians, bariatric surgeons, gastroenterologists, endocrinologists, bariatricians, nutritionists, behavioral psychologists, and exercise therapists. While surgery has historically been the only procedural intervention for the management of weight regain, TORe is gaining popularity as a less-invasive, safer alternative. Awareness of this procedure and the overall safety compared to traditional operative interventions is important to all these key stakeholders. Recognition of appropriate patients for TORe and referrals for the procedure are essential for wide-spread adoption.

The patient should be at the center of this multidisciplinary collaboration and decision-making process. The benefit to the patient, in terms of long-term outcomes, morbidity, mortality, quality of life, and cost should be a primary indicator driving the intervention. Patients with weight recidivism following surgery may be reluctant to undergo, or may not be a candidate for, re-operative intervention and should be presented with all available options. However, a lack of awareness of endoscopic revision as an efficacious and safe option among patients in the algorithm of weight regain is a major barrier for the implementation into practice.

Academic medical institutions are often centers of high-volume bariatric care, research, and training for providers specializing in the care of obesity. As a result, academic medical centers are important liaisons for this multi-disciplinary partnership and all the aforementioned stakeholders. These institutions are commonly leaders in researching and publishing scientific knowledge, thereby allowing dissemination of this knowledge at scientific meetings – a key step in wider adoption and awareness.

Surgical, gastrointestinal, and medical obesity societies are also critical to the dissemination, adoption, and coverage of new medical technology in obesity management. For TORe, these include, but are not limited to, the American Society for Gastrointestinal Endoscopy (ASGE), the Association of Bariatric Endoscopy (ABE), the American Gastroenterological Association (AGA), the American College of Gastroenterology (ACG), the Society of American and Endoscopic Surgeons (SAGES), the American Society for Metabolic and Bariatric Surgery (ASMBS), and The Obesity Society (TOS). Their collaboration and lobbying with government agencies and payers are essential to the success of this procedure.

Until insurance coverage is more consistent, TORe may be cost-prohibitive for patients and bariatric centers, limiting growth and case volume. Support from public and private institutions will be necessary in the interim to promote early adoption, train providers, and perform research. Finally, medical device companies are also major stakeholders in this process, and partnership will be essential throughout this journey.

● DIFFERENTIAL DIAGNOSIS

There are many unique challenges to the adoption of a new technology or technique that is not reimbursed in medical practice. First, training of proceduralists and demonstration of competency will be imperative for successful integration into a multidisciplinary program. Second, awareness of this intervention and the establishment of a referral base will be essential for adequate case volumes. Third, infrastructure is required to efficiently collect data to track operational and quality metrics required for early evaluation of the program. Eventually, these metrics can be shared between institutions for larger collaborations. Fourth, a lack of consistent insurance coverage leads to high costs at the level of the patient and institution. Procedures like TORe lack CPT codes and are deemed experimental which can limit availability to those patients able to pay out of pocket or institutions willing to incur a financial loss.

● DIAGNOSIS AND TREATMENT

In order to integrate new technology that is not reimbursed into clinical practice, data is the highest leverage requirement, as it is ultimately outcome metrics and cost that will be required for key stakeholders. Data also drives the development of consensus guidelines and standards of practice, which will collectively allow for widespread dissemination of accepted techniques and serve as the foundation for introducing new medical technology into practice. Value analysis committees would also look favorably on new technologies if a clear improvement in patient safety could be confirmed.

Significant barriers exist to the development of large data registries. First, there is currently no existing CPT code for the TORe procedure. As a result, medical centers are forced to use unlisted codes with variable reimbursement or surgical codes which may be considered fraud in certain states. The lack of a single accepted CPT code has led to institutional variation in documentation, thereby increasing the complexity of data gathering at the national and international levels. Without a single procedure-specific CPT code, it will be challenging to evaluate the medical, societal, and financial benefits of TORe at a population-wide level.

The development of societies such as the ABE, a subsidiary of the ASGE, has cultivated a collaboration between bariatric endoscopists, surgeons, medical institutions, and device companies. This collaboration has not only improved educational opportunities and training but has also served as the catalyst for the development of data registries, consensus guidelines and standards of practice, all of which will ultimately help in obtaining consistent insurance coverage.

● SCIENTIFIC PRINCIPLES AND EVIDENCE

A paucity of data exists as a framework for the implementation of new endoscopic techniques like TORe that are not reimbursed in medical practice. In many ways, these challenges parallel the early days of the laparoscopic surgical revolution, where procedures needed to be evaluated for safety and efficacy and also valued at a time when insurance coverage and coding were inconsistent. Similar to laparoscopic surgery versus open procedures, the endoscopic approach is less invasive, associated with decreased morbidity and reduced length of stay as compared to surgical approaches. From an economic standpoint, the endoscopic approach clearly offers a fiscal advantage. This framework can be extrapolated from the surgical literature. However, accurately assigning value for a particular endoscopic procedure is more nebulous and complex.[8]

Surgical revision for weight regain after RYGB varies widely between institutions, with approaches ranging from narrowing of the gastric pouch, complete resection of the gastrojejunal anastomosis, and/or lengthening of the bypassed limb. These procedures carry high morbidity and mortality, with complication rates ranging from 3.5% to 11.9%.[2] TORe offers a less invasive, safer approach with similar weight loss.[9]

While data is scarce in the comparison of these 2 approaches, one recent study showed similar weight loss at 1, 3, or 5 years following a surgical approach or TORe. However, the adverse event rate in the TORe group versus the surgery group were 6.5% versus 29.0%, respectively.[7] This study was limited by its small sample size but corroborated data from prior studies regarding the safety and efficacy of the TORe procedure.[5] Finally, while data is currently lacking, it can be extrapolated that TORe likely leads to reduced cost as compared to surgical revisions given its low adverse event rate and lack of hospital stay. Data is forthcoming.

Historical precedent exists for the implementation of new procedures in the surgical field, one example of which is laparoscopic sleeve gastrectomy. This operation has become the most common weight-loss procedure performed throughout the United States.[10] While early studies demonstrated lower morbidity compared to other weight loss procedures including RYGB, universal insurance coverage and broader acceptance were not immediate. The adoption of this procedure has grown exponentially in the last decade, in part due to large-scale, cooperative data tracking between multiple centers of excellence. These centers are mandated to track and share outcome metrics and, in turn, are preferentially designated to provide coverage for these procedures. Certain insurers including both private companies and the Centers for Medicare and Medicaid Services (CMS) require the Bariatric Surgery Center of Excellence (BSCOE) designation as a first step for inclusion in bariatric surgery networks and reimbursement. This designation and success in implementation was gained by wide-spread collaboration and lobbying to gather, process, and present data to payers and legislators.

● IMPLEMENTATION OF A SOLUTION

Implementation of a new procedure or technology in the medical field first requires clear, trackable metrics that can inform clinical outcomes and the cost of care delivery. When considering the incorporation of TORe in the treatment algorithm of weight recidivism following RYGB, key metrics should include metabolic outcomes, in addition to data on morbidity, mortality, adverse event rates, length of stay, procedure cost, and quality adjusted life years, for both surgical and endoscopic approaches. To clearly define these metrics, it is critical to align interests with key stakeholders including but not limited to primary care physicians, bariatric surgeons, gastroenterologists, endocrinologists, medical and surgical societies, and industry partnerships.

Medical and surgical societies are pivotal to foster this collaboration to create consensus standards of practice and guidelines among experts.

A roadmap forward for the incorporation of innovative techniques and technologies in practice can be informed by the laparoscopic revolution and procedures such as the sleeve gastrectomy. Similar to the adoption of early innovative surgical techniques, national societies should continue to focus on centralizing data collection and streamlining research, grant applications, and industry partnerships. This effort will ultimately lead to the development of standardized metrics and best practice patterns, in order to promote wider adoption and quality control. Additionally, it will be essential to develop referral networks and train providers in novel techniques in accordance with these goals. Advocacy by both patients and societies to legislatures and insurance companies will be important in raising awareness and promoting coverage. All of these efforts will also allow for registry creation and ultimately FDA-clearance and procedure-specific CPT codes.

It is important to acknowledge that this implementation strategy could inherently bias against underserved communities and those who are unable to pay out-of-pocket for procedures that are not covered by insurance. This bias will skew early data by selecting patients from certain races or higher socioeconomic backgrounds. As it is, obesity and adverse events from prior bariatric surgery are higher in communities of lower socioeconomic status.[11] Lack of access to safer and less invasive techniques such as TORe perpetuates engrained health care disparities. Access can, and should, be a key component of the financial support from institutions, industry partnerships, and federal grants to mitigate this inequality.

Key Steps in Change Management and Potential Pitfalls

Key Steps in Change Management

1. Identify clear metrics that can inform clinical outcomes and the cost of care delivery.
2. Understand both national and individual institutional difficulties in implementation, competing interests, costs, benefits, and risks with current alternative procedures.
3. Engage societies, device companies, and key stakeholders to collaborate on research, standardization, trials, and database development.
4. Establish a network of centers of excellence in a shared risk model with insurers to allow for early coverage while allowing for coordinated data gathering and trials.
5. Training of new physicians, practitioners, staff, and patients that can be facilitated via high volume centers based on consensus guidelines.
6. Publish work and approach FDA for wider authorization.
7. Obtain CPT code from CMS.
8. Empower advocacy by both patients and societies to legislators and insurance companies to gain awareness and coverage.

Potential Pitfalls

1. Not establishing central coordination of data collection and standards for coding, procedural approach, and education.
2. Not engaging in early discussions with private insurers and CMS regarding key metrics prior to obtaining insurance approval.
3. Not engaging with stakeholders both locally and nationally.
4. Not partnering with device companies for funding and collaboration in advocacy.
5. Broad implementation prior to standardization.

MEASURING OUTCOMES

Key metrics to monitor the effectiveness of the prior implementation strategy should include metabolic outcomes, in addition to data on morbidity, mortality, adverse event rates, length of stay, procedure cost, and quality adjusted life years, for both surgical and endoscopic approaches. Furthermore, longitudinal outcomes related to improvement in obesity-related comorbidities should also be followed. As above, the introduction of new techniques or technologies not consistently covered by insurance is fraught with inequity with respect to race and socioeconomic status. Monitoring demographic data to ensure equity of care to disadvantaged populations will be essential as utilization grows.

FOLLOW-UP AND MAINTENANCE

The implementation of new technologies and techniques that are not reimbursed is arduous. As demonstrated, widespread adoption is only feasible with partnership between major stakeholders and device companies, in addition to surgical and endoscopic societies. The development of key metrics, data registries, standards of practice are integral to ultimately achieve CPT codes and insurance approval. In the interim, support from public and private institutions may allow for early adoption, provider training, and research. TORe exemplifies this process. Early data has demonstrated improved safety and comparable weight loss to surgical interventions in the treatment of weight recidivism after RYGB, and its increased adoption can serve as a roadmap for other innovative technologies moving forward.

REFERENCES

1. Abu Dayyeh BK, Lautz DB, Thompson, CC. Gastrojejunal stoma diameter predicts weight regain after Rouxen-Y gastric bypass. *Clin Gastroenterol H*. 2011;9(3):228–233.
2. Tran DD, Nwokeabia ID, Purnell S, et al. Revision of Roux-En-Y gastric bypass for weight regain: a systematic review of techniques and outcomes. *Obes Surg*. 2016;26(7):1627–1634.
3. Schulman AR, Kumar N, Thompson CC. Transoral outlet reduction: a comparison of purse-string with interrupted stitch technique. *Gastrointest Endosc*. 2018;87(5):1222–1228.
4. Kumar N. Weight loss endoscopy: development, applications, and current status. *World J Gastroentero* 2016; 22(31):7069–7079.
5. Jirapinyo P., Kumar N, AlSamman MA, Thompson CC. Five-year outcomes of transoral outlet reduction for the treatment of weight regain after Roux-en-Y gastric bypass. *Gastrointest Endosc*. 2020;91(5):1067–1073.
6. Kumar N, Thompson CC. Comparison of a superficial suturing device with a full-thickness suturing device for transoral outlet reduction (with videos). *Gastrointest Endosc*. 2014;79(6):984–989.
7. Dolan RD, Jirapinyo P, Thompson CC. Endoscopic versus surgical gastrojejunal revision for weight regain in Rouxen-Y gastric bypass patients: 5-year safety and efficacy comparison. *Gastrointest Endosc*. 2021;94(5):945–950.
8. Savarise M, Senkowski C, eds. *Principles of Coding and Reimbursement for Surgeons. Coding for Laparoscopic Surgery*. Cham, Switzerland: Springer; 2017. http://ndl.ethernet.edu.et/bitstream/123456789/72650/1/140.pdf.pdf
9. Dolan RD, Schulman AR. Endoscopic approaches to obesity management. *Annu Rev Med*. 2021;73:423–438. doi: 10.1146/annurev-med-042320-125832
10. Bartosiak K, Różańska-Walędziak A, Walędziak M, Kowalewski P, Paśnik K, Janik MR. The safety and benefits of laparoscopic sleeve gastrectomy in elderly patients: a case-control study. *Obes Surg*. 2019;29(7):2233–2237.
11. Robertson BLA. *Obesity and Inequities*. WHO; 2014. https://apps.who.int/iris/bitstream/handle/10665/344619/9789289050487-eng.pdf

Consolidating OR Supply Chain to a Single Vendor

42

MARIAM MAKSUTOVA, JANET ABBRUZZESE, AND CHANDU VEMURI

Clinical Delivery Challenge

In today's medical landscape, a capitalist economy driven by entrepreneurial innovators provides a constant influx of new surgical tools and technologies. Hospital systems must balance medical advancement with financial sustainability, especially in the dynamic, high-stakes, and high revenue-generating setting of the operating room.[1] At our institution, system-wide value analysis and efforts toward surgical supply standardization revealed that, often, multiple products were used by different groups to accomplish the same goal. Even within provider groups performing the same procedure in the same way, we found that different products are often utilized. All the while, more products are being continually requested.

In a large healthcare system, it is not sustainable to continue in this way. Expenditures are high, reimbursements are decreasing, and margins are narrowing.[2] Hospitals must seize opportunities to safely reduce cost. A key strategic tactic is vendor consolidation. As in every industry, consolidating vendors in healthcare has multiple benefits including cost reduction through negotiated contracts and easier management of inventory. However, asking physicians to change products used in an operation for that purpose is not met with cheers, but rather trepidation that care will suffer. Resentment toward strategies that in any way focus on containing costs is common.[3] In this chapter, we discuss how vendor consolidation has the potential to result in high-quality care with satisfied, engaged stakeholders.

● WORKUP

To begin analyzing the relationship between product utilization and cost, it is important to build a knowledgeable team to define data parameters, critical metrics, and options for improvement. At our institution, 2 processes operate in parallel. The first brings together surgeons from every surgical subspecialty, surgical support staff, supply chain specialists, administrators, and other expert stakeholders to form the Value Analysis Team (VAT). This team works systematically to define the current state: What products are used in our operating rooms? How much of each is used and at what cost? What are the surgical outcomes for each? The VAT then works prospectively to oversee new product requests. The second process—the Clinical Supply Integration Project (CSIP) is physician initiated and focuses on existing product overlap. As part of the CSIP, a physician champion meets with the surgeons in their section to, similarly, identify what cases are being done, what supplies are being used, and so on. Additionally, CSIP physicians work to identify opportunities for consolidation in both disposable and non-disposable re-usable and non-re-usable items that exist within the current inventory. This information is then presented to the VAT. The overarching goal driving these processes is the identification of items for consolidation that would improve the cost profile while leaving the quality of care unaffected.

- Operational Metrics (Figure 42.1)
  - Usage
  - Price Index
  - Case Cost and Margin Data
  - Quality and Outcomes Data
- Process Tools
  - Value Analysis Team process to collect and analyze data
  - Clinical Supply Integration Project to identify products in-house

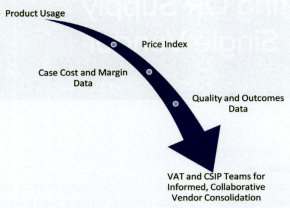

FIGURE 42.1 Key operational metric data needed for informed vendor consolidation processes.

Through VAT and CSIP initiatives, our institution underwent a large-scale process to standardize much of the supplies and equipment used in our operating rooms. In 2019, a potential opportunity for vendor consolidation was identified in Orthopedic surgery through CSIP. Hip and knee replacements are performed by a set group of providers at our institution. At that time, the University Hospital was using 2 vendors (vendor A and vendor B) for hip and knee implants. During the evaluation of these products, input from individuals involved at each step, from acquisition to utilization of the product was elicited and integral to successful vendor consolidation.

● DIFFERENTIAL DIAGNOSIS

We considered numerous potential causes for why providers may use several different companies' products to achieve the same result. These included:

- Surgeon preference and comfort level
- Push for new product acquisition by vendors
- Lack of a data-centered process for auditing existing inventory
- Limited communication about OR supplies between surgeons

● DIAGNOSIS AND TREATMENT

In our example, comprehensive operational metrics on hip and knee implants in Orthopedic surgery were collected. Market share for these products was broken down as follows: Hips – 60% vendor A, 40% vendor B; Knees – 85% vendor A, 15% vendor B. Analysis of benchmark pricing data placed the hospital in the 75th percentile compared to peer institutions. The goal established through CSIP was to be in the 25th percentile which, at the time, projected a savings of approximately $850,000.

The team comprised of orthopedic surgeons and supply chain staff met to review the data and discuss the merits of standardization, all the while emphasizing quality and safety as drivers. Physician champions were on hand to address preference and discuss vendor relationships. The products were subjected to a data-centered holistic review. Interestingly, in while attempting to consolidate, the group decided to test a third vendor. A limited evaluation trial was undertaken with implants from vendor C and ultimately the team decided that this would not be a useful addition or viable alternative. Furthermore, after reviewing the data between vendors A and B, no advantage to using products from both was identified. The decision was made to consolidate to vendor A and assess the price index to attain better pricing. Clinical team members focused on outcome data comparisons to ensure that there would be no impact to quality.

In 2020, a request for proposal resulted in an estimated savings of $805K with 90% commitment to one supplier. A contract with vendor A was executed in December 2020. The department is currently compliant with this one vendor for 93% market share and have exceeded $1.1 million in savings. Perhaps even more significantly, given a yearly spend in 2019 of $3.2 million, the first year's savings of $800K was a 25% reduction in cost.

● SCIENTIFIC PRINCIPLES AND EVIDENCE

The key principle to ensuring successful vendor consolidation is a transparent, inclusive, and objective process for auditing both existing inventory and new products. This process must be reproducible and widely applicable. At our institution—CSIP, a physician-initiated product review—and the VAT—a multidisciplinary committee of surgeons, nurses, infection prevention experts, analysts, finance directors, and others formed to collaboratively oversee the acquisition of surgical supplies—are excellent team-based solutions that meets the above criteria. Adhering to the core principle of advancing patient care, they obtain the objective usage data, cost data, and outcomes data necessary for informed decision making and carry out that decision-making with careful intentionality. Heavy physician engagement, including 2 VAT physician co-chairs, allows for consideration of practical factors from primary product users. Acknowledgment of such qualitative data results in better overall buy-in by enforcing that cost-cutting is not the only consideration in decision-making.

The most important information toward successful consolidation is data that reveals no true quality difference between 2 or more products. Outcomes data may come from vendors, be collected from published literature, or require a new investigation. Data-driven decision-making allows for differentiation between user preference and product superiority. In this way, we approach inventory through a standardized lens of health care value, defined as the best possible clinical outcome for the lowest possible price.

● IMPLEMENTING A SOLUTION

We implemented a transparent, objective process based on value and data analysis as described above. When a new product is requested, the requestor fills out a form consisting of questions about the product and why it is needed (Figure 42.2).

They then create a 5-minute pre-recorded video presentation in which they present a templated slide deck that includes information on the current product, the future product, the projected usage, the projected costs, and whether the request is for a new product adoption or a limited evaluation trial.

When time limited evaluations are performed, the surgical faculty present the results to the same VAT team for discussion of product approval (Figure 42.3). All stakeholders must be present for this presentation to review usage, cost, and quality. Attendance is important and increases the chances that a shared solution is well adopted. Furthermore, excellent attendance creates trust in the frameworks and builds collaboration that results in higher likelihood of success for future and adjunct projects (Table 42.1).

An inclusive process has many benefits including opportunities for rapid vendor consolidation for products used by all. For example, due to the collaborative and interdepartmental nature of our value analysis team, products that are not specialty-specific (drapes etc.) have, at times, been adopted by multiple departments. This additional route to product consolidation would not be an option for those working in departmental silos or those struggling with meeting attendance.

Once a decision is reached, it is critical that each team member returns to their respective departments to review the process with all individuals. Communicating why the decision was needed, explaining the objective approach followed, and highlighting downstream benefits will increase the odds that the change will be received positively and implemented widely. Without this transparency, some may assume that a decision was made based on cost alone, that quality of care was not considered, or that the relevant stakeholders were not involved. When this happens, change is slow or may be faced with overt or tacit opposition.

The primary pitfalls of vendor consolidation is the realization of these very assumptions. Without a dedicated and careful analysis, the consolidation may result in a decrement in quality of care, extreme

Serial Number:
Comments:
OR Lead:
Priority:
Request Date:
VA Assignment Date:
Site:
Service:
Submitter:
Submitter Email:
Submitter Phone:
Physician Requestor:
Physician Email:
Conflict of Interest:
Physician Assistant Email:
Physician End User:
Product Number:
Manufacturer Name:
Product Description:
Request Type:
Anticipated Annual Usage:
Packaging Details:
Latex Content:
Quoted Unit Price:
Frequent Users:
Anticipated Annual Usage:
Replace Existing Item:
Current Product Details:
Problems Solved by Product:
How Gap is Addressed currently?:
New Products ability to address the Gap:
Metrics for Success:
Anticipated Cost Savings:
Vendor Quote:
Product Brochure:
FDA 510(k):
Multiple Product Line Attachment:
Capital Approval:
Product Replacement:
Evidence to Support Claims:
Additional Materials:
Evaluation type:
Numner to Evaluate:
Training Education Required:

FIGURE 42.2 Sample new product request form.

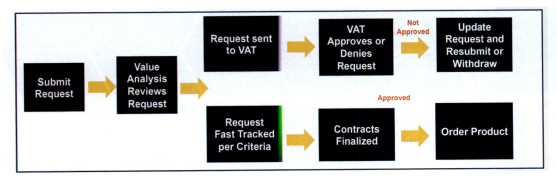

FIGURE 42.3 VAT team's standardized product approval process.

Table 42.1 Critical Elements in VAT Presentation for New Product Acquisition

Background: current product, new product with rationale
New Product Images/Video
Added Value Proposition: improved outcomes or decreased cost
Metrics of Success (for evaluation trials)
Financial Analysis: cost of current product, cost per use of new product, change in operational expenses if the new product was required taking into account expected usage
Vendor Consolidation: have all the users agree to switch to the new product, is this request in-line with consolidation efforts, are there other service lines that could also use this product

Key Steps in Change Management and Potential Pitfalls

Key Steps in Change Management

1. Build a knowledgeable and interdisciplinary team of relevant stakeholders.
2. Provide ample opportunities for physician involvement and participation.
3. Identify items for consolidation within current inventory and define the current state of OR purchasing.
4. Define a transparent, inclusive, and objective process for bringing in and assessing new products.
5. Rigorous data collection through avenues such as vendor information, published literature, and potential new investigations is paramount.
6. Ensure that decision-making is data driven.
7. Track resulting changes in number of products, cost, and clinical outcomes to monitor process success and identify areas for improvement.
8. Gather feedback from stakeholders to ensure their satisfaction with the process.

Potential Pitfalls

1. Failing to secure early buy-in from stakeholders may result in poor attendance, lack of communication, and/or lack of follow up.
2. Lack of transparency may lead to assumptions that decisions are made based on cost alone, that quality of care is not considered, or that the relevant stakeholders are not involved.
3. Lack of dedicated analysis may lead to decreased quality of care, extreme sacrifice for cost, and/or exclusion of important input from key parties.
4. Inability to track outcomes may mask instances where expected cost savings may not be achieved due to unintended effect on practice.

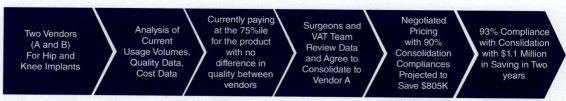

FIGURE 42.4 Single vendor consolidation by orthopedic surgery for hip and knee implants demonstrating $1.1 million in savings over 2 years.

sacrifice for cost, or exclude important input from key parties. A secondary pitfall may be that the expected cost savings is not realized despite an appropriate product consolidation due to lack of successful price renegotiation with the vendor or unintended effects on practice—such as when certain providers take more time to accomplish a procedure when they are unfamiliar with the consolidated products.

MEASURING OUTCOMES

The most obvious metric for the VAT's work in vendor consolidation is the reduction in the number of products used for the same purpose. This is monitored by service line leads in the implementation and maintenance phase of CSIP work. Additionally, it is important to elicit whether vendor consolidation resulted in a better negotiated price and vital to track any resulting changes in clinical outcomes. In the example presented in this chapter, savings exceeding $1.1 million to date were accompanied by no discernable changes to the clinical care provided. (Figure 42.4) Furthermore, it is important to gather feedback from stakeholders to ensure their satisfaction with the process, which ensures longevity of the solution.

FOLLOW-UP AND MAINTENANCE

Success of consolidation depends on diligent follow through and follow up. As described above once the decision is made to consolidate a particular product, the execution depends on participant buy in, outcomes monitoring, skillful negotiation with remaining vendors, and accountable inventory management. Follow-up should focus on relinquishment of the passed-over product, monitoring for unforeseen consequences of the chosen product, and tracking user satisfaction. Careful tracking of financial effects may include assessment of continued cost saving and opportunities for contract renegotiation.

REFERENCES

1. Rutter TW, Brown ACD. Contemporary operating room management. *Adv Anesth*. 1994;11:173–214.
2. Childers CP, Maggard-Gibbons M. Understanding costs of care in the operating room. *JAMA Surg*. 2018;153(4):e176233.
3. Engelman DT, Boyle EM, Benjamin EM. Addressing the imperative to evolve the hospital new product value analysis process. *J Thorac Cardiovasc Surg*. 2018;155(2):682–685.

When Healthcare Systems Become Their Own Insurer

43

SEAN MICHAEL O'NEILL AND STEVEN R. CRAIN

Clinical Delivery Challenge

Mid-State Health (MSH) is based in a metropolitan region of 3 million people and includes a quaternary care, 800-bed teaching hospital in addition to 5 regional hospitals, all of which have surgical capabilities and are located within a 3-hour drive. Physicians are employed by the MSH Medical Group, a for-profit entity formally affiliated with the MSH health system. Surgical services span all specialties and include 400 surgeons performing a total of 80,000 inpatient and outpatient operations and procedures per year. MSH's financial position is consistently strong, with a $500 million positive margin on $4 billion in revenue for the most recent fiscal year, and a history of similar performance. The health insurance market is stably concentrated, with MSH's primary payer covering 80% of patients, including those with Medicare and Medicaid plans.

While successful, MSH does face competition from City Central Hospital (CCH), which is the top hospital in the state and city in national rankings and outperforms MSH's flagship location in both patient volume and revenue. However, at a system level, MSH has higher patient volume and revenue due to its greater presence across the wider region.

With the goals of achieving sustainable dominance in the local healthcare market and surpassing CCH in regard to reputational quality, the MSH Board of Directors has approved a bold and ambitious plan. They will create MSH Health Plan, in partnership with their leading health insurer, with the goal of establishing fully-capitated status for 80% of their patient population within 5 years. From the Board's perspective, they are not only seeking to "lock in" patients to an MSH-exclusive health plan, but are counting on the capitated incentive structure to drive large-scale improvements in quality, safety, patient satisfaction, and health promotion. The partner health insurer, Stateside Group, has been increasingly utilizing claims data to exert pressure on health systems to limit costs and improve quality, and they see this partnership as a way to explicitly embed themselves within the healthcare delivery system itself.

Dr. Jeannette Clark, a neurosurgeon, is the Chief of Surgery at MSH's flagship hospital and Vice President for Surgical Services across the MSH system. The Board expects MSH's surgical services to transition from a model in which more care is rewarded, to one in which better care is rewarded. What can she do to prepare for the future?

Can a single organization provide clinical care and, at the same time, manage the financial risk associated with that care? Healthcare systems that are "self-insured" attempt to do exactly that. Having direct control over both revenue from and spending on a finite set of patients allows them to invest in delivering the highest value care. The healthier these patients are and the fewer downstream complications they experience, the better off the patients and the healthcare system will be. Traditional fee-for-service healthcare systems have incentives to focus on highly reimbursed procedures while minimizing cost—delivering value is not a necessary condition for success. However, what might happen if a fee-for-service system attempts to become self-insuring? And what are the implications for surgical leaders?

Kaiser Permanente is the largest and longest-established such self-insuring system, and has been studied extensively as a model for how these incentives can result in transformational change and high-quality care.[1-5] Over 100 traditional healthcare systems have attempted to become at least partially self-insured, through a variety of mechanisms.[6,7] The revenue and liabilities for even moderately-sized self-insured

282 SECTION 9 • Improving Value of Care

systems are typically $1 billion to $3 billion annually, which implies a staggering amount of financial risk for a new entrant, particularly if the goal is to become fully self-insured.[6] Perhaps not surprisingly, many of these new plans fail within several years.[6,7] Consequently, healthcare systems that attempt this strategy often do so through risk-mitigating partnerships with an existing large health insurer, and continue to provide care to patients covered by third-party payers, rather than aiming for capitation of their entire patient population.[6,7]

What does this mean for surgical care? While they are a different concept, some of the lessons learned from Accountable Care Organizations (ACOs) are salient, in that ACOs attempt to engage healthcare delivery systems to bear some of the financial risk of low-value care. Initial analyses suggest that the ACO concept has had very little impact on surgical care at all,[8,9] at least in part due to a focus on chronic care rather than surgical services.[10] However, as surgery includes many of the highest cost procedures, surgical leaders will need to thoughtfully consider how their services fit in a self-insured, value-driven system.

In the case described in this chapter, we will trace the journey of a traditional, fee-for-service healthcare system as it attempts to become a self-insuring healthcare system, and highlight approaches that surgical leaders can take to drive clinical and organizational success in the midst of such a large-scale change program.

● WORKUP

Transitioning from a traditional healthcare system to becoming a self-insured, one could reasonably be characterized as a large-scale change. There are no consensus guidelines for such an undertaking. As such, the lessons learned from large corporations are likely the most apt guide for success in such a dramatic and transformative change as going from a fee-for-services healthcare system to a self-insured one. Scott Keller and Bill Schaninger have decades of experience in management consulting specifically focused on implementing large-scale change initiatives. They recently developed a systematic framework, described in "Beyond Performance 2.0: A Proven Approach to Leading Large-Scale Change," based on data from thousands of organizations, for how to maximize the chances of success. The most basic lesson from their work is that organizational *performance* and organizational *health* must be equally emphasized. We will utilize their framework and findings to guide the choices of leaders in surgery facing this challenge.

The first task will be to develop a clear and compelling vision for how surgical services fit in with this new self-insured future. At a high level, this vision will be some form of the best that existing self-insured health systems have achieved. Because the health system will now collect payment from patients ahead of time rather than after the fact, they are paying the health system to keep them healthy for the future, rather than for addressing problems as they arise. For surgical services, that means that simply doing more surgery is not better, unless it improves overall health and well-being, or prevents or mitigates downstream consequences of disease. Certainly, surgical services delivered with high rates of complications or at excessive cost run counter to this mission, so greater emphasis will need to be placed on prudent financial stewardship, outcomes tracking and continuous quality improvement. Reinforcing this vision that more surgery is not necessarily better, it is very likely that surgeons will eventually be compensated through a salary model, rather than the traditional productivity-based model.

With an eye toward the long-term organizational health of the surgical workforce, it is critical that **surgeon-leaders are placed on the system's top-level team that is managing the transition. The vision for the future of surgery should be a collaborative effort** with the most influential internal surgeon-leaders. This group should develop a unified vision and learn to tell that story in a personalized way—to convey to people, authentically, what it will mean to them if this transition is successful. For example, "If this really works, I will never have to worry about losing money or RVUs when I tell a patient not to have an operation. I will be able to really focus on what's best for the patient." can't believe that won't have to worry about missing RVU targets every time I recommend a patient not have an operation." Overall, the goal of this first stage—involving multiple surgeons in top transitional teams and developing and communicating a clear and compelling vision for the future—is to establish that this transition is something that is done *with* surgeons, rather than something that is done *to* surgeons. Concerns that are not elicited at this stage are certain to arise as major barriers down the road. The lack of surgeon involvement in the early ACO experience underscores the real danger that these profound changes may occur without meaningful involvement or contribution from surgeons.[10]

Next, leaders must **assess their department's readiness to achieve the vision of the future**, and **identify which skillsets and backgrounds should be emphasized for workforce recruitment, retention, and promotion**. Two major issues will become immediately apparent. First, what is the current compensation model? Most likely, surgeons are compensated relative to their clinical productivity. This model reinforces a deeper mindset that is nearly universal in procedural fields—that "busy is better"—the more I do, the more I get paid. Even in systems on a salaried model, this mindset can be deep-rooted. However, to achieve the hoped-for gains in quality of care in surgery, a different mindset—"better is better"—must take root, and will need to be reinforced with a matching compensation model. If higher volumes of care continue to be rewarded without a commensurate requirement for the value of that care, the self-insured model for surgical services simply does not make sense.[9] This is, understandably, likely to be the most disruptive issue for surgeons in the transition to a self-insured system. Second, how willing, experienced, and committed is the surgical workforce in regard to outcome measurement and continuous improvement? If there are gaps in any of those areas, they must be prioritized for recruitment, retention and promotion.

● DIFFERENTIAL DIAGNOSIS

At this point, Dr. Clark has involved influential surgeon-leaders throughout the health system in creating a vision for the future of MSH Surgery within a self-insured system, begun to communicate what a successful transition would mean to her, and all of the surgeon-leaders have done the same. She has long been personally familiar with and thrived as a result of the productivity-based compensation model at MSH. She admits that it is challenging to understand how the most productive surgeons in the system—who drive significant revenue in the present state—would ever submit to a salaried or a value-based care compensation model. Finally, she has identified several small, but currently disconnected groups of providers and nurses within the system (but in different clinical divisions) with deep experience in surgical quality improvement and research. She draws a 2×2 table (Compensation Model × Improvement Workforce) to understand where MSH Surgery is, and where they need to go. Investments must be made in building resources and expertise in continuous improvement, but more importantly, managing the transition away from the "busy is better" mindset is likely to be the most significant challenge of the entire process (Figure 43.1).

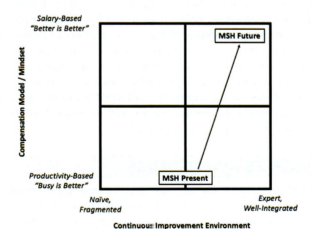

FIGURE 43.1 Key organizational characteristics to drive high performance in self-insured healthcare systems (compensation model and continuous improvement environment).

DIAGNOSIS AND TREATMENT

Having now identified the most critical gaps between present and future, leaders must now build a plan to close those gaps. Most crucially, authentic mechanisms for ongoing two-way communication of the strategy and feedback on its implementation must be established. For skill gaps in the workforce, leaders should make specific changes to recruitment, onboarding, and promotion processes. By attracting, retaining, and elevating surgeons, nurses, administrators and leaders who both believe in the goal of continuous improvement and have the background and experience to execute it, leaders will begin to slowly but steadily change the culture of their organization. Leaders need to intentionally plan for continuously eliciting and addressing barriers of all types. This process will take years—most insidiously, even if large-scale structural and personnel changes are made, latent and oppositional mindsets can be very challenging to uproot.

The greatest challenge for surgical leaders will be to create a new mindset and culture. Surgeons and staff who disagree with the new initiative are likely to leave the health system, which may induce significant disruptions to clinical services. This is why involving influential surgeon-leaders from the very beginning is so important. While some surgeons will never accept the new model and some will be highly enthusiastic, the vast majority will want to find a way to make their practice work in a self-insured world. However, if these staff feel uninvolved with the transition process and that their perspectives are not listened to or valued, the risk of widespread staff departures increases greatly.

Having stemmed the tide of staff turnover with robust and authentic communication and involvement in the process, and planning to recruit staff with the skills and mindset to help surgical services thrive in the self-insured environment, the next most critical long-term investment to make will be in persistently retelling the narrative for the future state through onboarding, training, and the regular course of work. If the top surgical leaders, and all departmental, divisional, and group leaders can internalize the narrative that the self-insured model will allow the health system to create a better, healthier, and safer system for all involved, including patients and staff, and then consistently re-tell why this is meaningful and important at every opportunity—meetings, emails, training, onboarding, and in the midst of unexpected crises and problems—it will start to reinforce the change in mindset needed to thrive in the future.

Dr. Clark first spent 1-on-1 time in dialogue with all of her top surgeon-leaders to elicit their perspectives and help draft a narrative for how MSH Surgery would transition to and thrive in the self-insured future state. She then organized a retreat with all of these surgeon-leaders and staff surgeons, in addition to key departmental leaders in nursing, allied health, finance, and human resources to not only communicate the vision and elicit concerns but also to establish that success in the self-insured future will only come through a unified, coordinated team effort, rather than through a thousand individual strivings. Specific plans for recruiting surgeons, nurses, and administrators with experience in self-insured health systems and with a mindset for and experience in continuous improvement were instituted. The narrative for where and why MSH Surgery is going in the future was reinforced in regular communications from all surgeon-leaders through individual conversations, meeting agendas, emails, and even branding and signage. She (with her staff) dedicated numerous half day, focused retreats at all MSH locations and with all surgical divisions to establish authentic two-way modes of communication and feedback, knowing that these connections would be essential going forward as the project progressed.

SCIENTIFIC PRINCIPLES AND EVIDENCE

Despite the Kaiser Health Plan's status as the second-largest private health insurer in the United States in 2021, with an 8% national market share and $107 billion in direct premiums, Kaiser has been self-insured from its beginnings more than 80 years ago. Very little rigorous study has been made of how traditional health systems may transition to becoming a self-insured system. To inform our present question, however, in addition to the broader quality improvement literature, there is a recent case study series of health systems starting their own insurance plans as well as lessons learned from across large organizations undergoing dramatic changes in the management literature.

Allan Baumgarten has published a focused series of reports[6,7] on provider-sponsored health plans (PSHPs), which include more than 140 health insurance plans initiated by or exclusively affiliated with specific health care systems. The recent track record is challenging, as many of the more than 40 plans initiated since 2010 have already gone out of business, typically within just a few years.[6,7] Due to the substantial financial risk inherent in transitioning to becoming a self-insured system, the most common recent trend is for health systems to form joint ventures with existing large-scale health insurers.[7] He identifies that the key to success is to deliver on the value proposition of providing higher-quality care than competitors, allowing the system to charge less for insurance premiums as they attract a larger population and a more balanced risk pool. This is, however, a long-term strategy that must maintain financial viability amidst local competition, unstable individual markets, and pricing challenges, as well as begin to produce significant improvements through new-found excellence in clinical coordination and improvement. Due to these daunting challenges, very few of the 40 PSHPs initiated since 2010 were identified as promising or likely to succeed.[6]

Given these dire odds and steep challenges, it is reasonable to look to studies of large-scale organizational change to glean useful principles and lessons. More so than any specific quality improvement method or clinical focus, leaders in healthcare systems attempting to transition from a traditional to a self-insured model will need to lead by engaging the majority of their workforce to believe in and work toward achieving the vision of the future state. Keller and Schaninger's work is based on decades of experience in management consulting, hundreds of data-driven case studies of change implementation, and focused surveys of more than 5,000 executives across more than 2,000 organizations. They emphasize that while the performance aspects of such a change—solving the problems of pricing, risk management, and competition, to name a few—are important, the organizational health aspects of the change—rooting out harmful mindsets, facilitating ownership, collaboration, and personalization of the process, and reshaping the work environment to foster both the change and workforce well-being—are just as critical to long-term success. Organizational Performance can be thought of as "what" a health system does—in a self-insuring health system, this includes not just delivering clinical care, but managing and pricing the risk of health insurance plans. Organizational Health is "how" a health system does what it does—how does it align the workforce toward achieving the promise of high-value care, how does it execute on achieving that promise, and how does it renew itself and its workforce to adapt when competitive markets change?

● IMPLEMENTATION OF A SOLUTION

Having established the vision, engaged key surgical and non-clinical leaders, and developed a plan for transitioning to a salaried staff model with robust capabilities for continuous clinical improvement, the task of implementing the plan depends on maintaining the engagement of surgical leaders through robust two-way communication, continuing to identify and mobilize influential leaders, and modifying and adapting the plan as unexpected issues arise. Perhaps most importantly, however, is the task of leading by example, and making this large-scale change personal. If this will require a salary model, be the first to change your compensation structure. Be transparent and fair, and be honest and authentic about the dramatic change that this represents. Short-term inefficiencies may result from maintaining productivity-based compensation levels in a salaried model once the incentives for high productivity are removed. Specialized incentives may be necessary to maintain stability and minimize workforce disruption as the groundwork is laid for a new culture aligned toward high-value surgical care, not high-volume surgical care. Attempts to reduce compensation at this stage may seem financially sensible, but they are likely to hamper the sustainability of the entire project.[6] At all phases of the process, maintaining robust communication, leading by example, re-emphasizing the vision and narrative, building a workforce aligned to the future state, and making it clear that this self-insurance transition is something that is being done *with* surgeons rather than *to* surgeons are the key elements for realizing success.

Pitfalls of the process for surgical leaders are numerous. First, failing to either engage influential surgeon-leaders or to place them on the highest-level teams in charge of directing the effort may result in widespread ambivalence or resentment toward the project. Similarly, the surgical leaders placed highly within the health system must maintain their "seat at the table" and remain deeply engaged in the overall process.

SECTION 9 • Improving Value of Care

There are many issues beyond surgical care that are potential pitfalls, including insurance product development, sales, marketing and pricing, chronic care coordination, and many others. While surgical leaders may not be tasked with managing these issues, it is essential that they are deeply engaged with how the overall health system transition is proceeding. It is not without good reason that so few of these ventures in the last 10 years have been successful.

If involvement, communication, and engagement is low, staff departures and disruptive turnover may result; competitors may sense discontent and draw key surgeons, leaders and staff away. Even with a stable workforce, mindsets and culture are deep rooted, and influence every clinical decision, whether realized or not. Specific efforts must be made to identify and consistently root out ways of thinking that are counter to a value-based clinical delivery model. A failure to communicate the process early, often, and with authenticity will also alienate the workforce from the process. A failure to invest in clinical quality improvement expertise will limit the ability of the system to realize the gains in safety, efficiency, and value that are promised in a self-insured model. Moreover, a tremendous pitfall is to lose focus or energy on the long-term goal.

Key Steps in Change Management and Potential Pitfalls

Key Steps in Change Management

1. Involve surgeon-leaders at the highest levels of the health system from the beginning.
2. Develop a vision for the future of surgery in the new system, with a broad group of surgeon-leaders.
3. Vision should emphasize the high-value, health-promoting care.
4. Identify gaps in skills and backgrounds needed to achieve the future vision.
   - Continuous quality improvement
   - Outcome measurement
   - Collaborative work style
   - Belief in the value-based care model
5. Identify ways to reinforce the new model through compensation.
   - Plan for a long-term transition to a salaried model
   - Plan for short-term inefficiencies to minimize staff disruption and defections to competitors
   - Set expectations in recruitment of new staff
   - Measure surgical services in a value-based framework
6. Recruit, retain, and promote staff based on the needs of the future.
7. Maintain robust, authentic, two-way communication throughout the process.
   - Lead by example
   - Personalize the narrative of the future
8. Plan to maintain energy and focus on the transition for many years.

Potential Pitfalls

1. Not involving a broad group of surgeon-leaders from the very beginning.
2. Developing a vision that does not align with influential surgeon-leaders' perspectives.
3. Not authentically or effectively communicating the vision to the workforce.
4. Not leading by example or making the changes personal, sowing division between leadership and staff.
5. Not planning for workforce disruptions or competitors' strategies.
6. Not identifying deep-seated mindsets the reinforce volume-based care.
7. Failing to build, cultivate, and prioritize continuous clinical quality improvement.
8. Failing to monitor outcomes in a value-based framework (quality of care, long-term population health, and cost).
9. Failing to stay engaged with overall system leadership—is the system-wide project succeeding or failing?
10. Losing energy and focus over time.

Transitioning from a traditional fee-for-service healthcare system to a fully-capitated self-insured system is not a months-long or even years-long process—it is a generational shift, and leaders should plan to maintain a focus on the transition for many, many years.

● MEASURING OUTCOMES

The overall clinical goal of a health care system transitioning to a self-insured model must be to capitalize on the financial incentives to deliver high-value, health-promoting healthcare services. While surgical services are likely to be less involved in preventive and chronic care efforts, surgical leaders must pay very close attention to avoidable complications, readmissions and returns to emergency care. Performance on these measures should be presented in a regular, transparent, and blame-free manner that will foster and energize forward-looking improvement work. Opportunities to develop and implement larger-scale improvement projects arising from these metrics should be encouraged and supported.[4,5]

Ultimately, the mark of success for surgeon-leaders in a self-insured system is whether the program is contributing to, or detracting from, the overall health system's goal of delivering high-value health care services. In a traditional model, while surgical services are typically the costliest, they are also the most financially rewarding, which creates ample opportunity for positive margins on surgery alone. In a self-insured model, surgical services will likely still remain the costliest services, but leaders will have to keep in mind that all payments have already been received up front through capitation. Thus, assessing a financial margin on surgical services will no longer be a meaningful metric, as the premiums from non-surgical patients will contribute to the care of surgical patients. This reinforces the need to measure and assess the value of surgical services—benchmarking costs against competitors and historical controls, measuring the cost of avoidable downstream complications, and building in measures of surgical patients' overall health and satisfaction.

● FOLLOW-UP AND MAINTENANCE

As mentioned earlier, a transition from a traditional fee-for-service healthcare system to a self-insured healthcare system is bound to be a long, perhaps even generational process. All of the strategic elements described here—involving surgeons in top leadership, reinforcing the vision and narrative to change mindsets and culture, reinforcing behavior with a new compensation model, recruiting and cultivating a workforce capable of achieving the vision, and adapting to new challenges as they arise—must eventually be hard-wired into the system. Making compensation, recruitment, communication, and collaborative improvement processes permanent and self-reinforcing is the final task for the surgical leader in this transition. In all likelihood, the surgeon-leaders present at the beginning of the transition will have turned over leadership by the time the process has reached its original goals. However, no less energy and focus on the process can be afforded for the leaders that follow, which should be a prime consideration when promoting and recruiting the next generation of leaders. It is a fallacy to think that the work of change and improvement in a healthcare delivery organization is ever "complete" or "finished". The process of implementing, measuring, adapting, re-implementing, re-measuring, re-adapting, and on and on—never ends.

● CONCLUSION

While clear examples of success are few and far between, it is becoming ever more apparent that the only financially sustainable future for healthcare in the Unites States will be one in which high-value—rather than high-volume—care is most rewarded. Therefore, whether it comes through self-insuring systems, provider-sponsored health plans, ACOs, or increasingly detailed preauthorization processes and stringent payment systems, we can only expect that the entities that manage the financial risk of healthcare—typically, government and third-party insurers—and the healthcare systems that actually deliver services and drive costs will become ever more closely integrated.

REFERENCES

1. Schilling L, Chase A, Kehrli S, Liu AY, Stiefel M, Brentari R. Kaiser Permanente's performance improvement system, part 1: from benchmarking to executing on strategic priorities. *Jt Comm J Qual Patient Saf.* 2010; 36(11):484–498. doi: 10.1016/s1553-7250(10)36072-7
2. Schilling L, Deas D, Jedlinsky M, Aronoff D, Fershtman J, Wali A. Kaiser Permanente's performance improvement system, part 2: developing a value framework. *Jt Comm J Qual Patient Saf.* 2010;36(12):552–560. doi: 10.1016/s1553-7250(10)36083-1
3. Schilling L, Dearing JW, Staley P, Harvey P, Fahey L, Kuruppu F. Kaiser Permanente's performance improvement system, part 4: creating a learning organization. *Jt Comm J Qual Patient Saf.* 2011;37(12):532–543. doi: 10.1016/s1553-7250(11)37069-9
4. Liu VX, Rosas E, Hwang J, et al. Enhanced recovery after surgery program implementation in 2 surgical populations in an integrated health care delivery system. *JAMA Surg.* 2017;152(7):e171032. doi: 10.1001/jamasurg.2017.1032
5. Parrish AB, O'Neill SM, Crain SR, et al. An enhanced recovery after surgery (ERAS) protocol for ambulatory anorectal surgery reduced postoperative pain and unplanned returns to care after discharge. *World J Surg.* 2018;42(7):1929–1938. doi: 10.1007/s00268-017-4414-8
6. Baumgarten A. *Analysis of Integrated Delivery Systems and New Provider-Sponsored Health Plans.* Princeton, NJ: Robert Wood Johnson Foundation; 2017.
7. "New Provider-Sponsored Health Plans: Joint Ventures Are Now the Preferred Strategy," Health Affairs Blog, February 23, 2018. doi: 10.1377/hblog20180216.720494. Available at https://www.healthaffairs.org/do/10.1377/forefront.20180216.720494/full/
8. Nathan H, Thumma JR, Ryan AM, Dimick JB. Early impact of medicare accountable care organizations on inpatient surgical spending. *Ann Surg.* 2019;269(2):191–196.
9. Brooke BS. Achieving high-value surgical care through accountable care organizations: are the risks worth the Rewards? *Ann Surg.* 2019;269(2):197–198. doi: 10.1097/SLA.0000000000003070
10. Dupree JM, Patel K, Singer SJ, et al. Attention to surgeons and surgical care is largely missing from early medicare accountable care organizations. *Health Aff (Millwood).* 2014;33(6):972–979.

SUGGESTED READING

Keller S, Schaninger B. *Beyond Performance 2.0: A Proven Approach to Leading Large-Scale Change.* Hoboken, NJ: John Wiley & Sons, Inc; 2019.

Bate P, Mendel P, Robert G. *Organizing for Quality: The Improvement Journeys of Leading Hospitals in Europe and the United States.* Abingdon, UK: Radcliffe Publishing, Ltd; 2008.

Kotter J. *Leading Change.* Boston, MA: Harvard Business School Press; 1996.

INDEX

Page numbers followed by '*f*' indicate figures; those followed by '*t*' indicate tables.

A

Academic health centers (AHCs), 116
Access to care
  change management, steps for, 12–13
  decision variables and constraints, 11
  distribution of ambulatory care across practice, 11
  follow-up and maintenance, 13
  measurement of variation in clinic visits, 13
  potential pitfalls and threats to equity, 12–13
  solution for improving, 12
  telehealth uses, 12
Accountable Care Organizations (ACOs), 121–122, 130, 250, 282
  administrative teams, 251
  driver diagram, 251, 252*f*
  follow-up and maintenance, 255
  health outcomes and care patterns, 251
  leadership awareness of, 251
  management pitfalls, 254
  performance of, 250
  programs, 250
  quality improvement, 253
  surgeon participation within, 250
  transformation teams, 253
Acute Hospital Care at Home programs, 35
Advanced practice providers (APPs), 28
Affiliations, 121
Agency for Healthcare Research and Quality (AHRQ), 173, 238
Ambulatory block time
  causes for underutilization, 88
  change management strategies and pitfalls, 91
  coordinating clearances and scheduling for surgery, 87*f*
  Gemba walks, 88, 90
  implementation of strategy to improve, 90–91
  LEAN thinking, 89–90
  outcome measurement, 91
  process mapping, 88–90, 89*f*
  scheduling and schedulers' efficiency, 86, 88–89, 92
Ambulatory care visits, 9, 9*f*, 10*f*
  challenges, 10–11
  changes in ambulatory care schedules, 10
  data sources, 9–10
  differential uptake of, 10
  influencing factors, 11
  institution-wide and surgical practice, 10*f*
  key stakeholders, identification, 9
  provider scheduling in outpatient clinics and, 11
Ambulatory surgery center (ASC), 63, 66, 193
  block time utilization at, 64
  criteria for surgical candidacy, 72
  hospital admission rate after, 71
  implementation of Plan-Do-Study-Act (PDSA) cycles, 72
  leadership, 70, 72
  life-threatening complications at, 69–71
  management of complications at, 70–71, 73*f*
  operational metrics, 69–70, 70*f*
  outcome and process metrics, 72–73
  outpatient procedures, 65
  pitfalls related to, 73
  Postanesthesia Care Unit (PACU) criteria for safe discharge, 72
  process management, 70*f*
American College of Surgeons (ACS), 149
American Commission on Cancer, 219
American Gastroenterological Association, 270
American Society for Gastrointestinal Endoscopy, 270
American Society of Anesthesiologists, 266
American Society of Metabolic and Bariatric Surgery, 149
Anesthesia review, 87
Athenahealth Physician Sentiment Index 2021, 127
Atrium Health, 121
  ACS NSQIP Collaborative 5-year outcome trends, 122*f*
  clinical optimization program, 123
  Collaborative Physician Alliance, 126
  culture commitments, 126
  general surgery service line, 123
  healthcare delivery model, 126–127
  incentives and engagement of general surgeons, 126
  Medical Group Surgery Care Division, 126
  Physician Connection Line (PCL), 125
  referral patterns, 121–122
  stakeholder group, 126
Atrium Health Levine Cancer Institute Metrics Reports, 123, 123*t*–125*t*

B

Baptist Health System, 246
Bariatric surgery, 75–77

Index

Bariatric Surgery Center of Excellence, 272
Best practice alert (BPA), 66, 67f
Binding arbitration process, 258
Body-Q score, 83
Breast Oncology Service Line, 205
British Medical Journal, 220
Bundled care payment models (BCPMs), 141
Bundled payments, 246
  for care improvement, 143
  programs, 243
Burnout, 196

C

Care Beyond Walls and Wires remote monitoring
    program, 20
Care elements, 155
Centers for Medicare and Medicaid Services (CMS),
    143, 246, 253, 272
Clinical delivery challenge
  ambulatory operating room block time, 86
  for avoiding life-threatening complications at ASC, 69
  brand and reputation of AHCs, 116
  coordinating care and referrals across affiliates, 131
  dissemination of quality standards in hospital
    networks, 107
  home monitoring, 79
  Hospital-at-Home (HaH) program, 33
  of insufficient inpatient OR capacity, 63–64, 64f
  losing market share of hospitals, 95
  lower acuity facility, 75
  in operating rooms, 48
  patient length of stay, 33
  surgical care delivery, 24
  surgical care in rural environments, 3
  transfer management program, 19
  transitioning out of hospital, 137
  value-based surgical care, 42
  volume–outcome relationship, 101
Clinically Integrated Network (CIN), 121–122, 130
Clinical Supply Integration Project (CSIP), 275
Clinic visits, 9
Commission on Cancer accreditation, 213
Complex surgical programs, 141
Complex time-sensitive cases, 55
  accommodation of elective cases, 59
  adaptation, 56
  in cancer care, 57
  change management strategies and potential
    pitfalls, 58
  conservation, 56
  factors detrimental to, 56
  operating room (OR) access, 57
  optimal active medical management, 57
  outcomes, measurement of, 59
  preparation, 56

  reallocation, 56
  reasonable alternatives, 57
  resource management, 56
  substitution, 56
  triage system, 56–58
Comprehensive Cancer Center, 217
Comprehensive Care for Joint Replacement Model, 243,
    246
Consumer Assessment of Healthcare Providers and
    Systems, 46
Coordinating care and referrals across affiliates
  change management and pitfalls, 134–135
  management plan, 134–135
  outcome measurements, 135
  performance intelligence framework, 133
  RE-AIM framework, 134
  review of data, 131–132
  virtual video-based visits, 135
COVID-19 pandemic, 19, 55, 215, 238
  complex time-sensitive cases on, 55–56
  Home Hospital (HH) care model, 84
  interhospital transfer programs and policies on, 19
  telemedicine uses, 44, 46
critical access hospitals, 4–5, 102
cumulative sum (CUSUM) charts, 186
Current Procedural Terminology (CPT) code, 269

D

Decision-making process, 266
Deep vein thrombosis (DVT), 170
Define-Measure-Analyze-Improve-Control (DMAIC),
    173
  methodology, 149
  process, 155
  quality improvement, 149
Destination programs, 141–142
  change management steps, 144
  pitfalls, 144
  value of program, 145
Dilated gastrojejunal anastomosis, 269f
Diversifying committees, 234

E

Electronic health record (EHR), 27, 151
  based transfer management solutions, 21
Electronic medical records (EMRs), 48, 88, 198
  based decision tools, 266
  systems, 142
Emergency departments (EDs)
  care for postoperative complications, 42–43
  odds of returning post-surgery to, 45
Emergency Medical Treatment and Labor Act
    (EMTALA), 21
Emotion, 167

"Emotion and the Art of Negotiation," 167
Enhanced Patient Clinical Streamlining (EPACS)
 Program, 209
Enhanced recovery after surgery (ERAS) programs,
 33–34
Environmental services (EVS)
 personnel, 191
 staff, 191
Episode-based bundled payment model, 244

F
Federal Aviation Administration (FAA), 158
Fee-for-service (FFS)
 model, 141
 system, 141
Financial pressures, 166
Fishbone diagram, 184f
Food and Drug Administration (FDA), 269

G
Gastro-jejunostomy, 269
Geisinger Bariatric Dashboard, 154
Gemba walks, 88, 90

H
Healthcare delivery, organizational changes in
 acceleration, 128
 analyze and approach, 127–128
 aspire, 128
 assessment, 128–129
 aware, 128
 change management and pitfalls, 129
 performance metrics, 129–130
 project management action plan, 128–129
Healthcare Equity Consult Service (HECS), 233
Healthcare intervention measurement, 29f
 behavior/social needs outcome, 28–29
 healthcare costs and utilization, 29
 health impacts, 29
 process measures, 28
 provider outcomes, 29
Healthcare systems, 142, 144, 281
Healthcare utilization, 46
Health Equity Implementation Framework, 227f
Health outcomes, in United States, 24
Hepatocellular carcinoma (HCC), 220
High-functioning teams, 195
High-quality surgical care, 189
High-reliability industries, 158
High-volume hospitals, 183
High-volume surgeons, 183
Home Hospital (HH) care models, 79
 bariatric HH program, 79

benefits, 80–81
challenges in implementing, 81
change management strategies and pitfalls, 83
components of care, 79–81
effectiveness of, 82
enhanced recovery after surgery (ERAS) protocols, 82
experiences, 84
implementation of, 81–82
insurance coverage, 84
Johns Hopkins' toolkit, 82
outcome measurement, 83–84
perioperative HH program, 80t
potential cost savings, 82–83
surgical, 82, 84
Horizontal differentiation, 132
Horizontal integration, 132
Hospital-at-Home (HaH) program, 33
 change management strategies, 39
 criteria for establishing, 37t
 follow-up and maintenance, 39
 forecasting and developing predictive models,
  33–34, 34t
 impact of, 36
 at Johns Hopkins Hospital, 34–35
 network of support, 35f
 at OHSU, Portland, 36–38
 outcome measurement, 39
 patient and health system benefits of, 36t
 patient screening for, 38t
 pitfalls, 39
 relative costs, 36
 in rural environment, 38
 successful, 35
Hospital consolidation, 98, 101
Hospital discharge planning, 42. See also Post-discharge
  care
Hospital markets, 95. See also Losing market share,
  hospital
Hospital networks, 102, 105
Hospital outpatient departments (HOPDs), 63, 66
 block time utilization at, 64
Hospital readmissions, 14
Hospital transfer centers, 21
Hospital Without Walls program, 35–36

I
Implementation process, 228
Improve Care Now for inflammatory bowel disease, 117
Infrastructure and structural challenges, 166
Inner setting, 228
Inpatient and outpatient facility utilization, 63, 63f
Inpatient OR capacity, optimization of, 65f
 ASC/HOPD preparedness, 65
 barriers to outpatient case movement to alternative
  sites, 64

Inpatient OR capacity, optimization of (*Continued*)
  change management strategies and pitfalls, 66–67
  multidisciplinary work group, 64
  operational metrics, 64
  Plan-Do-Check-Act (PDCA) cycles, implementation of, 67
  principle for reframing outpatient case scheduling, 65
  "Right Case, Right Place," implementing, 65, 67
Inpatient preoperative evaluation team, 51
Institution-specific operational metrics, 64
International Affairs and Best Practice Guidelines, 207
Intervention characteristics, 228
Ishikawa diagram, 184

J

Judgment, 178

L

Laparoscopic sleeve gastrectomy, revolution/procedures, 272
LEAN thinking, 89–90
Leapfrog Group, 101
Length of stay (LOS), 150
  external data, 150
  internal analysis, 150
Life expectancy, in United States, 24
Local multihospital system (LMS), differentiation/integration, 132, 132*f*
Losing market share, hospital
  ambulatory arena, 98
  care delivery modalities and, 98
  causes, 97
  change management strategies and pitfalls, 99
  context of hospital consolidation, 98
  external analysis, 95–96, 96*t*
  internal analysis, 96, 97*t*
  opportunities for growth and market share protection, 99
  strategies to overcome, 97–99
Lower acuity facility
  acuity exclusion criteria, 76, 78
  change management strategies and pitfalls, 77
  decentralization, 76
  operational metrics, 75
  patient allocation to, 76
  procedure types, 75
  realignment of surgical cases and its outcome, 77–78
  site of care optimization, challenge, 75–78
Low-risk surgical procedures, 264*t*
  CPT billing codes, 264*t*
  follow-up and maintenance, 268
  management pitfalls, 267
  preoperative tests, 263, 264*t*
  procedure, 264*t*

quantitative and qualitative approaches, 265
  surgical specialty, 264*t*
Low-volume hospital, 101
  capabilities, 102
  change management strategies and pitfalls, 104–105
  hospital network formation impacts, 102–103, 103*f*
  measures to optimizing care and outcomes, 104–105
  mission and service, 102
  in the Netherlands, 102
  procedure case-mix and volume, 101–102
  quality and safety concerns with, 102, 105
  strategies to avoid low-volume surgery in, 104
  in United States, 101

M

"Making Every Contact Count" program, 25
MBSAQIP Registry, 151, 154
Medical specialists, 150
  cardiologists, 150
  nephrologists, 150
  pharmacists, 150
  pulmonologists, 150
Medicare beneficiaries, 263
Metabolic and Bariatric Surgery Accreditation and Quality Improvement Program (MBSAQIP), 76–77, 149, 270
Michigan Surgical and Health Optimization Program, 26
Michigan Value Collaborative (MVC), 266
Mid-State Health (MSH), 281
Mobile apps for postoperative surveillance, 44–46
Morbidity conference, 233
Mortality conference, 233
Multidisciplinary care, 217
  coordination, 217

N

National Academy of Medicine, 149
National Healthcare Safety Network (NHSN), 111
National Surgical Quality Improvement Program (NSQIP), 46, 70, 122
Negotiation, 167
  pitfalls, 168
  steps of, 167–168
  success of, 169
New health network associates, exporting brand to, 116
  brand use, 117, 119
  change management strategies and pitfalls, 119
  Licensing agreement and Conditions of Use (COU), 118
  networking/affiliation work, measures, 119
  quality, evaluation, 117
  quality and safety assessment, 117–118
  resources and culture, evaluation, 117
  strategies to protect brand, 118

Nontechnical skills deficits, 180
No Surprises Act, 258

O

On-demand virtual health care, 20
Operating rooms scheduling model, 48
  allocation, 48
  case-leveling system, 49, 50t
  change management strategies and potential
    pitfalls, 53
  first case on-time start, 49, 51f
  first come, first served model, 48, 54
  flexibility in, 53
  operational metrics, 48, 49t, 51–52
  operational team, 48, 53
  outcomes, 53–54
  schedule optimization, 53–54, 54f
  turnaround time, 48, 51–52, 52f
Operative block time, optimization, 63
Organizational conditions, 195
Outer setting, 228
Out-of-network billing, 256
  common insurance plans, 258
  follow-up and maintenance, 260
  management pitfalls, 259
  in surgical episodes, 257t
Outreach activities and referrals for new network
    affiliates. See also Atrium Health
  affiliated general surgery group, 126
  incentives and engagement of general
    surgeons, 126
  in-network referrals, 121
  organizational changes for, 127–129
  outcome measurements, 129–130
  priorities for, 126–127
  referral patterns, review, 121–125
  stakeholders, assessment, 126

P

Pancreatic cancer, diagnosis
  differential diagnosis, 4
  endoscopic retrograde cholangiopancreatography
    (ERCP), 3–4
  endoscopic ultrasound (EUS), 3
  magnetic resonance imaging/magnetic resonance
    cholangiopancreatography (MRI/MRCP), 3
  pancreatic protocol CT scan, 3
  in rural setting, 3–4
  surgical oncology follow-up, 5
  and treatment, 4
    pancreaticohepatojejunostomy, 5
  tumor marker CA 19-9 expression, 3
Pareto principle (80/20 rule), 173
Patient Aligned Care Teams (PACTs), 133–134

Patient-centered benefits, 220
Patient education
  post-discharge care, 42–43
  wound care instructions, 43–44
Patient journey from clinic to OR, 86f–87f
  data sources, 87–88
Peds National Surgical Quality Improvement
    Program, 117
Performance intelligence, 133
Perioperative Enhancement Team (POET), 26
Picker Institute and the Commonwealth Fund, 207
Picker's 8 principles, patient-centered care, 208f
Plan-Do-Study-Act, 29, 173
Post-discharge care
  clinical outcomes, 46
  communications, 44
  determinants of, 43
  preoperative counseling, 44
  remote patient monitoring, 44–46
  telemedicine uses, 44–46
  wound care instructions, 43–44
Post-discharge telephone communications, 44
Postoperative complications management, 42–43.
    See also Post-discharge care
Postoperative readmissions, 14
Postsurgical ED visits and readmissions
  based on unmet social needs, 16
  change management to unplanned readmission
    reduction, 16–17
  comorbid conditions, 15
  evaluation and transparency outcomes, 17
  implementation of an intervention, 16–18
  improvement in care delivery, 15–16
  patient-level factors, 15
  pitfalls, 16–17
  planned vs unplanned readmissions, 14–15
  social needs assessment, 16
  solution to unplanned readmissions for nonurgent
    postsurgical complications, 15–16
  stakeholder collaboration in, 15
  transitional care programs, 15–16
Preoperative Anesthesia and Surgical Screening
    (PASS), 26
Preoperative Assessment, Consultation, and Treatment
    (PACT) clinic, 51
Preoperative counseling, 44
Prescription Drug Monitoring Programs, 151
Process
  of care measures, 170
  improvement methodologies, 173
  mapping, 88–90, 89f, 171
Proficiency-based curriculum, 161
Proficiency-based privileging schema,
    162f
Pulmonary embolism (PE), 170

Q

Qualitative data collection, 174
Quality measurement, 181
Quality & Patient Safety department, 180
Quality standards in hospital networks, dissemination, 107–108
  analysis and approach, 112
  areas for improvement, 111
  aware and aspire, 112
  challenges in implementing quality standards, 109, 111
  change management strategies, 112–114, 112f
  components and patient outcomes, utilization, 113
  equity in essential supplies, 113–114
  implementation of support processes, 113
  opportunities for reeducation, 114
  outcome measurement, 114
  process measures, 108, 108t
  quality standard outcomes, 109, 110f
  stakeholders, 108–109
  tracking of care, 109
Quantitative data metrics, 189

R

Reach, Effectiveness, Adoption, Implementation, and Maintenance (RE-AIM), 134
Reconciliation model, 248
Referral
  algorithm, 209
  centers, 21
  patterns, data sources, 121–125
Remote patient monitoring programs, 20
Robotic technology, 157
Roux-en-Y Gastric Bypass (RYGB), 269
Rural hospitals
  network in rural and tertiary surgical teams, 6
  select procedures done in, 4–5
  spectrum of care in, 4
  surgical procedures in, 5
  workup and management of surgical problems in, 5–6
Rural stoicism, 6
RVU conversion factors, 258

S

Service line development and maintenance, 210
Site of care optimization, 75–77
Six Sigma, 173
Skills
  nontechnical, 178
  technical, 178–179
Social determinants of health (SDoH), 14–15
Spatial differentiation, 132
Statistical process controls (SPC), 186
Stroke triage, 20
Structured exercise bariatric surgery program, 26

Substituting medical therapy, 56
Surgeon-specific factors, 185
Surgical care delivery, 24, 238
  conceptual model, 24–25, 25f
  constraints in, 25–26
  healthcare intervention measurement, 28–29
  improvement strategies, 27–28, 28f
  iterative testing, evaluation, and revision, 29
  Michigan Surgical and Health Optimization Program, 26
  PASS clinic model, 26
  perioperative period in, 26–27
  referral to nonmedical needs assistance program, 26
  reimbursement schedules, 25–26
  in rural environments, 3
  screening evaluation, 26
  screening for modifiable health behaviors and unmet social needs, 25
  for smoking-related diseases, 27
Surgical complications, 42
Surgical culture, 197
Surgical hospital-at-home programs, 82
Surgical procedure, steps in, 159f
Surgical Review Corporation, 149
Surgical site infections (SSIs), 42, 107
  diagnosis and treatment, 44
  patient's risk for developing, 45–46
  postoperative, 45
  prevention bundles, 111
System-wide Anti-Racism Oversight Committee, 233

T

Teachable moment, 26
Teamwork processes, 192
Technical deficits, 180
Telehealth/videoconferencing, 4
Telemedicine, 44–46
Tertiary centers, 5–6
Thyroidectomy, 69
  assessment, candidacy for outpatient, 69–71
  contraindications to outpatient, 72f
Time-sensitive elective cases, prediction of, 55
Transfer management programs
  capacity management strategies, 20, 22
  at clinician level, 21
  electronic health record-based solutions, 21
  EMTALA directions for interhospital transfers, 21
  factors contributing to capacity issues, 20
  follow-up and maintenance, 22
  implementation outcomes, 22
  pitfalls in initiating transfers, 22
  resources allocation/implementing operational change, 19
  strategies to improve, 20–21

Transitional Care Programs, 15
Transitioning out of hospital
    change management and pitfalls, 139–140
    connectedness with community health workers, 139
    delivery of care, 138
    discharge planning, 138
    Institute for Healthcare Improvement's, 139
    outcome measurement, 140
    patient monitoring, 138
    social or behavioral health needs, 138
Transoral outlet reduction endoscopy (TORe), 269
    gastric bypass anatomy, 270
    incorporation of innovative techniques, 272
    management pitfalls, 273
    not reimbursed, 271
    surgical revision for, 271
Triple-phase computerized tomography scan, 217
"Turf wars," 165
Tuskegee Syphilis Study, 226

U
Unequal distribution, clinical care, 11

V
Value Analysis Team (VAT), 275
    management and potential pitfalls, 279
    presentation for new product, 279t
    for standardized product approval, 279f
    transparent, objective process, 277
    in vendor consolidation, 280f
Value-based care, 206
Vascular
    procedures, 165
    surgery, 166, 169
    Surgery Limb Salvage Clinic, 225
Vendor consolidation processes, 276f
Vertical differentiation, 132
Vertical integration, 132
Veteran's Affairs system, 263
Veterans Health Administration (VHA), 133–134
VTE chemoprophylaxis, 171, 171f
VTE process, 172

W
Well-reimbursed specialty surgery care, 239
Willis-Knighton Health System, 104